T0263992

Challenging Issues in Women's Health Care

Guest Editor

KATHLEEN KENNEDY, MD

OBSTETRICS AND GYNECOLOGY CLINICS OF NORTH AMERICA

www.obgyn.theclinics.com

Consulting Editor
WILLIAM F. RAYBURN, MD, MBA

December 2009 • Volume 36 • Number 4

SAUNDERS an imprint of ELSEVIER, Inc.

W.B. SAUNDERS COMPANY

A Division of Elsevier Inc.

Elsevier, Inc. • 1600 John F. Kennedy Blvd. • Suite 1800 • Philadelphia, PA 19103-2899

http://www.theclinics.com

OBSTETRICS AND GYNECOLOGY CLINICS OF NORTH AMERICA Volume 36, Number 4
December 2009 ISSN 0889-8545, ISBN-13: 978-1-4377-1693-1, ISBN-10: 1-4377-1693-8

Editor: Carla Holloway

© **2009 Elsevier** ■ **All rights reserved.**

This journal and the individual contributions contained in it are protected under copyright by Elsevier, and the following terms and conditions apply to their use:

Photocopying

Single photocopies of single articles may be made for personal use as allowed by national copyright laws. Permission of the Publisher and payment of a fee is required for all other photocopying, including multiple or systematic copying, copying for advertising or promotional purposes, resale, and all forms of document delivery. Special rates are available for educational institutions that wish to make photocopies for non-profit educational classroom use. For information on how to seek permission visit www.elsevier.com/permissions or call: (+44) 1865 843830 (UK)/(+1) 215 239 3804 (USA).

Derivative Works

Subscribers may reproduce tables of contents or prepare lists of articles including abstracts for internal circulation within their institutions. Permission of the Publisher is required for resale or distribution outside the institution. Permission of the Publisher is required for all other derivative works, including compilations and translations (please consult www.elsevier.com/permissions).

Electronic Storage or Usage

Permission of the Publisher is required to store or use electronically any material contained in this journal, including any article or part of an article (please consult www.elsevier.com/permissions). Except as outlined above, no part of this publication may be reproduced, stored in a retrieval system or transmitted in any form or by any means, electronic, mechanical, photocopying, recording or otherwise, without prior written permission of the Publisher.

Notice

No responsibility is assumed by the Publisher for any injury and/or damage to persons or property as a matter of products liability, negligence or otherwise, or from any use or operation of any methods, products, instructions or ideas contained in the material herein. Because of rapid advances in the medical sciences, in particular, independent verification of diagnoses and drug dosages should be made.

Although all advertising material is expected to conform to ethical (medical) standards, inclusion in this publication does not constitute a guarantee or endorsement of the quality or value of such product or of the claims made of it by its manufacturer.

Obstetrics and Gynecology Clinics (ISSN 0889-8545) is published quarterly by Elsevier Inc., 360 Park Avenue South, New York, NY 10010-1710. Months of issue are March, June, September, and December. Periodicals postage paid at New York, NY, and additional mailing offices. Subscription price per year is $257.00 (US individuals), $431.00 (US institutions), $130.00 (US students), $309.00 (Canadian individuals), $544.00 (Canadian institutions), $191.00 (Canadian students), $376.00 (foreign individuals), $544.00 (foreign institutions), and $191.00 (foreign students). To receive student/resident rate, orders must be accompanied by name of affiliated institution, date of term, and the signature of program/residency coordinator on institution letterhead. Orders will be billed at individual rate until proof of status is received. Foreign air speed delivery is included in all *Clinics* subscription prices. All prices are subject to change without notice. POSTMASTER: Send address changes to *Obstetrics and Gynecology Clinics*, Elsevier Health Sciences Division, Subscription Customer Service, 3251 Riverport Lane, Maryland Heights, MO 63043. **Customer Service: Telephone: 1-800-654-2452 (U.S. and Canada); 314-447-8871(outside U.S. and Canada). Fax: 314-447-8029. E-mail: journals customerservice-usa@elsevier.com (for print support); journalsonlinesupport-usa@elsevier.com (for online support).**

Reprints. For copies of 100 or more of articles in this publication, please contact the Commercial Reprints Department, Elsevier Inc., 360 Park Avenue South, New York, New York 10010-1710. Tel.: 212-633-3818; Fax: 212-462-1935; E-mail: reprints@elsevier.com.

Obstetrics and Gynecology Clinics of North America is also published in Spanish by McGraw-Hill Interamericana Editores S.A., P.O. Box 5-237, 06500, Mexico; in Portuguese by Reichmann and Affonso Editores, Rio de Janeiro, Brazil; and in Greek by Paschalidis Medical Publications, Athens, Greece.

Obstetrics and Gynecology Clinics of North America is covered in MEDLINE/PubMed (Index Medicus), Excerpta Medica, Current Concepts/Clinical Medicine, Science Citation Index, BIOSIS, CINAHL, and ISI/BIOMED.

Printed and bound by CPI Group (UK) Ltd, Croydon, CR0 4YY

Transferred to Digital Print 2011

GOAL STATEMENT

The goal of *Obstetrics and Gynecology Clinics of North America* is to keep practicing physicians up to date with current clinical practice in OB/GYN by providing timely articles reviewing the state of the art in patient care.

ACCREDITATION

The *Obstetrics and Gynecology Clinics of North America* is planned and implemented in accordance with the Essential Areas and Policies of the Accreditation Council for Continuing Medical Education (ACCME) through the joint sponsorship of the University of Virginia School of Medicine and Elsevier. The University of Virginia School of Medicine is accredited by the ACCME to provide continuing medical education for physicians.

The University of Virginia School of Medicine designates this educational activity for a maximum of 15 *AMA PRA Category 1 Credits*™ for each issue, 60 credits per year. Physicians should only claim credit commensurate with the extent of their participation in the activity.

The American Medical Association has determined that physicians not licensed in the US who participate in this CME activity are eligible for a maximum of 15 *AMA PRA Category 1 Credits*™ for each issue, 60 credits per year.

Category 1 credit can be earned by reading the text material, taking the CME examination online at http://www.theclinics.com/home/cme, and completing the evaluation. After taking the test, you will be required to review any and all incorrect answers. Following completion of the test and evaluation, your credit will be awarded and you may print your certificate.

FACULTY DISCLOSURE/CONFLICT OF INTEREST

The University of Virginia School of Medicine, as an ACCME accredited provider, endorses and strives to comply with the Accreditation Council for Continuing Medical Education (ACCME) Standards of Commercial Support, Commonwealth of Virginia statutes, University of Virginia policies and procedures, and associated federal and private regulations and guidelines on the need for disclosure and monitoring of proprietary and financial interests that may affect the scientific integrity and balance of content delivered in continuing medical education activities under our auspices.

The University of Virginia School of Medicine requires that all CME activities accredited through this institution be developed independently and be scientifically rigorous, balanced and objective in the presentation/discussion of its content, theories and practices.

All authors/editors participating in an accredited CME activity are expected to disclose to the readers relevant financial relationships with commercial entities occurring within the past 12 months (such as grants or research support, employee, consultant, stock holder, member of speakers bureau, etc.). The University of Virginia School of Medicine will employ appropriate mechanisms to resolve potential conflicts of interest to maintain the standards of fair and balanced education to the reader. Questions about specific strategies can be directed to the Office of Continuing Medical Education, University of Virginia School of Medicine, Charlottesville, Virginia.

The faculty and staff of the University of Virginia Office of Continuing Medical Education have no financial affiliations to disclose.

The authors/editors listed below have identified no professional or financial affiliations for themselves or their spouse/partner:
Brittany B. Albright, BS; Jan Born, PhD; Judith R. Davidson, PhD; Amy C. Denham, MD, MPH; Linda S. Efferen, MD; Eve Espey, MD, MPH; Heather Flynn, PhD; David V. Hamilton, MD, MA; Julie E. Heringhausen, BSN; Carla Holloway (Acquisitions Editor); William Irvin, MD (Test Author); Kathleen Kennedy, MD (Guest Editor); Nina Kohn, MBA, MA; Maria Muzik, MD, MS; William F. Rayburn, MD, MBA (Guest Editor); Virginia C. Reichter, NP; Lori E. Ross, PhD; Vickie Seltzer, MD; Diane K. Shrier, MD; Lydia A. Shrier, MPH; Simone Vigod, MD, FRCPC; Carolyn Voss, MD; Ullrich Wagner, PhD; Amy Weil, MD; and Adam J. Zolotor, MD, MPH.

The authors/editors listed below identified the following professional or financial affiliations for themselves or their spouse/partner:
Anita H. Clayton, MD is an industry funded research/investigator for BioSante Pharmaceuticals, Boehringer-Ingelheim, Bristol Myers Squibb, and Eli Lilly & Co.; is on the Advisory Committee/Board for Boehringer-Ingelheim, Bristol Myers Squibb, and Eli Lilly & Co.; is a consultant for Boehringer-Ingelheim; and, is on the Speakers' Bureau for Eli Lilly & Co.
Sheila M. Marcus, MD is a consultant for Up To Date.
David Mischoulon, MD, PhD is on the Speakers Bureau for MGH Academy/Reed Elsevier, Nordic Naturals, and Pamlab; is an industry funded research/investigator for Nordic Naturals, Laxdale (Amarin), Ganeden, Cederroth, and SwissMedica; is a consultant for Pamlab and Bristol Meyers Squibb; and receives royalties from Back Bay Scientific.
Tony Ogburn, MD is a consultant for Schering-Plough.
Meir Steiner, MD, PhD, FRCPC is a consultant for Wyeth Pharmaceuticals, Bayer Shering Pharmaceuticals, Astra-Zeneca, Azevan Pharmaceuticals, and Servier; has grants from Canadian Institutes of Health Research, Physicians Services Inc.; has research support from Wyeth Pharmaceuticals, Astra-Zeneca, Lundbeck, and Eli Lilly; and, receives honoraria from Azevan Pharmaceuticals and Bayer Shering Pharmaceuticals.

Disclosure of Discussion of non-FDA approved uses for pharmaceutical products and/or medical devices:

The University of Virginia School of Medicine, as an ACCME provider, requires that all faculty presenters identify and disclose any off-label uses for pharmaceutical and medical device products. The University of Virginia School of Medicine recommends that each physician fully review all the available data on new products or procedures prior to clinical use.

TO ENROLL

To enroll in the Obstetrics and Gynecology Clinics of North America Continuing Medical Education program, call customer service at 1-800-654-2452 or visit us online at www.theclinics.com/home/cme. The CME program is available to subscribers for an additional fee of $195.00

Contributors

CONSULTING EDITOR

WILLIAM F. RAYBURN, MD, MBA
Randolph Seligman Professor and Chair, Department of Obstetrics and Gynecology,
Chief of Staff, University Hospital, University of New Mexico Health Science Center,
Albuquerque, New Mexico

GUEST EDITOR

KATHLEEN KENNEDY, MD
Associate Professor, Department of Obstetrics and Gynecology, University
of New Mexico School of Medicine, Albuquerque, New Mexico

AUTHORS

BRITTANY B. ALBRIGHT, BS
University of New Mexico School of Medicine, University of New Mexico, Albuquerque,
New Mexico

JAN BORN, PhD
Department of Neuroendocrinology, University of Lübeck, Germany

ANITA H. CLAYTON, MD
David V. Wilson Professor of Psychiatry and Neurobehavioral Sciences, Professor
of Clinical Obstetrics and Gynecology, University of Virginia, Charlottesville, Virginia

JUDITH R. DAVIDSON, PhD
Adjunct, Assistant Professor, Departments of Psychology and Oncology; Queen's
University, Clinical Psychologist, Kingston Family Health Team, Kingston, Ontario, Canada

AMY C. DENHAM, MD, MPH
Assistant Professor of Family Medicine, Department of Family Medicine, University
of North Carolina School of Medicine, Chapel Hill, North Carolina

LINDA S. EFFEREN, MD, FACP, FCCP, FCCM
Senior Vice President and Chief Medical Officer; South Nassau Community Hospital,
Oceanside, New York; Associate Professor of Clinical Medicine, Department of Medicine,
Albert Einstein College of Medicine, Bronx, New York

EVE ESPEY, MD, MPH
Associate Professor, Department of Obstetrics and Gynecology, Associate Dean
of Student Affairs, Office of Students Services, University of New Mexico School
of Medicine, Albuquerque, New Mexico

HEATHER FLYNN, PhD
Assistant Professor, Department of Psychiatry, University of Michigan, Ann Arbor, Michigan

DAVID V. HAMILTON, MD, MA
Fellow, Department of Psychiatry and Neurobehavioral Sciences, Institute for Law, Psychiatry, and Public Policy, University of Virginia, Charlottesville, Virginia

JULIE E. HERINGHAUSEN, BSN
Medical Student, Medical School University of Michigan, Ann Arbor, Michigan

NINA KOHN, MBA, MA
Biostatistics Unit, North Shore Long Island Jewish Research Institute, Manhasset, New York

SHEILA M. MARCUS, MD
Clinical Professor, Department of Psychiatry, Child and Adolescent Psychiatry, University of Michigan, Ann Arbor, Michigan

DAVID MISCHOULON, MD, PhD
Director of Research, Depression Clinical and Research Program, Department of Psychiatry, Massachusetts General Hospital; Associate Professor of Psychiatry, Harvard Medical School, Boston, Massachusetts

MARIA MUZIK, MD, MS
Assistant Professor, Department of Psychiatry, University of Michigan, Ann Arbor, Michigan

TONY OGBURN, MD
Associate Professor, Residency Program Director, Department of Obstetrics and Gynecology, University of New Mexico School of Medicine, Albuquerque, New Mexico

WILLIAM F. RAYBURN, MD, MBA
Randolph Seligman Professor and Chair, Department of Obstetrics and Gynecology, Chief of Staff, University Hospital, University of New Mexico Health Science Center, Albuquerque, New Mexico

VIRGINIA CULLEN REICHERT, NP
Assistant Director of Nursing, Stony Brook University Medical Center, Stony Brook, New York

LORI E. ROSS, PhD
Social Equity and Health Research Section, Centre for Addiction and Mental Health; Assistant Professor, Department of Psychiatry, University of Toronto; Toronto, Ontario, Canada

VICKI SELTZER, MD
Chairman Emeritus, Obsterics and Gynecology, North Shore University Hospital and Long Island Jewish Medical Center, Old Westbury, New York

DIANE K. SHRIER, MD
Clinical Professor of Psychiatry and of Pediatrics, Department of Psychiatry and Behavioral Sciences, George Washington University Medical Center, Washington, DC

LYDIA A. SHRIER, MD, MPH
Director of Clinic-based Research, Division of Adolescent/Young Adult Medicine,
Children's Hospital; Assistant Professor of Pediatrics, Department of Pediatrics,
Harvard Medical School, Boston, Massachusetts

MEIR STEINER, MD, PhD, FRCPC
Department of Psychiatry and Behavioural Neurosciences, Department of Obstetrics and
Gynecology, McMaster University, Women's Health Concerns Clinic, St. Joseph's
Healthcare, Hamilton, Ontario, Canada

SIMONE N. VIGOD, MD, FRCPC
Department of Psychiatry, Women's College Hospital; Lecturer, Department of Psychiatry, University of Toronto, Toronto, Ontario, Canada

CAROLYN VOSS, MD
Professor, Department of Internal Medicine, Executive Director of Ambulatory Care,
University of New Mexico Health Sciences Center, Albuquerque, New Mexico

ULLRICH WAGNER, PhD
School of Psychology, Bangor University, Bangor, Gwynedd, United Kingdom

AMY WEIL, MD
Associate Professor of Medicine and Social Medicine, Department of Medicine,
Division of General Medicine and Epidemiology, University of North Carolina School
of Medicine, Co-Director, Beacon Child and Family Program, University of North Carolina
School of Medicine, Chapel Hill, North Carolina

ADAM J. ZOLOTOR, MD, MPH
Assistant Professor of Family Medicine, Department of Family Medicine, University
of North Carolina School of Medicine, Chapel Hill, North Carolina

Contents

> The recognition that women have different health care needs than men has enabled changes to take place in clinical care, research, and education of women's health. Providing health care coverage to all women must be a high priority. Research must address the differences between men and women and how they respond to disease and treatment. The physician workforce needs to be expanded; physicians should be well trained to provide comprehensive health care to women. Strategies, such as those used in comprehensive centers of women's health and women's health residencies, can improve education and increase the number of women in academia.

> Beginning in the past century and continuing to evolve into the twenty-first century, there have been dramatic changes in women's work and personal/family lives within the United States. These changes have particularly affected white, middle-class women and women in medicine and other professions. Physicians in fields whose practitioners are predominantly female and/or who treat primarily women and families need to be aware of the scope and nature of these changes and to recognize that their own personal experiences and values might differ from those of women of different generations as well as different socioeconomic and cultural backgrounds.

> Prevalence studies show that 1 in 5 women experience an episode of major depressive disorder during their lifetime. The peripartum period is a prime time for symptom exacerbation and relapse of depressive episodes. Health care providers, specifically those in obstetric care, should be aware of: (1) the frequency of depression in pregnant and postpartum women; (2) signs, symptoms, and appropriate screening methods; and (3) the health risks for the mother and growing fetus if depression is

undetected or untreated. Because management of depressed peripartum women also includes care of a growing fetus or breastfeeding infant, treatment may be complex and requires input from a multidisciplinary team, including an obstetrician, psychiatrist, and pediatrician, to provide optimal care.

The popularity of natural or "alternative" remedies to treat medical and psychiatric disorders has accelerated dramatically over the past decade, in the United States and worldwide. This article reviews the evidence for clinical efficacy, active ingredients, mechanisms of action, recommended dosages, and toxicities of the 3 best-studied putative natural antidepressants, St. John's wort (hypericum), S-adenosyl methionine, and the Ω-3 fatty acids eicosapentaenoic acid and docosahexaenoic acid. Despite growing evidence for efficacy and safety, more comprehensive studies are required before these remedies can be recommended as safe and effective alternatives or adjuncts to conventional psychotropic agents. There are limited data regarding safety in pregnancy and during lactation, and caution is therefore recommended in women who are pregnant or breastfeeding.

Nocturnal sleep is characterized by a unique pattern of endocrine activity, which comprises reciprocal influences on the hypothalamo-pituitary-adrenal (HPA) and the somatotropic system. During early sleep, when slow wave sleep (SWS) prevails, HPA secretory activity is suppressed whereas growth hormone (GH) release reaches a maximum; this pattern is reversed during late sleep when rapid eye movement (REM) sleep predominates. SWS benefits the consolidation of hippocampus-dependent declarative memories, whereas REM sleep improves amygdala-dependent emotional memories and procedural skill memories involving striato-cortical circuitry. Manipulation of plasma cortisol and GH concentration during sleep revealed a primary role of HPA activity for memory consolidation. Pituitary-adrenal inhibition during SWS sleep represents a prerequisite for efficient consolidation of declarative memory; increased cortisol during late REM sleep seems to protect from an overshooting consolidation of emotional memories.

This article describes the circumstances under which women may develop insomnia and the various treatment options, including hypnotic medication and nonpharmacologic approaches. The efficacy and safety of these treatments are reviewed. The choice of treatment depends on the nature of the insomnia, the stage of a woman's life, the presence of medical or mental health conditions, the availability of treatments, and personal preference.

For immediate, short-term relief of acute insomnia, hypnotic medication, especially the nonbenzodiazepines (zolpidem, zopiclone, eszopiclone) are options. For chronic insomnia, insomnia-specific cognitive and behavioral therapies are generally the interventions of choice.

RELATED INTEREST

Psychiatric Clinics of North America June 2010 (Vol. 33, Issue 2)
Women's Mental Health
Susan G. Kornstein, MD and Anita H. Clayton, MD, *Guest Editors*
www.psych.theclinics.com

THE CLINICS ARE NOW AVAILABLE ONLINE!

Access your subscription at:
www.theclinics.com

Foreword

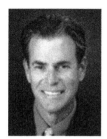

William F. Rayburn, MD, MBA
Consulting Editor

"Challenging Issues in Women's Health Care," guest edited by Kathleen Kennedy, MD, reflects the expanding role of obstetrician-gynecologists in optimizing women's health. Dr. Kennedy and I reviewed all of the other *Clinics* to identify papers of interest relating to psychosocial challenges we often encounter that, while not related directly to obstetrics and gynecology, are linked to the needs of many patients. Given the outstanding quality of those authors' recent manuscripts and their importance to obstetrics and gynecology, Dr. Kennedy and I believe that these select articles could be combined and presented here for the benefit of our readership.

The content of this issue encompasses the detection and initial management of common disorders that afflict women but are nongynecologic in primary origin. For example, depression and sleep disturbances are common patient complaints encountered daily in clinical practice. Because most reproductive-aged women depend on their physician for a full range of services, obstetrician-gynecologists increasingly hear such nongynecologic complaints and are asked to initiate some form of treatment.

Certain sections of this special issue cover topics that have a major prevention component, such as substance use. Updated information on substance use stresses various techniques that can easily be used in practice to promote smoking cessation and to discourage unhealthful alcohol and illicit drug abuse. These sections cannot be ignored because obstetrician-gynecologists can make an important difference, depending on the physician's engagement.

An example of a commonly-encountered challenging issue that rarely occurs as a single disorder is sexual dysfunction. Difficulty with both arousal and desire are intertwined, as is a lack of orgasm and arousal. The obstetrician-gynecologist's roles in assessing sexual dysfunction, initiating treatment, and making appropriate referrals are crucial because our patients often view their sexuality as an important quality-of-life issue.

Another malady addressed openly in this issue involves intermittent mood or physical symptoms associated with menstrual cycles. A constellation of symptoms includes depression, anger, irritability, anxiety, social withdrawal, somatic symptoms,

Obstet Gynecol Clin N Am 36 (2009) xv–xvi
doi:10.1016/j.ogc.2009.10.012
0889-8545/09/$ – see front matter © 2009 Elsevier Inc. All rights reserved.

breast tenderness, abdominal bloating, headache, and swelling of the extremities. Half of affected women find their symptoms to be tolerable, while the remainder find their symptoms troubling and seek care, more often from a gynecologist than from a psychiatrist. Those with a severe premenstrual syndrome or premenstrual dysphoric disorder require special attention that is well outlined here.

Violence against women, especially by domestic partners, is a major public health issue with significant social, economic, and health ramifications. It occurs in every ethnic, cultural, religious, educational, and economic group. Children, pregnant women, the elderly, and others with disabilities are especially vulnerable. As described in this issue, obstetricians-gynecologists need to be familiar with community resources and with laws and regulations that establish reporting requirements by health providers.

I am grateful to the dedicated individuals who updated their contributions for this special issue. Common conditions described in this unique issue by many experts outside our field are addressed candidly and sensitively within the context of screening and initial management. It is rewarding to continue collaborating with repeat contributors and to again call upon their expertise and knowledge. This collection provides a solid foundation for the modern evaluation and, if necessary, management of such challenging issues.

William F. Rayburn, MD, MBA
Department of Obstetrics and Gynocology
University of New Mexico School of Medicine
MSC10 5580, 1 University of New Mexico
Albuquerque, NM 87131-0001, USA

E-mail address:
wrayburn@salud.unm.edu

Preface

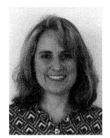

Kathleen Kennedy, MD
Guest Editor

Women's health care embraces the entire spectrum of a woman's life. Over the past century, women have been impacted most dramatically by changes in work, personal, and family life. Women's mental and psychosocial health and well-being must take into account the social, economic, and political issues surrounding women. Personal problems and stress often affect a woman's life and the social roles she plays. For this reason, challenging issues often arise in women's health care as a result of a woman's unique physiology and response to personal concerns.

In an office setting, challenging health concerns for women can be very tough and time-consuming for providers. Many obstetrician-gynecologists are insufficiently trained to handle complex psychosocial issues in women's care. Thus, for the first time, we embarked on a mission to combine the finest articles on topics that address difficult psychosocial conditions in women's health that either bring patients to the office or that are revealed from discussions in an office setting. We searched expert literature from other *Clinics of North America* issues to explore information that would be of interest to women's health care providers.

In this issue, the authors of each article were requested to update and critique their literature and reference information. In addition, the authors redirected the content of their articles to encompass the obstetrician-gynecologist perspective. We began with articles addressing global concerns. These include Dr. Tony Ogburn's article regarding the barriers to women's health and Dr. Diane Shrier's overview of psychosocial aspects of women's lives.

Epidemiologic data indicate that major depression is approximately twice as common in women as in men. Because the first onset of depression peaks during childbearing years, we invited Dr. Maria Muzik, an authority on the mental health of mothers of young children, to present her article on depression and childbearing. Dr. David Mischoulon explains the natural remedies for treatment of depression. Women are also twice as likely as men to suffer from sleep disturbances and insomnia. We approached Dr. Jan Born and Dr. Judith Davidson to share their expertise on this topic. Because understanding and recognizing intimate partner violence is critical to caring

Obstet Gynecol Clin N Am 36 (2009) xvii–xviii
doi:10.1016/j.ogc.2009.10.013   obgyn.theclinics.com
0889-8545/09/$ – see front matter © 2009 Elsevier Inc. All rights reserved.

for women, we invited Dr. Adam Zolotor, who is widely recognized in the field of intimate partner violence, to contribute. While research suggests that sexual dysfunction is common, exploring this concern is difficult for many providers. Dr. Anita Clayton was approached to include her excellent critique on female sexual dysfunction. While addiction in women has increased over the years, identification and treatment of addiction are still deficient. The article by Virginia Cullen Reichert, NP highlights tobacco dependence in women. This is followed by a comprehensive addition by Brittany Albright and Dr. William Rayburn about substance abuse. Finally, premenstrual dysphoric disorder affects 3% to 8% of premenopausal women. Dr. Simone Vigod enlightens readers with her expertise in understanding and treating premenstrual dysphoric disorder.

Because some psychosocial and medical issues are more common in women than in men, the obstetrician-gynecologist must stay current on these topics to provide optimal care to patients. Providing this collection of diverse and pertinent current literature regarding difficult issues in women's health care will, hopefully, offer some ease and assistance in approaching these concerns with patients.

Kathleen Kennedy, MD
Department of Obstetrics and Gynecology
University of New Mexico School of Medicine
MSC10 5580; 1 University of New Mexico
Albuquerque, NM 87131-0001, USA

E-mail address:
kakennedy@salud.unm.edu

Barriers to Women's Health: Why is It So Hard for Women to Stay Healthy?

Tony Ogburn, MD[a],*, Carolyn Voss, MD[b],
Eve Espey, MD, MPH[c]

KEYWORDS

- Women's health care • Women's health education
- Health care access • Women's health research

Of all the forms of inequality, injustice in health care is the most shocking and inhumane.

—Dr Martin Luther King, Jr

Health care in the United States is often touted as the best in the world. It certainly is the most expensive. Expenditures on health care exceeded $2.2 trillion, or $7421 per capita, in 2007. Health care spending accounted for 16.2% of the gross domestic product in the United States, ranking first in the world.[1] Despite greater spending on health care, the United States ranks thirty-seventh out of 191 countries in overall health, according to the World Health Organization.[2] France is number one in health rankings, yet spends less than 10% of its gross domestic product on health care. Other countries that spend less than the United States but have higher health rankings include the United Kingdom, Italy, and Germany.[2] By 2018, health care spending in the United States is projected to exceed $4 trillion and account for 20.3% of the country's gross domestic product.[1]

Many people think that the United States health care system is in crisis and the topic is a source of frequent public debate. Most Americans believe that Congress should

This is an updated version of the article "Barriers to Women's Health: Why Is It So Hard for Women to stay Healthy?," which appeared in *Medical Clinics of North America* (Volume 92, Issue 5, September 2008).

[a] Department of Obstetrics and Gynecology, University of New Mexico School of Medicine, MSC 10 5580, 1 University of New Mexico, Albuquerque, NM 87131–0001, USA
[b] Department of Internal Medicine, University of New Mexico Health Sciences Center, MSC10 5550, 1 University of New Mexico, Albuquerque, NM 87131–0001, USA
[c] Department of Obstetrics and Gynecology, Office of Student Services, University of New Mexico School of Medicine, MSC 08 4700, 1 University of New Mexico, Albuquerque, NM 87131, USA
* Corresponding author.
E-mail address: jogburn@salud.unm.edu (T. Ogburn).

Obstet Gynecol Clin N Am 36 (2009) 737–752
doi:10.1016/j.ogc.2009.10.007
0889-8545/09/$ – see front matter © 2009 Elsevier Inc. All rights reserved.

pass health care reform legislation: 41% state that legislation should be passed this year and 30% state that it should happen but not necessarily this year.[3] Leading up to the last presidential election, all the major candidates indicated that health care reform was a priority for the country. Health care reform has taken a leading role in the agenda of the Obama administration and the current Congress. Opinions about the reasons for the crisis are varied and there is little consensus on solutions. Unfortunately, the crisis in health disproportionately affects women. This article discusses several of the main issues in health care including lack of health care coverage and access to care, underfunded research in women's health, and the fragmentation of women's health care among medical specialties. Potential solutions to improve the health of women in the United States are explored.

ACCESS TO CARE

Millions of Americans lack adequate access to health care. The uninsured have minimal access except for emergency services and the underinsured face barriers that impede optimal health.

The Uninsured

The United States is the only developed country in the world that does not provide universal health coverage for its population. Instead, a mix of employer-based health insurance and government programs, including Medicare and Medicaid, cover only approximately 85% of the population. It is estimated that 45 million people are uninsured in the United States.[4] Most of the uninsured are in working families (81%).[4] They typically work in small businesses, the service industry, or in blue collar positions that do not offer employer-sponsored insurance. Medicaid and the State Children's Health Insurance Program (SCHIP) provide coverage for some many, but the programs' eligibility requirements exclude many of the working poor. Seventy-nine percent of the uninsured are citizens.[4]

The number of uninsured people has risen steadily in the United States for much of the past decade. Between 2004 and 2006, 3 million more people became uninsured.[5] Recently, there has been a decrease in the number of uninsured by approximately 1.2 million because of the increased coverage by government programs, such as SCHIP.[4] Unfortunately, since 2000 there has been an increase in workers that do not have access to employer-sponsored insurance. In 2000, 12.8% of workers were uninsured, increasing to 14.9% in 2007.[6]

Several factors explain the steady rise. Despite an employer-based health care system, one third of businesses in the United States do not offer health care coverage to their employees.[7] This lack of coverage disproportionately affects employees in small businesses: in the time period 2000 to 2005, over 250,000 small businesses stopped providing coverage.[8] Increased costs were the primary reason for discontinuing health care benefits. Costs to employers rose at three to four times the rate of inflation over the past decade.[7]

Even if insurance is offered, employee contributions to premiums have increased dramatically, which makes health insurance unaffordable for many. The annual cost of coverage for a family of four exceeded $12,000 in 2006 and the employee contribution rose to $3300.[7] Considering a minimum wage worker earns approximately $11,000 per year, it is clear why many workers choose not to participate in employer-sponsored programs.

Government programs cover many Americans. Additionally, about 25% of the uninsured are eligible for coverage by Medicaid or SCHIP but are not enrolled.[5]

A lack of awareness of eligibility and cumbersome enrollment procedures play a role in preventing more eligible individuals from participating. In addition, policies requiring re-enrollment every 6 to 12 months result in loss of coverage. Individuals who remain eligible are disenrolled because of these procedural barriers.

Of the remaining uninsured people, approximately 56% are not eligible for public programs, usually because their incomes exceed eligibility requirements. Eligibility is based on percentage of the federal poverty level. In 2006, the federal poverty level was defined as an income of $20,614 for a family of four. Typically, programs for children and pregnant women (and in some states for family planning services) have income requirements of approximately 200% of the federal poverty level.[4] Experts estimate that a family needs an income of greater than 300% of federal poverty level to afford health care coverage if they were purchasing it directly in the marketplace.

The health impact of being uninsured is significant and affects women in many ways. Women with health coverage are more likely to obtain appropriate preventive, primary, and specialty care.[9] Approximately 38% of women have employer-based insurance in their own name, whereas 25% of women have dependent coverage. Dependent insurance in the spouse's name makes a woman vulnerable to a loss of coverage when divorced or widowed.

Eighteen percent of women are uninsured. Uninsured women are less likely to have had a visit with a provider in the past year (67%), compared with women with either private insurance (90%) or public insurance (Medicaid [88%] and Medicare [93%]).[10] In addition, they are more likely than women with insurance to report not having a current Pap smear, not filling a prescription because of cost, and having no regular physician.[9] Uninsured women with serious or chronic conditions are less likely to receive the care they need.[11] The Institute of Medicine estimates that 18,000 excess deaths occur among individuals under age 65 attributable to lack of health coverage.[11]

The Underinsured

Even women with insurance face barriers to health care. One in six women with private health insurance and one in three women with Medicaid report that, because they could not afford it, they postponed or went without needed health care services in the previous year.[10] Access to medications, specialty care, and needed procedures may be limited in several ways including copays, capping the scope of drug coverage, and limiting the number of prescriptions for which a patient is eligible. These restrictions disproportionately impact lower income women.

Prescription contraceptive coverage provides an example of limitations placed on women's access to needed health care. Most insurance companies allow only a 1 month's supply of medications, requiring copay each month. One study found that overall women pay a greater proportion of the costs of contraceptives compared with other prescription medications. Women with private insurance paid approximately 60% of the total cost of oral contraceptives, compared with typical out-of-pocket costs for noncontraceptive medications of only 33%.[12] In addition to increased costs, receiving only 1 month of pills at a time is a barrier to pill continuation. Dispensing 6 months or 1 year's supply of pills allows women to comply better with the pill regimen.

Many insurance companies do not cover all available methods of contraception. A 2001 survey found that whereas 98% of insured employees had general prescription coverage, only 41% had coverage of all available reversible contraceptive methods.[13] Women's access to the most effective methods, such as use of intrauterine devices and implants, are often excluded because of high up-front costs. Such an approach is short-sighted because these methods are the most cost effective after approximately 1 year of use. The practice of limiting coverage of contraceptives is discriminatory because contraceptives are one of the most commonly used prescription drugs among younger Americans and they are used only by women. There is an increasing trend to legislate contraceptive coverage or "contraceptive equity." Twenty-seven states have enacted laws that require insurers that provide prescription drug coverage to cover contraceptives.

Federal law requires that insurers of federal employees provide comprehensive contraceptive coverage.[14] Federal legislation entitled "Putting Prevention First" has been introduced that would mandate contraceptive coverage for all insured women nationally, but the proposal has made little headway to date.

Many insurance plans have high deductibles for or completely exclude specific services. The Hyde amendment, enacted in its initial version in 1976, forbids the use of federal funds for abortion except in the case of rape, incest, or physical endangerment of the mother's life.[15] This proscription includes individuals covered by Medicaid, Medicare, the military, and the Indian Health Service. More than 7 million women who rely on Medicaid do not have access to federal support for abortion care, although they are typically poor and the least likely to afford services out of pocket. Similarly, some insurance plans exclude abortion except in certain circumstances, such as rape and endangerment of the mother's life. Abortion is one of the most common medical procedures for women. There is no common procedure that is excluded for males. In spite of the federal ban on abortion funding, 17 states allow the use of state funds to pay for all or most abortions for Medicaid enrollees.[16]

Solutions to Access Issues

Several strategies may improve access to care. Many agree that universal health care coverage is desirable, although the specifics of implementation are hotly debated. A single-payer system has the significant advantage of decreasing total administrative costs. In 2004, these costs accounted for 31% of health care expenditures in the United States compared with only 16.7% in Canada, a country with a single payer, national health insurance program.[17] Physicians for a National Health Plan, an organization representing more than 15,000 physicians, medical students, and other health care professionals in the United States, estimates that the savings from decreased administrative costs of a single-payer system could cover all Americans without increasing overall costs.[18]

Others advocate for universal care through employee-individual or employer mandates. Massachusetts enacted a law in 2006 that required all individuals to purchase health care or be subjected to fines. Two years after implementation it seemed that the program was successful in increasing coverage for the uninsured but costs were a significant issue.[19]

The uncertainty regarding the best approach to health care reform can be illustrated by the intense debate the topic has generated as the Obama administration and 111th Congress address the issue. A detailed analysis of all of the proposals is beyond the scope of this article, but options being considered include employer and individual mandates, health care exchanges, a public option, and premium subsidies.[20] Central themes of the reform efforts include providing coverage for the uninsured, improving quality of care for all, and controlling the rapidly increasing cost of health care.[20]

In 2008, the American College of Obstetricians and Gynecologists proposed a health care reform plan that calls for universal health coverage that promotes prevention, especially prenatal care and contraception; continuity of care; and a medical home and core services for women.[21] The American College of Obstetricians and

Gynecologists further states that health coverage should be accessible and affordable to everyone in the United States, regardless of citizenship or residency status.

Given the widespread attention that health care issues are receiving from politicians at all levels, professional organizations, and the public, it is apparent that health care reform is needed in the United States. There is general agreement that such reform should provide coverage for all Americans while maintaining quality of care. Given the lack of consensus on how to achieve these goals, however, significant reform may not occur in the next few years.

Other strategies should be used in the short term. Continuation and expansion of programs, such as the Medicaid waiver program, would provide coverage for some services. This program allows states to extend family planning services to certain groups as long as the program is budget neutral or results in overall cost savings.[22] These programs typically extend services to women; services offered are based on income requirements at or near 200% of poverty level. Such programs increase the number of family planning providers, increase accessibility, decrease unintended pregnancy, and provide overall costs savings.[23]

Targeted efforts, such as provider and patient education about the availability of Medicaid coverage, could increase the participation of women who are eligible but have not enrolled.

RESEARCH IN WOMEN'S HEALTH

Research in women's health is critical to improving the health status of women, to reducing the incidence of disease, to providing optimal treatments, and to improving quality of life. Women have traditionally been excluded or marginalized from most medical research. Women's health research historically encompasses disease involving the reproductive tract including pregnancy-related issues and reproductive health. Other conditions, such as cardiovascular disease and infectious diseases, were studied in men, and results were applied to women with the incorrect assumption that women were the same as men except for the reproductive tract. Researchers have found that wide variations exist between women and men in their responses to disease and treatments, including HIV infection, urinary incontinence, cardiovascular disease, pain response, and mental illness.[24] Although the past two decades have seen improvements in women's health research, much remains to be accomplished.

History of Women in Clinical Research

Policies that were formed as recently as the 1980s excluded or limited the involvement of women in clinical trials. These policies derived from concerns about female vulnerability, ethical and legal concerns, and a presumption that research risk outweighed the benefits.[25] Such policies seem misguided in retrospect, but they were intended to protect women, especially during pregnancy. In the 1960s and 1970s, the disastrous experiences with thalidomide, the shield, and diethylstilbestrol created a protectionist atmosphere that went too far in its reach. Pregnant women, and by extension reproductive-aged women who might unknowingly be pregnant, were included as a category of "vulnerable populations" for purposes of research along with prisoners and mentally disabled persons.

In 1985, the Public Health Service issued a report from its Task Force on Women's Health that identified areas for improvement including women's health research.[26] In response to the report, the National Institutes of Health (NIH) established guidelines in 1986 that encouraged inclusion of women in clinical research. Minorities were included in 1987.[27] Despite these guidelines, concerns persisted that women and minorities remained underrepresented in research. In 1990, the Government Accountability Office (GAO) published the results of an investigation reporting that the NIH had made little progress in achieving its goals of increased inclusion of women and minorities in research.

In response to the GAO report and other publicity, changes occurred in the 1990s. In 1991, the Office of Women's Health (OWH) was established in the Department of Health and Human Services with a mission to "provide leadership to promote health equity for women and girls through sex/gender-specific approaches."[28] In addition, the Office of Research on Women's Health (ORWH) was established at the NIH in 1990.[29] One of the main functions of the ORWH is to "coordinate and serve as a focal point for women's health research funded by the NIH."

Most important was the passage of the NIH Revitalization Act of 1993, which was signed into law by President Clinton in 1994. This act put into law existing NIH policies and guidelines with several key differences. It required that (1) the NIH ensures that all women and minorities are included in all research, (2) women and minorities are included in all phase III trials in adequate numbers to allow for valid analyses of differences in intervention effect, (3) cost is not allowed as an acceptable reason for excluding these groups, and (4) the NIH initiates programs and support for outreach efforts to recruit and retain women and minorities and their subpopulations as volunteers in clinical trials.[27] These requirements were a significant step forward in expanding and improving women's health research.

The Food and Drug Administration

In 1977 the Food and Drug Administration (FDA) issued guidelines limiting the participation of broadly defined "women of childbearing potential" in drug research. This was in part caused by concerns arising from the diethylstilbestrol and thalidomide experiences. Women's participation was limited to phase III trials, and then only after animal reproductive studies and phase I and II trials were completed. Because manufacturers were not required to perform animal reproductive studies, women continued to be excluded from the latter stage trials.[25]

Responding to changes at the NIH, the FDA issued revised guidelines in 1993. The new policy strongly encouraged the inclusion of representatives of both genders in drug trials in numbers adequate to allow the detection of clinically significant gender differences in drug response. It also encouraged the analysis of gender differences as a part of new drug applications. The regulations stopped short of requiring women's participation.[30]

In 1998, a new regulation required the separate presentation of safety and efficacy data for men and women in new drug applications, but it did not require discussion or analysis of these data. The 1998 regulation also required the tabulation of study participants by gender in new drug applications annual reports.

Overall, the regulations have had a positive impact. A GAO report issued in 2001 found that adequate numbers of women were included in pivotal trials on drug efficacy. Concern was expressed, however, that early, small-scale studies to determine toxicity and dosing levels had a low proportion of women; concern was also expressed that the data available from studies were not optimally analyzed to explore potential gender differences in dosing and that the FDA lacked appropriate oversight capability to ensure compliance with the regulations regarding women in research.[31]

Future Directions

The establishment of regulations at the NIH and FDA and the formation of the ORWH and the OWH has led to significant improvements in women's health research. In addition to the FDA and NIH, other government agencies have offices or divisions of women's health including the Centers for Disease Control and Prevention, Health Resources and Administration, and the Agency for Healthcare Research and Quality.

Efforts must be made to maintain the gains of the last two decades and to ensure that the existing gaps are filled in. The work of the OWH and others has been successful in increasing the number of studies on women's health. For example, the number of applications for NIH Research Project Grants (RO1) funding and other types of project grants for women's health research increased by 48% from 1989 to 1990 to 1999 to 2000, nearly double the 25% increase for all applications.[32]

Funding for women's research agencies must continue and expand. Unfortunately, from 2006 to 2009 funding for women's health offices at federal agencies remained flat or grew only modestly. The OWH budget increased from $28 to $30 million, whereas the OWHR at the NIH remained the same at $40.9 million. Overall, this level of funding amounted to a decrease when taking inflation into account.[33] Projections for fiscal year 2010 include minimal increases for both offices. Furthermore, only offices at the NIH and the Substance Abuse and Mental Health Administration are authorized by statute. Offices in such agencies as the Centers for Disease Control and Prevention and FDA are at risk each budget cycle. The Women's Health Office Act, introduced in the House and Senate in 2007 and reintroduced in the House in 2009, provides for statutory authorization of women's health offices in the other federal health agencies including the FDA, Health and Human Services, and Agency for Healthcare Research and Quality.

In addition to adequate funding, research must be designed to ensure not only participation by adequate numbers of women but also to account for inherent gender differences and the impact that these differences may have on study results. Studies should be designed and implemented so that results can be analyzed by gender to determine if differences do exist for women.[34,35] These tenets are critical for studies on conditions that affect both genders, such as cardiovascular disease. For example, the Multiple Risk Factor Intervention Trial, a study of the relationship between heart disease, cholesterol, and behavioral factors, included women only in the observational arm. The experimental arm was comprised of 13,000 men, making it impossible to draw conclusions about women from the results of this study.[36]

Women in Academics

Limitations in women's health research and policy may derive from the lack of women in positions of influence. Efforts should be made to increase the number of women in the biomedical sciences. Women's health research may languish in the absence of women on university faculties. Female researchers are more likely to investigate diseases in women and tend to ask scientific questions differently.[37] One of the main activities of the ORWH is the promotion of women in the biomedical sciences to achieve a critical mass of female researchers. One example of an initiative that works is the "re-entry program." This program enables fully trained researchers to participate on a grant after taking time off for family or personal needs.

Other approaches include the recruitment of more women into NIH postdoctoral fellowships and career development workshops and seminars designed to encourage and assist women in applying for research funding.[32] These efforts have achieved a degree of success measured by an increase of 84% in the number of research awards to women compared with a 49% increase for men in the decade since implementation.

Despite these gains, there is room for improvement. Although roughly equal numbers of women and men enter medical school, women who choose to enter academic medicine are less likely to be promoted or serve in leadership positions.[38] Women are less likely to achieve the rank of full professor and have their own laboratory space and grant support early in their careers, and have lower salaries than men with similar experience and academic rank.[39] A multifaceted approach is necessary to decrease these inequities. Continued monitoring of women's progress is essential to ensure that persistent inequities are identified. Women must be effectively mentored in the early and middle portions of their careers by senior faculty. Men in senior leadership roles must be trained and encouraged to provide effective leadership to women, because insufficient numbers of senior female faculty are available to fulfill the need. Professional organizations should encourage participation by women and ensure their systems provide the support needed for women to succeed.

Additionally, career paths should be more flexible. Stringent timelines for promotion and tenure may be a barrier to women who are more likely than men to work fewer hours and take extended periods of leave. This variation should be accommodated and pathways devised that allow women to progress in academia while fulfilling other personal obligations.

WHO ARE WOMEN'S HEALTH PHYSICIANS?

"Women's health" is a broad term that lacks clear definition. Historically, women's health focused on reproductive tract conditions, such as pregnancy, contraception, disorders of the menstrual cycle, and menopause. Broader definitions have emerged in recent years as women's health is defined as encompassing a broad range of issues. There are major differences in how men and women develop and handle disease that must be considered. In addition, there are different challenges faced by men and women, such as social and economic factors that affect health.

As women's health has become more complex, so has the role of the women's health care provider. Unfortunately, no consensus exists about who should be the primary provider of health care to women. As a result, care is typically fragmented, which results in gaps in the provision of preventive services and acute and chronic care.

What Health Care Services do Women Need?

Ideally, women need a physician who can provide gender-specific needs, such as obstetric care, cervical and breast cancer screening, contraception, and menopausal care. In addition, they need the broader range of preventive services including colon cancer screening, lipid screening, and immunizations. Ideally, their provider is able to provide general acute care for common conditions, such as urinary tract infections, upper respiratory infections, and sexual transmitted diseases, and common chronic conditions, such as hypertension, diabetes, and asthma. Finally, women need a provider who is able to address behavioral and psychosocial issues, such as smoking cessation and domestic violence.

Who Provides Care?

Three specialties typically provide primary care to women: (1) internists, (2) obstetrician-gynecologists, and (3) family medicine physicians, and nurse practitioners and physician assistants trained in these disciplines (a group whose role becomes ever more important as the primary care physician workforce continues its rapid decline in number). All three specialties have advocated for being the primary care providers for women. Susan Fryhofer, then president of the American College of Physicians, in a column in the *ACP-ASIM Observer* entitled "Why doctors of internal medicine are the best choice for women's health," stated that internists were most suited to provide care for women because they could provide not only gender-specific needs, such as breast and cervical cancer screening, but also care for other complex disorders, such as colon cancer, heart disease, and diabetes.[40]

Hal Lawrence, vice president for Practice Activities at the American College of Obstetrician-Gynecologists, writes that "Ob/Gyns are best suited to be a women's ongoing physician since they can provide care across her life time including caring for menstrual disorders in the adolescent, pregnancy related care and contraception in the reproductive years, and deal with issues such as heart disease prevention and bone health during the menopausal years. Throughout the lifespan Ob/Gyns can provide wellness promotion, education, preventive services, and initiate the detection of gynecologic and nongynecologic health issues."[41]

The Future of Family Medicine project, an organization commissioned by seven national family medicine organizations, advocates that family medicine physicians are positioned to provide a medical home to patients and provide a "basket of services" that includes acute and chronic care, preventive services, and maternity care.[42]

In reality, the evidence indicates that none of the specialties provides optimal comprehensive care for women. Reports consistently indicate that obstetrician-gynecologists provide gender-specific services at higher rates than other primary care physicians but that all specialties do poorly providing gender-neutral preventive services.

A recent study using data from the 2000 National Health Interview Survey found that women who saw a gynecologist were more likely to have gender-specific preventive services, such as Pap smear, mammography, and clinical breast examination, than if they only saw a general medical physician.[43] Seeing both types of providers did not increase the chances of obtaining these services. For gender-neutral services including colorectal cancer screening, diet counseling, and exercise counseling, rates of screening did not differ between patients who saw a gynecologist or general medicine physician. Higher rates of each service were seen, however, if a patient saw both types of provider. Unfortunately, overall rates of screening for these services were low no matter what type or types of provider were seen. For example, colorectal cancer screening rates were 39% for general medical physicians, 44% for gynecologists, and 46% for patients who used both.

A study using data from the National Ambulatory Care Survey found that internists and family medicine physicians were more likely to provide gender-neutral services, such as cholesterol screening, whereas obstetrician-gynecologists were more likely to provide gender-specific services. Again, provision of gender-neutral services was low among all specialties.[44] In another study using the National Ambulatory Care Survey database, patients seeing an obstetrician-gynecologist for a preventive care visit had a clinical breast examination performed 87% of the time. Rates were much lower for internists (33%) and family medicine physicians (45%).[45]

A telephone survey of women in the Baltimore area found that women using both an obstetrician-gynecologist and a generalist physician received more appropriate preventive services than those seeing a generalist alone.[46]

A study based on claims made to a large Midwestern health plan found that women were much more likely to have a Pap smear or mammogram if seen by an obstetrician-gynecologist compared with an internal medicine physician. They did not look at gender-neutral services.[47]

Even if one of the three specialties was able to provide the comprehensive care that women need, none is positioned to be the sole provider of women's health care. There are not enough obstetrician-gynecologists, family medicine physicians, or internists to provide all the primary care that women need now or in the future. Of the physicians completing residency training in internal medicine each year, about 80% subspecialize and approximately 10% become hospitalists, leaving only about 10% to provide general internal medicine or primary care. Family medicine residency positions have decreased from 2920 positions offered in 2003 to 2535 in 2009.[48] Of these positions, only 91% were filled through the Match, and only 42.2% were filled by United States graduates. The number of positions in obstetrics and gynecology has remained stable for many years at approximately 1150. Approximately 10% of obstetrics and gynecology graduates subspecialize.

Strategies for Improvement

Multiple approaches must be used to ensure optimal care for women. With the current workforce, no single specialty is able to provide the services needed.

A collaborative approach is needed where providers in all three specialties can provide the basics of care and coordinate needed care that is beyond their expertise.

Undergraduate Medical Education

A recent survey of United States medical schools using the Association of American Medical Colleges' Curriculum Management and Information Tool found that few schools offer interdisciplinary women's health courses or clerkships or include gender-specific information in their curricula.[49] They found that having a formal women's health program at the institution or having a female dean were positively correlated with inclusion of women's health in the curriculum. Another survey in 2001 found that only 44% of schools had a women's health curriculum, although an additional 18% were in the process of developing one.[50] The authors suggested that ensuring that women's health has an "academic home" with resources provided for faculty training in women's health was a key to success.

Undergraduate medical education must integrate comprehensive women's health into the curricula so that all graduates have the knowledge and skill set to provide the basics of care. All medical students should graduate with an understanding of the specific health needs of women, a knowledge base that includes the gender differences, and have the technical skills to provide care including performing a pelvic examination.

In addition to improving education in women's health care, the number graduates must be increased. The American Association of Medical Colleges recommends increasing the number of graduates by 30% over 2002 levels by 2012.[51] The American Association of Medical Colleges also recommends increasing residency positions to accommodate the proposed increase in medical school graduates. The Council on Graduate Medical Education, authorized by Congress in 1986 to provide an ongoing assessment of physician workforce trends, training issues, and financing policies, and to recommend appropriate federal and private sector efforts to address identified needs, reported in 2005 that the United States faces a shortage of 85,000 physicians by 2020 and that the number of physicians entering residency training should be increased by 3000 per year by 2015.[52] Health care reform must address this impending shortage and ensure that appropriate increases in residency training positions are authorized and funded.

Graduate Medical Education

Current program requirements for internal medicine residents regarding women's health are general. They require that residents "receive instruction and clinical experience in the prevention, counseling, detection, and diagnosis and treatment of gender-specific diseases of men and women." In addition residents must "have sufficient instruction and clinical experience in office gynecology" and "be instructed in the indications, contraindications, complications, limitations, and interpretations of findings and develop technical proficiency in... pap smear and endocervical culture."[53] There are no specified criteria for what diseases must be covered or a minimum number of examinations to achieve proficiency. These requirements provide great latitude for programs in how they provide instruction in women's health and assess competency. A survey of internal medicine program directors in 2004 found that more than one third thought most of their residents did not achieve competency in evaluating and treating common conditions, such as vaginitis, domestic violence, and contraception.[54] The American Board of Internal Medicine requires "competency" in performing a Pap smear for board certification and specifies that a resident must be an active participant in at least five procedures.[55] A study of internal medicine residents found that those performing more than 10 Pap smears were far more likely to feel confident to perform the procedure.[56]

Family medicine program requirements specify that residents must receive instruction and clinical experience in women's health but do not specify how this is to be accomplished or set specific criteria for competency.[57] As with internal medicine, these requirements may by interpreted and implemented in many ways by individual training programs.

The concern for obstetrician-gynecologists is not lack of competency in gender-specific care, such as cervical and breast cancer screening, but instead it is their competency in gender-neutral conditions that may be deficient. Previous program requirements in obstetrics and gynecology specified that residents must have at least 6 months of instruction and experience in primary and preventive care and that this training can occur in obstetrics and gynecology continuity and high-risk obstetrics clinics and in internal medicine clinics or rotations in the emergency department. Program requirements implemented in 2008 do not require a specified amount of time in primary care but specify that educational experiences in primary care should take place throughout the residency and may occur in a variety of settings including continuity clinics and high-risk obstetrics clinics.[58] Again, a fair amount of latitude exists in how extensive or comprehensive training may be. It is also questionable how applicable primary and preventive care experience in a high-risk obstetrics clinic is to the general, nonpregnant population.

A recent Presidential task force at the American College of Obstetricians and Gynecologist addressed the role of obstetrician-gynecologists in the provision of primary care. It recommended that, at a minimum, obstetrician-gynecologists should be able to provide screening, prevention, diagnosis, and management of common health issues that affect all women. Management may include appropriate referral, initiation of treatment accompanied by referral, or full continual management, depending on the expertise of the provider.

All three specialties must ensure that graduates have the core skills needed to provide basic primary care for women. Internists and family medicine physicians should be able to provide gender-specific care including Pap smears and breast examinations to their female patients. Obstetrician-gynecologists should be able to appropriately screen patients for the full range of preventive services. All obstetrician-gynecologists likely will not have the interest, expertise, or time to provide ongoing care for chronic illness, but they should be able to screen for such conditions and refer appropriately. They may also be in the position of providing a "medical home" for many women, providing care within their scope of practice, and coordinating the remainder of a patient's care.

Women's health residencies and fellowships are an interdisciplinary approach to train physicians that are specialist in comprehensive women's health excluding obstetrics. Programs usually are based in an internal medicine department and trainees typically complete rotations in obstetrics and gynecology and other pertinent clinical rotations, such as sports medicine, behavioral health, and breast clinics. Currently, there are 10 residencies and 22 fellowship programs in the United States. Although such programs do not yet train large number of providers, they may in the future as the need for comprehensive women's health providers increases and interest in this type of practice grows. In addition, such programs may be a source for leaders in the field of women's health.

Comprehensive Women's Health Centers

In 1996, the US Department of Health and Human Services OWH established the National Centers of Excellence in Women's Health (CoEs). Located in academic medical centers around the country, the CoEs program works to establish and evaluate a new model health care system that unites state-of-the-art health care services addressing all of a woman's needs, gender-based research, public and professional education and training, community linkages for health services and programs, and leadership positions for women in academic medicine.[59] The potential success of such centers is well documented. At the University of Michigan, where a program was established in the early 1990s and received designation as a CoE in 1997, there have been notable improvements in patient care and research, increased recruitment and promotion of women faculty, and increased inclusion of women's health issues in the curriculum. Since the program's inception, the ranks of senior women faculty have increased by 182% compared with 26% for men and tenured women faculty grew by 108% compared with an increase of 9% for men.[60] The Office of Women's Health has four other innovative programs designed to provide comprehensive, interdisciplinary, integrated care for women including National Community Centers of Excellence in Women's Health and Rural Frontier Women's Health Coordinating Centers.

SUMMARY

Women's health care has made great strides in the past two decades. The recognition that women have different health care needs than men has enabled changes to take place in clinical care, research, and education. Much remains to be done. Providing health care coverage to all women must be a high priority. Research must be adequately funded and continue to address the differences that exist between men and women and how they respond to disease and treatment. The physician workforce needs to be expanded and physicians should be well trained to provide comprehensive health care to women. Strategies, such as used in Comprehensive Centers of Women's Health and women's health residencies, should be used to ensure improved education and increases in the numbers of women in the ranks of academia.

REFERENCES

1. Centers for Medicare and Medicaid. National health expenditure data fact sheet. Available at: http://www.cms.hhs.gov/NationalHealthExpendData/25_NHE_Fact_Sheet.asp#TopOfPage. Accessed August 24, 2009.

2. World Health Organization. The world health report 2000 – health systems: improving performance. Available at: http://www.who.int/whr/2000/en/whr00_en. pdf. Accessed August 24, 2009.

3. Poll Gallup. Available at: http://www.gallup.com/poll/121883/Most-U.S.-Want-Health care-Reform-Vary-Urgency.aspx. Accessed August 24, 2009.

4. Kaiser Family Foundation. The uninsured: a primer 2008. Available at: http://www. kff.org/uninsured/upload/7451-04.pdf. Accessed August 24, 2009.

5. Kaiser Family Foundation Commission on the Uninsured. Characteristics of the uninsured: who is eligible for public coverage and who needs help affording coverage? Available at: http://www.kff.org/uninsured/upload/7613.pdf. Accessed August 24, 2009.

6. Kaiser Family Foundation Commission on the Uninsured. The fraying link between work and health insurance: trends in employer-sponsored insurance for employees, 2000–2007. Available at: http://www.kff.org/uninsured/upload/7840. pdf. Accessed August 24, 2009.

7. The Henry J. Kaiser Family Foundation. Employee health benefits: 2007 annual survey. Available at: http://www.kff.org/insurance/7672/index.cfm. Accessed August 24, 2009.

8. The Henry J. Kaiser Family Foundation. The uninsured: a primer, key facts about Americans without health insurance. Available at: http://www.kff.org/uninsured/. Accessed August 24, 2009.

9. The Henry J. Kaiser Family Foundation Women's health insurance coverage. 2007. Available at: http://www.kff.org/womenshealth/upload/6000_06.pdf. Accessed August 24, 2009.

10. The Henry J. Kaiser Family Foundation. Women and health care, a national profile. Available at: http://www.kff.org/womenshealth/whp070705pkg.cfm. Accessed August 24, 2009.

11. Institute of Medicine of the National Academes. Uninsurance facts and figures: the uninsured are sicker and die sooner. Available at: http://www.iom.edu/ uninsured. Accessed August 24, 2009.

12. Phillips K, Stotland N, Liang S, et al. Out of pocket expenses for oral contraceptives and number of packs per purchase. J Am Med Womens Assoc 2004;59: 36–42.

13. The Guttmacher Institute. Report on public policy special analysis: the cost of contraceptive insurance coverage, vol. 6, number 1, 2003. Available at: http:// guttmacher.org/pubs/tgr/06/1/gr060112.html. Accessed August 25, 2009.

14. The Guttmacher Institute. State policies in brief. Insurance coverage of contraceptives. Available at: http://www.guttmacher.org/statecenter/spibs/spib_ICC. pdf. Accessed August 24, 2009.

15. The Guttmacher Institute. Policy review: the heart of the matter: public funding of abortion for poor women in the United States. Available at: http://www.guttmacher. org/pubs/gpr/10/1/gpr100112.html. Accessed August 24, 2009.

16. Guttmacher Institute. Guttmacher state policies in brief: state abortion policies. Available at: http://www.guttmacher.org/statecenter/spibs/spib_OAL.pdf. Accessed August 24, 2009.

17. Woolhandler S, Campbell T, Himmelstein D. Costs of health care administration in the United States and Canada. N Engl J Med 2003;349:768–75.

18. Physicians for a National Health Plan. Single-payer national health insurance. Available at: http://www.pnhp.org/facts/single_payer_resources.php. Accessed August 25, 2009.

19. Kaiser Family Foundation. Massachusetts health care reform: two years later. Available at: http://www.kff.org/uninsured/upload/7777.pdf. Accessed August 25, 2009.

20. The Henry J Kaiser Family Foundation. Presidential candidate health care reform proposals: a side by side comparison. Available at: http://www.health08.org/side byside_results.cfm?c=5&;c=11&c=16. Accessed July 14, 2008.

21. American College of Obstetricians and Gynecologists. Health care for women, health care for all. A reform agenda Available at: http://www.acog.org/depart ments/govtrel/HCFWHCFA-ReformPrinciples.pdf. Accessed August 25, 2009.

22. Espey E, Cosgrove E, Ogburn T. Family planning American style: why it's so hard to control birth in the US. Obstet Gynecol Clin North Am 2007;34:1–17.

23. Gold R. Doing more for less: study says state Medicaid family planning expansions are cost-effective. Available at: http://www.guttmacher.org/pubs/journals/gr070101.html. Accessed August 25, 2009.

24. Pinn V. Sex and gender factors in medical studies: implications for health and clinical practice. JAMA 2003;289:397–400.

25. Johnson T, Fee E. Women's health research: a historical perspective. In: Haseltine F, editor. Women's health research: a medical and policy primer. Washington, DC: American Pyschiatric Press; 1997. p. 27–46.

26. United States Public Health Service. Women's health. Report of the Public Health Service Task Force on women's health issues. Public Health Rep 1985;100(1):73–106.

27. Office of Research on Women's Health. Inclusion of women in research. Available at: http://orwh.od.nih.gov/inclusion.html. Accessed August 25, 2009.

28. Office of Women's Health. About us. Available at: http://www.4woman.gov/owh/index.cfm. Accessed August 25, 2009.

29. Office of Research on Women's Health. About ORWH. Available at: http://orwh.od.nih.gov/about.html. Accessed August 25, 2009.

30. Food and Drug Administration. Guideline for the study and evaluation of gender differences in the clinical evaluation of drugs. Fed Regist 1993;58(139):39406–16.

31. Government accountability office. Women's health: women sufficiently represented in new drug testing but FDA oversight needs improvement 2001. GAO Report # 01–754 Available at: http://www.gao.gov/new.items/d01754.pdf. Accessed August 31, 2009.

32. Stone J, Pinn V, Rudick J, et al. Report from the NIH Office of Research on women's health: evaluation of the first 10 years of the office of research on women's health at the National Institutes of Health: selected findings. J Womens Health 2006;15(3):234–47.

33. Society of Women's Health Research. Issue: federal funding of women's health research. Available at: http://www.womenshealthresearch.org/site/PageSer ver?pagename=policy_issues_funding. Accessed September 1, 2009.

34. Pinn V. Research on women's health: progress and opportunities. JAMA 2005;294:1407–10.

35. Institute of Medicine. Exploring the biological contributions to human health: does sex matter? 2001. Available at: http://www.nap.edu/catalog/10028.html. Accessed August 25, 2009.

36. Moncher K, Douglas P. Importance of and barriers to including women in clinical trials. In: Legato M, editor. Principles of gender specific medicine. New York: Elsevier Academic Press; 2004. p. 275–82.

37. Haseltine F. Formula for change: examining the glass ceiling. In: Haseltine F, editor. Women's health research: a medical and policy primer. Washington, DC: American Pyschiatric Press; 1997. p. 225–30.
38. Nonnemaker L. Women physicians in academic medicine: new insights from cohort studies. N Engl J Med 2000;342:399–405.
39. Hamel M, Ingelfinger J, Phimster E, et al. Women in academic medicine: progress and challenges. N Engl J Med 2006;355(3):310–2.
40. Fryhofer SA. Why doctors of internal medicine are the best choice for women's health. ACP-ASIM Observer 2000;20(5):8.
41. Lawrence HA. Women's ongoing physician? Her Ob/Gyn. Ob Gyn News 2008; 43(2):11.
42. Martin JC, Avant RF, Bowman MA, et al. Future of Family Medicine Leadership Committee. The future of family medicine: a collaborative project of the family medicine community. Ann Fam Med 2004;2(Suppl 1):S3–32.
43. Lewis B, Halm E, Marcus S, et al. Preventive services use among women seen by gynecologists, general medical physicians, or both. Obstet Gynecol 2008;111: 945–52.
44. Scholle S, Chang J, Harman J, et al. Trends in women's health services by type of provider seen: data from the 1985 and 1997–98 NAMCS. Womens Health Issues 2002;12(4):165–77.
45. Wallace A, MacKenzie T, Weeks W. Women's primary care providers and breast cancer screening: who's following the guidelines? Am J Obstet Gynecol 2006; 194:744–8.
46. Henderson J, Weisman C, Grason H. Womens health issues. Womens Health Issues 2002;12:138–49.
47. Lurie N, Slater J, McGovern P, et al. Preventive care for women: does the sex of the physician matter? N Engl J Med 1992;329:478–82.
48. National Residency Matching Program. Results and data: 2009 main residency match. Washington, DC: National Residency Matching Program; 2009.
49. Henrich J, Viscoli C. What do medical schools teach about women's health and gender differences? Acad Med 2006;81:476–82.
50. Keitt S, Wagner C, Tong C, et al. Positioning women's health curricula in US medical schools. MedGenMed 2003;5(2):40.
51. American Association of Medical Colleges. AAMC statement on the physician workforce. Available at: http://www.aamc.org/workforce/workforceposition.pdf. Accessed September 1, 2009.
52. Council on graduate medical education. Physician workforce policy guidelines for the United States, 2000–2020. Sixteenth report. January, 2005. Available at: http://www.cogme.gov/16.pdf.
53. Accreditation Council for Graduate Medical Education. Internal medicine program requirements. Available at: http://www.acgme.org/acWebsite/down loads/RRC_progReq/140_im_07012007.pdf. Accessed September 1, 2009.
54. Spencer A, Kern L. Primary care program directors' perceptions of women's health education: a gap in graduate medical education persists. J Womens Health 2008;17:549–56.
55. American Board of Internal Medicine. General requirements. Available at: http://www.abim.org/certification/policies/imss/im.aspx#procedures. Accessed September 1, 2009.
56. Chew R, Chew L, Bradley K. The association between numbers of Pap smears performed and self-reported confidence in an internal medicine residency. J Womens Health 2006;15:928–33.

57. Accreditation Council for Graduate Medical Education. Family medicine program requirements. Available at: http://www.acgme.org/acWebsite/downloads/RRC_progReq/120pr07012007.pdf. Accessed September 1, 2009.

58. Accreditation Council for Graduate Medical Education. Obstetrics and gynecology program requirements. Available at: http://www.acgme.org/acWebsite/downloads/RRC_progReq/220obstetricsandgynecology01012008.pdf. Accessed September 1, 2009.

59. Office of Women's Health. National centers of excellence in women's health. Available at: http://www.4woman.gov/coe/. Accessed September 1, 2009.

60. Rogers J, Johnson T, Warner P, et al. Building a sustainable women's health program: the Michigan model. J Womens Health 2007;16(6):919–25.

Psychosocial Aspects of Women's Lives: Work and Family/ Personal Life and Life Cycle Issues

Diane K. Shrier, MD[a],*, Lydia A. Shrier, MD, MPH[b,c]

KEYWORDS

• Women • Work/Life • Family • Life cycle

Beginning in the past century and continuing to evolve into the twenty-first century, there have been dramatic changes in work and personal/family lives within the United States. These changes, although strongly affecting men and children, have impacted most dramatically on women's lives, particularly white, middle-class women[1–3] and women in medicine and other professions. Physicians in fields whose practitioners are now predominantly female and/or who treat primarily women and families (obstetrics/gynecology, pediatrics, women's health, and child/adolescent psychiatrists) need to be aware of the scope and nature of these changes. They also need to recognize that their own personal experiences and values might differ from those of women of different generations as well as different socioeconomic and cultural backgrounds.

Traditionally, women's normative life cycle was viewed as tied to the reproductive aspects of their lives. Although there has been remarkably little written about the stages of women's lives,[4–6] anecdotal and statistical material demonstrate that women's adult lives have become increasingly complex with the multiple dimensions of biology, family, and work interacting and influencing each other[3] and variations as to life choices and the timing of major career and family events. As noted by Anne Seiden,[7] women's lives could be envisioned more like "a 'life pretzel' in which the

This is an updated version of the article "Psychosocial Aspects of Women's Lives: Work, Family, and Life Cycle Issues," which appeared in *Psychiatric Clinics of North America* (Volume 26, Issue 3, September 2003).

[a] Department of Psychiatry and Behavioral Sciences, George Washington University Medical Center, 2300 Eye Street, NW, Washington, DC 20037, USA
[b] Division of Adolescent/Young Adult Medicine, Children's Hospital, Boston, MA 02115, USA
[c] Department of Pediatrics, Harvard Medical School, Boston, MA, USA
* Corresponding author. 1616 18th Street, Suite 104, Washington, DC 20009.
E-mail address: diane.shrier.med.64@aya.yale.edu (D.K. Shrier).

Obstet Gynecol Clin N Am 36 (2009) 753–769
doi:10.1016/j.ogc.2009.10.009
0889-8545/09/$ – see front matter © 2009 Elsevier Inc. All rights reserved.

obgyn.theclinics.com

biologic-reproductive circle, the family-marital circle, and the educational-vocational circle are all bound together," interacting, overlapping, sometimes enhancing and sometimes conflicting with one another. Ellen Cook and colleagues[8] suggest that because women's work life and career decisions are inextricably embedded in their life contexts, an ecological model may provide a more comprehensive and flexible view of women's career development. Women (and men) exist and behave within a social environment, act in response to that environment, and their actions influence the environment. Person-environment interactions are shaped by how individuals perceive and understand them.

Societal norms in the United States have shifted dramatically from the expectation before the 1970s that women's primary, and often exclusive and preferred, roles were to revolve around the private, domestic sphere as mother and wife. Currently, women's normative adult roles have broadened to include work, although there is a considerable variation as to how and when and whether the domestic and work roles will take place over the course of a woman's life.[9] Some women defer marriage and children until well established in their careers. Others marry young and simultaneously establish career identities and roles as wives and mothers. Others defer their careers or work lives until their children are in school or outside of the home. Still other women focus on career and economic self-sufficiency, choosing to remain single or child free—a choice less likely to be made by men in similar careers.[3]

Economically disadvantaged women, lesbians, and women from ethnic minorities (especially African Americans), have worked outside the home out of financial necessity since at least the Industrial Revolution of the mid-nineteenth century.[10] Before World War II, society viewed paid employment outside the home for women who did not need to work to help support their families as temporary and preliminary to their main job as wife and mother. Employment opportunities for women were limited primarily to domestic service, factory work, social work, nursing, and teaching. During World War II when large numbers of men were drafted or volunteered for military service, women temporarily joined the paid labor force in large numbers as a patriotic duty. Most middle-class white women returned to their unpaid family, domestic, and volunteer responsibilities after the men came back from war and took over their former jobs as the family breadwinners.

Beginning in the 1960s, as part of the second-wave women's movement, dramatic changes began to occur in the work and family lives of women, especially middle-class, white, heterosexual women, with a broadening of work opportunities and aspirations and changes in societal expectations about the roles of women.[3] In the 1940s and 1950s, 95% of women married, the vast majority of married women had several children, and only one-third of women were in the paid labor force. Two-thirds of women expressed a preference not to work outside the home after marriage. By 1979 only 5% of women expressed such a preference. Currently, 95% of women work outside the home for at least part of their adult lives, most by choice and because of societal expectation, others for financial necessity. In fact, less than 3% of families are in traditional marriages in which the man is the sole breadwinner and the woman remains at home full time.[9] In 1975, 47% of women with children younger than 18 and 39% of women with children younger than 6 were in the paid workforce. By 2005, 71% of women with children younger than 18 (a decline from 73% in 2000) and 62% of women with children younger than 6 were employed.[11]

Motherhood continues to be considered as central to the adult identities of women, whereas fatherhood is not viewed as central to men's adult identities.[12] With some exceptions, males continue to experience their primary role as worker, with marriage and children not taken into account in regard to their timing and choices of career and life planning. Women's biologic clocks and greater limitations on fertility to their 20s and 30s and, with fertility treatments now extending into their early 40s, are far more likely than men to consider marriage and parenthood's impact on career aspirations and timing. Those women who are childless by choice or by circumstance face the challenge of dealing with the continuing societal expectation that motherhood is "essential, normal, and natural for all women" and that "whatever else they do with their lives, women are expected to become mothers."[12]

According to Cook and colleagues,[8] traditional male model assumptions have been applied to women's career development including that (1) work and family roles are distinct; (2) individualism and autonomy are highly valued; (3) work is the central focus of one's life; (4) one's career trajectory is linear, continuous, progressive, and rational; (5) opportunity is egalitarian and hard work is rewarded. Instead, most women and some men (including many men in Generation X and younger), endorse the importance of work and family/personal life balance.[13] Addressing factors of importance to women may enhance career development and satisfaction of both sexes. In the alternative work/life model more suitable for women (and men), (1) multiple life roles are often inextricably intertwined and cannot be considered in isolation; (2) many women's decisions are guided by consideration of relationships and the principles of collectivism, interdependence, and collaboration; (3) in general, women in the workforce bear most of the household and familial executive and actual responsibilities and prioritize family over work considerations in making career decisions; (4) women are more likely than men to interrupt, resume, change the course, and alter the pace of their careers to accommodate other concerns, such as having and raising children, caring for elders, and negotiating structural barriers[14]; and (5) gender discrimination and sexual harassment pervade many aspects of women's careers and create disparities in organizational supports, pay, advancement, success, and satisfaction.[15–17]

Especially for women, whose biologic clocks have a narrower window than men, peak childbearing years overlap with the peak career-building years and most work settings do not accommodate the flexibility needed to integrate work and family/personal lives.[18] In addition, Americans have been working increasingly longer hours over the past 3 decades, with adverse affects on family and leisure time, sleeping, eating, and stress-related emotional and physical disorders.[19] Americans work an average of 2 months more a year than citizens of France and West Germany who have mandatory 6 weeks of annual leave.[19] Distinctions between private and public lives have been blurred through new technologies that create the expectations of constant availability through cell phones, e-mail, text messaging, and call waiting. Up to 40% of adults surveyed felt stressed or burned out by excessive workloads and inadequate personal and family time.[20] Employed mothers suffered in greater numbers than other workers, particularly those with preschool-age children, reporting even higher levels of stress related to inadequate time for their families.[20,21]

Recently, some women who can afford to do so have chosen to take time out from their careers, reduce their hours, or work for themselves to spend more time caring for their children, and there has been increased interest by corporations and academic and medical institutions to find ways to retain women through more flexible, family-friendly changes in the workplace environment and culture[22–25] or to plan for ways for women who have taken time off to return to the same workplace.[26,27] In addition, workplaces that pay attention to work-life balance have a competitive advantage, more productive and satisfied workers, and higher rates of retention.[20,28]

Although more men currently share household and child care and elder care responsibilities than in previous generations, women continue to carry a disproportionate share—a second shift, including most women physicians.[29,30] Women's family roles involving care of children and ill, disabled, or elderly relatives are more likely to intrude upon their paid employment mentally or in actuality. Women are more likely to "have two simultaneous roles, whereas men are allowed to have sequential roles," generally deferring "family roles to the evening after work"[10] or weekends. Although some women may suffer from role strain, conflict, or overload, research also shows that women who combine multiple roles are physically and emotionally among the healthiest in contrast to those who do one role exclusively.[10]

Since the 1960s, women have increasingly experienced lower rates of marriage, higher rates of divorce, later age at marrying, and fewer children and, with women living on average more than a decade longer than men, many women can anticipate spending many years of their adult lives single and alone. The divorce rate since the 1960s has risen to, and remained at, approximately half the marriage rate. There is increasing societal acceptance of single women bearing or adopting children, including never married, divorced, or lesbians, whether alone or with the support of a partner or extended family or friends. Deferring childbearing or choosing not to have children has also become a choice made by some women or couples, whereas small families with one or, at most, two children has become the norm, especially for women with professional careers.[3]

GENDER DISCRIMINATION, SEXUAL HARASSMENT, TOKENISM, AND MICROINEQUITIES

Despite the increasing range of opportunities for women and the passage of federal and state legislation prohibiting gender discrimination in the workplace, women continue to earn lower wages than men of comparable levels of education and skills. In 2005, women's median earnings were still only 81% of men's overall, including 89% for African Americans and 88% for Hispanics, whereas males from these minority groups suffer additional racial or ethnic discrimination.[11] In addition, most women continue to be employed in female-dominated and lower-status positions such as sales, administrative support, social work, and teaching. Even among women in the professions, including medicine, law, business, science, and technology, they remain significantly underrepresented in positions of leadership with the authority to determine policies pertaining to compensation and work conditions.[25,31,32]

Although the more egregious and blatantly illegal forms of gender discrimination and sexual harassment are alleged to have diminished in frequency, a series of studies in a wide variety of workplace settings continue to demonstrate the persistence of more subtle forms, such as gender stereotyping, microinequities, tokenism, and milder but significant forms of discrimination and harassment.[2,15–17,31] Gender discrimination in the workplace became illegal in the United States after Congress passed the Civil Rights Act in 1964. Since 1972, Education Amendments have prohibited gender and other forms of discrimination by education programs that received federal funding. Sexual harassment, a subcategory of gender discrimination, was defined in 1980 by the Equal Employment Opportunity Commission (EEOC) as "unwelcome sexual advances, requests for sexual favors, and other verbal or physical conduct of a sexual nature" affecting the terms or conditions of employment or advancement. Two types of sexual harassment have subsequently been recognized on the basis of case law. Quid pro quo harassment involves the exchange of a job benefit for expressed or implied sexual favors. Hostile work environment results when there is a frequent, repetitive, and continuous offensive pattern by supervisors, clients, or coworkers that adversely affects the terms of conditions of employment or education.[15,16]

Tokenism

Tokenism "is the practice of hiring or appointing a token number of people from under-represented groups to deflect criticism or comply with affirmative action rules" (http://www.Answer.com). Tokenism occurs for women when they comprise less than 15% of the workforce in a particular work setting, which continues to be the case at the highest ranks in most professions, including medicine.[3] Each "token" woman is viewed as a representative of all women. Some research suggests that tokenism has adverse effects on token women, whereas other research challenges those findings. Examples of the alleged adverse impact would include experiences where mistakes made by a white male are perceived as an individual error, whereas mistakes made by the token woman are often viewed as evidence that women "should not have been hired and are bound to fail."[33] Token positions are often stressful and highly visible. The token woman's individual behavior and characteristics may be distorted to fit stereotypes, such as "seductress," "bitch," "mother," or "kid sister." The token woman may be subject to unwelcome and derogatory sexist humor and there may be a focus on her physical appearance and clothing rather than on her work performance.[33,34] She may be the only woman in meetings or other group settings and her contributions may be ignored or interrupted and only heard when subsequently presented by a male coworker.

If the token woman's performance is outstanding, her achievements may threaten some of her traditional male coworkers who may feel humiliated at being "bested" by a woman. The token woman may then be retaliated against and either isolated from sources of information and the workplace social network or further criticized as a workaholic or as overly aggressive for behaviors that would be admired in her male coworkers. Token women may attempt to gain acceptance and avoid being mistreated in a number of ways. Some may become "queen bees," undermining and not supporting the achievements of other women in the workplace. Some may dress and behave in stereotypically ultrafeminine ways, minimize their own competence, and allow their male coworkers to take credit for their achievements. Others may dress in a more masculine fashion, act like one of the guys, and downplay their feminine side.[3,34]

The research that challenges the alleged adverse impact of tokenism on women finds that a token woman may experience a sense of enhanced well-being in a male-dominated profession or job. She may feel (and be) a pioneer and experience a high sense of achievement. By working in a male-dominated field, her work may be more highly valued by society and she may achieve higher economic benefits and status.[35]

Microinequities

Microinequities are subtle forms of gender discrimination. They may not reach the threshold for illegality "but negatively impact morale, job performance, and opportunities for promotion and training."[35] Examples of microinequities experienced by women include slights and visibility problems, being left out of informal and formal networks at work, devaluation of work based on gender, being discouraged from applying for career opportunities or exploited by credit being given to others for her work, and not being considered for a promotion or for awards.[35] The effects of these microinequities can be cumulative, can occur unexpectedly and only intermittently, and over time can undermine the woman's internal sense of competence.

Microinequities can be particularly difficult to address directly without the woman being misrepresented as overly sensitive.

Sequelae of Gender Discrimination and Sexual Harassment

Self-report surveys and case reports in the literature consistently demonstrate various significant physical and mental health and work performance sequelae for a substantial minority of women exposed over time to even the less severe forms of gender discrimination, harassment, tokenism, or microinequities.[36] The most common sequelae are depressive and anxiety disorders and a range of acute somatic symptoms that are new or represent the exacerbation or recurrence of previous disorders or symptoms. Headaches, rashes, gastrointestinal and genitourinary complaints, sexual dysfunction, and substance use are reported. Interpersonal relationships at work and with family and friends may be adversely affected. There may be significant economic costs to the woman and her employer. Absences from work, decline in work performance, or decisions to take another job are common reactions to workplace discrimination or harassment. Women who complain to supervisors, file formal complaints within the workplace or with the EEOC, or take legal action against their employer run the risk of retaliation, even though retaliation is against the law. They may be fired, blackballed from obtaining other work in their field, or reassigned to less significant work. They are often discredited, ostracized, and disbelieved by coworkers, experiences that lead over time to loss of self-esteem and an undermining of their professional identity. Legal remedies are uncertain, take many years, and can be highly costly financially, emotionally, and physically.[37]

Health Professionals

Health professionals, especially those in leadership positions and those who are in fields or specialties predominately female or who treat women, need to be well informed about overt and subtle forms of gender discrimination, including sexual harassment. Some physicians misunderstand the woman's posttraumatic symptoms as the cause rather than the consequence of their discrimination experiences. Other clinicians, whether out of ignorance or personal prejudices, may further compound the woman's trauma by ignoring indications that the woman has indeed experienced discrimination, by providing stigmatizing diagnoses and by communicating disbelieving attitudes to the patient, employer, and legal setting.[38] They need to be careful not to retaliate against women who make formal complaints or take legal action. Even those institutions that pride themselves on being a gender neutral meritocracy need to be aware of the research demonstrating the ongoing impact of gender-based discrimination on women's careers.[31,32]

OTHER WORK PROBLEMS AND WORK INHIBITIONS

Some researchers and theoreticians have emphasized a variety of primarily internally driven work problems and inhibitions experienced by women.[39] Others have focused attention on the need for the traditional workplace itself to change to accommodate women's strengths and skills.[40–43] In regard to intrapsychic issues, individual case studies and some empiric research have demonstrated women's greater tendency to attribute success and achievements to luck or to relationships with others rather than to innate ability. Other case studies describe some women's fear that high achievement will lead to loss of highly valued relationships, rejection or retaliation, or being viewed as deviant. And finally, case studies have described women with inhibition of competition and assertiveness out of fear and guilt of harming others or of surpassing a devalued mother.[35,43]

AN ALTERNATIVE, NONDEFICIT MODEL

Some scholars have moved to an alternative nondeficit model of female development as different from traditional models of male development.[41,43] Interpersonal relationships are viewed as central to a woman's sense of identity and self-worth, and women are more likely than men to be encouraged to develop their caregiving and affiliative skills from early on in life. Research by faculty at the Sloan School of Management at Massachusetts Institute of Technology (MIT) has demonstrated the beneficial effect of employers moving away from the traditional male authoritarian, hierarchical workplace model with clear separation of public and private life.[42] Incorporating and valuing caregiving and affiliative skills developed in the private sphere and better integrating public and private spheres are shown to have a positive effect on employee satisfaction in the workplace, economic benefits to the employer, an overall reduction of stress, and improved balancing of work and a personal life.[42] Such workplace changes have been slow in coming and are still not widespread among places of employment. In the interim, women often struggle with internal and external mixed messages to be independent and achieving as well as attending to the needs of family and friends. Some researchers and theoreticians see women as often being better at "attending to the needs of others than identifying and claiming their own needs … especially [if she] is attempting to establish her career at a time when she is also parenting and being a wife."[35]

THE SANDWICH GENERATION

As women marry and bear children later than in previous generations and as their parents benefit from increases in longevity into their 80s and 90s, more women (and men) are faced with simultaneously attending to work, children, and elderly relatives. What has been called the "Sandwich Generation" has primary responsibility for the care of dependent children and elderly relatives, often in combination with working outside the home.[44] Even if full-time domestic help can be hired for children and elderly relatives, the executive responsibilities for finding and supervising such care and the resultant emotional and physical stresses are more likely to fall on women.[3,45]

Women have traditionally borne these caregiving responsibilities, place a high value on interpersonal relationships, and find it harder than men to compartmentalize and delegate those caregiving tasks. "Women are especially stressed by situations that are beyond their control and by those in which they perceive themselves to be responsible for the well-being of others … failure causes a marked lowering of self-esteem."[35] The problems are compounded by the reduced availability of competent caregivers owing to greater opportunity for women to obtain more lucrative nontraditional employment outside the domestic sphere. The time, financial strain, and emotional energy involved in elder care may overwhelm a woman's emotional and physical resources. The caregiver may feel emotionally drained, overwhelmed, and become physically ill herself. She may find it difficult to discriminate between the necessary realistic requirements of caring for an elderly ill parent and guilt-driven excessive demands.[45] New geriatric specialists have arisen to provide assistance to the caregiver and elderly relative in making a range of complex social, economic, and health decisions. Some employers offer such assistance as part of the benefits they provide to their employees. The impact of these caregiving responsibilities is compounded by the absence of a societal systemic network of universal health care, child care, mandatory paid parental leave, respite for caregivers, and systems of elder care available in other industrialized nations.[3]

WOMEN IN MEDICINE

A successful class action suit filed by the National Organization for Women in 1970 against every US medical school forced compliance with the Civil Rights Act of 1964 prohibiting gender and race/ethnic discrimination in the workplace. By 1975 the numbers of women in medicine had more than tripled and continued to climb so that by 2005 there was parity between men and women entering medical school and in the early stages of their careers.[46] Despite these gains, women physicians continue to be far less likely than their male counterparts to hold positions of authority and leadership in all aspects of the medical profession.[47] Women in academic medicine are far less likely to achieve tenure and the higher faculty ranks despite equal levels of competence and satisfaction,[48,49] even in fields such as obstetrics/gynecology and pediatrics where most practitioners are women. Similar situations exist among PhDs, business, law, and other fields of science and technology.[26,31,32] Women also leave academic medicine at higher rates and lower faculty ranks[50] resulting in substantial costs to medical centers,[51] scientific enterprise, and global competitiveness.[31] This is not primarily because of a pipeline issue or inadequate career mentoring. Institutional and societal supports that take into account the gendered nature of career development, considering both work and family roles and environments and both individual characteristics and social factors, are likely to be more effective in retaining women in academic medicine and other professional leadership roles than supports that focus solely on work-related career issues.[52]

THE CHANGING CULTURE OF MEDICINE

There are growing concerns about the changing nature of the practice of medicine and the culture of medical institutions that have an adverse impact on men, but even more so on women. These changes have contributed to increased levels of physician dissatisfaction, burnout, and feeling unsupported and isolated.[53] Although physicians have always worked hard, caring relationships with patients, teaching of students and trainees, and collaboration with colleagues have generally made the profession a satisfying one. More recently, with the advent of managed care, large group practices, rising costs of professional liability insurance and malpractice litigation, unsubsidized medical education with subsequent high debt, and financial pressures on academic institutions, there has been an increased focus on generating income through grants and clinical care at the expense of education and teaching. All of these factors have shifted medicine into more of a profit-making business venture. Physicians in clinical practice are pressed to see more patients for less time and need to spend more time on paperwork and hire more staff to deal with insurance companies at the expense of patient care. The importance of the doctor-patient relationship in healing and in physician satisfaction is often neglected, although there have been recent efforts to reverse that trend.[54–56] Although rates of depression in physicians are the same as for men and women matched by age in other professions, suicide rates are substantially higher. Male physicians are about one-and-a-half times and female physicians three to four times more likely to commit suicide than their age-matched peers.[57] A 2003 American Foundation for Suicide Prevention consensus statement notes that the current "culture of medicine accords low priority to physician mental health" with punitive barriers to their seeking help.[57] As noted earlier, caring, collaborative, and affiliative relationships may be more central to a woman's identity and development[8] than the traditional male hierarchical model of independence, competition, and individual success. Women, like the "canary in the mine," may be more sensitive to or may more readily recognize the current dysfunctional relational aspects of the culture in practice and institutional medicine.[52]

A number of academic medical institutions have responded to these concerns and have developed programs, on the basis of research findings, to better support faculty, students, and practitioners' "ability to function at their highest potential."[52–57] Examples include the National Initiative on Gender, Culture, and Leadership in Medicine to identify effective supports for faculty and students,[52] the Physician Work Life Study,[54] the Women Physicians' Health Study,[58] faculty development and medical student programs that include more family-friendly work/life environments,[24,59,60] and Faculty and Physician Wellness programs to create a more nurturing environment and nonpunitive access to recognition and treatment of disorders and impairments (University of Virginia School of Medicine, Vanderbilt University School of Medicine, and Massachusetts Physician Health Program).[57] All these programs and many others are geared to providing emotional and social, as well as professional, supports to physicians and other health care professionals and trainees.[22,47,55,56] These initiatives parallel work life programs being created in businesses, universities, and other professions.[28] The initiative for these developments often came from concerns raised by and about women and families and work/life balance but were subsequently recognized to create a more effective, productive, and satisfying work environment for men as well as women.[20,23,24,47,57]

THREE RESEARCH PARADIGMS ON WOMEN'S WORK

Before the second wave women's movement of the 1960s, 1970s, and beyond, research on work and career focused almost exclusively on the experiences of men, as occurred similarly in other domains such as physical and mental health. Research on women's work, whether paid or unpaid, and the combining of work and family roles were largely neglected and not regarded as subjects worthy of serious investigation. From the 1970s to the present, through the influence of the women's movement, research on women's work and family roles has increased substantially, particularly by researchers from the fields of sociology (especially family studies), psychology, and organizational behavior. The focus of this research could be divided into three distinct but overlapping phases or paradigms. The first, from 1975 to 1984, emphasized what was called "women's role expansion," the second (which continues) involves "multiple competing roles," and the third is "work-family convergence."[9]

Research with an Emphasis on Women's Role Expansion—1975 to 1984

The initial research on women's work and family lives focused on women expanding their roles from the traditional ones of wife, mother, and unpaid domestic responsibilities, ignored any possible changes to men's roles, and assumed that the changes were likely to produce adverse effects. Thus, research questions addressed the possible harm of the dramatic increase of women's participation in the paid workforce on children, spouse, and women themselves. Despite continuing societal expectations to the contrary, repeated studies have demonstrated that even children younger than 6—who are assumed to be most at risk—suffered no adverse emotional, cognitive, or social conditions if they were cared for by competent nonmaternal alternative caregivers, including group daycare.[61] The problem remains a societal issue in that the United States continues to be the only industrialized nation not to provide subsidized and sufficient quantities of quality child care with national policies, adequate pay, and requirements for training and for child caregiver:child ratios according to the age of the child. Nor are there national policies for mandatory paid parental leaves. The myth persists that maternal care is the best form of child care—except for poor women, especially women of color, and welfare mothers.[11]

Research on Multiple Competing Roles and Comparisons between Women and Men—1984 to Present

The second phase of research, which continues to the present, compares men and women. The assumption is made that work and family are competing or conflicting roles, that combining work and family are women's issues, that all families are heterosexual and also have children. This myth that work and family roles are in conflict persists despite evidence to the contrary that many women (and men) experience work and family as mutually enriching and beneficial, rather than a source of conflict.[60,62,63] A number of studies have been done on role conflict, role overload, and role strain, again the assumption being made that these issues only pertain to women. Research does show widespread role conflict, overload, and strain for women, but this is largely the result of conflicting internal and external expectations experienced by the women studied.[35]

Role conflict

Role conflict refers to the "psychological effects of being faced with two or more sets of incompatible expectations or demands."[35] The expectation is that the woman will be fully committed to work, using the traditional male model, and also be required to give her highest priority to family, using the traditional female model. Most women in paid employment who were studied experience role conflict. However, the conflict is reduced when the woman had a supportive spouse, children beyond the preschool years, high income, and less hassle and stress and more flexibility on the job.[2,3,18,62]

Role overload or strain

Role overload or role strain is similar to role conflict but refers to the difficulties in meeting the demands of career and marriage, especially with children, without giving short shrift to either role. Insistence on meeting the highest standards for domestic and work life without setting priorities (eg, gourmet meals, spotless housekeeping while producing high-quality work outside the home) is likely to result in role overload or strain. Some women feel the internal need to prove themselves as wives, mothers, and workers at the same levels as women who have chosen to focus their efforts on one role or the other. The strain is intensified by the difficulties in finding and keeping quality child care, lack of support from spouse or extended families, and lack of opportunity for socializing and personal time.[35]

Research on Work-Family Role Convergence—Current Paradigm

The third and current research phase and paradigm is called work-family role convergence. Career and work "is now widely recognized as an appropriate, normative, healthy, and intrinsically rewarding aspect of women's and men's adult lives."[9] Similarly, connections with family, domestic partners, spouse, children, and other sources of social networks and supports are now widely recognized as an integral and healthy part of people's lives. There is considerable variation on how families manage combining work and family (especially when there are children). Although there is still an inequity in the division of labor, whether by choice or tradition or other factors, men's participation (especially among middle-class and more highly educated families) has continued to increase since 1970. Currently, on average, "men in dual-earner families do 34% of the housework and larger percentages of the parenting, with a sizable number close to 50–50 in both areas."[9] Studies show that dual-career couples with a more equitable sharing of work and family responsibilities report greater marital satisfaction and stability.[11] There has been research specifically on gay and lesbian couples, domestic unmarried partners, families who have experienced divorce, and extended families raising children, but these variations will not be the focus of this article. Such variations on "traditional" families now comprise most families in the United States and all are capable of raising psychologically healthy children if the needs of children are made a priority.

INDIVIDUAL COPING STRATEGIES FOR DEALING WITH ROLE CONFLICT OR OVERLOAD

Women have used a variety of coping strategies to deal with potential role conflict or overload.[2,3,10,35] Some women have made choices to eliminate roles and remained unmarried or childless, unlike men in comparably demanding careers. Other women have taken a sequential approach to paid employment and childbearing by first establishing a career before having children or having children early and then resuming work. Other women (and their partners) who choose to combine family and career simultaneously may increase or decrease their work hours or responsibilities (depending on the age and developmental needs of their children), or accept lower and simpler standards for housekeeping and meals, or delegate certain roles to paid others or to relatives. Some women use the traditional male approach of compartmentalizing and focusing attention on one role at a time. Some may use one role to excuse herself from other role responsibilities by just being "too busy" or may limit social relationships to others with similar attitudes toward combining career, marriage, and children, thus feeling more supported in her choices. Other women attempt the "superwoman" solution and try to handle all roles simultaneously by working harder, faster, and in a more highly efficient and organized fashion. In a minority of families, both parents negotiate sharing of responsibilities for work, home, and children. Other strategies include intrapsychic changes, altering "one's personal attitudes toward the role."[35] By use of cognitive-behavioral approaches, such as cognitive reframing, relaxation exercises, meditation, and other stress-reduction techniques, including consciously setting aside time for exercise, hobbies, and pleasurable leisure time for herself, the woman may be able to reduce her emotional distress responses.[3,35]

ENRICHING AND REINFORCING MULTIPLE ROLES

Although some women experience combining career and family simultaneously as a conflict of roles and responsibilities, many others find that multiple roles can be enriching and may reinforce, rather than disrupt, each role and other aspects of the women's lives.[3,62] Research demonstrates that women who are employed "report better physical and psychological health than women who are not employed, as well as the women experiencing enhanced financial independence."[62] Women who combine multiple roles (work and family) are physically healthier and are more likely to have a greater sense of well-being and happiness than women who have only career or family roles.[9] Women in their middle years who do not have preschool-age children report the highest feeling of well-being when they have all three roles of wife, mother, and paid worker, whereas women having only one of these roles report the least satisfaction and feelings of well-being.[10] Shifting gears between work and family may provide psychological protection and alleviate stress. Satisfactions in one role may counteract disappointments in the other.[10] However, at the same time, a number of factors increase the likelihood of women suffering from stress-related somatic and emotional disorders, such as anxiety and depression. These factors include women being likely to work in jobs where they have less control over work hours and content, having difficulty obtaining and keeping adequate child care, and experiencing confusion over their own internalized roles and values.[2,3]

WORKPLACE INSTITUTIONAL STRATEGIES AND PROGRAMS

Initial efforts within the workplace to enable workers to feel less stressed were focused on the establishment of Employee Assistance Programs (EAP) to which workers could be referred and educational programs on stress management techniques as though the problem was that of the individual worker. More recently, greater attention has been paid by some workplaces to design strategies to enable workers to better integrate work and personal lives.[18,22,23,28] A minority of organizations and researchers have moved away from assuming that the problems with role conflict, strain, and overload in attempting to combine career and family or a personal life need to be resolved by the individual woman (and her partner and family).[47] Some researchers have developed more creative workplace models to enable men and women to better integrate work and family in ways that benefit the workplace and personal lives.[28,42,64,65] In addition, various institutional changes have helped some workers, especially women, maintain a better balance between family and work.[18,28] Included are employee benefits, such as paid or unpaid personal days for family responsibilities, assistance in locating services for child care or elder care, job sharing, and flex time.[10,18,23]

MIDLIFE AND BEYOND TO OLD AGE

Midlife is defined as 45 to 65 years overlapping with old age, although increasingly euphemisms are substituted for both periods of life—seniors, empty nesters, prime timers. Old age is increasingly divided into three periods: the young-old, ages 60 to 75; the old-old, ages 75 to 85; and the oldest-old, from the late 80s and beyond. Psychological, interpersonal, health, and economic issues for women are different for each of these periods and there is tremendous interindividual variability owing to social class, birth cohort, ethnicity, and health.[66]

In 1900, women were on average only likely to live to age 47, with many dying in childbirth or during their childbearing years. Currently, increasing numbers of women (and men) can anticipate living into their 80s and beyond. Those who have borne and raised children are finding that only a small percentage of their lives will include child care responsibilities with an increasing number of years spent "postmaternal" or free from caring for children. If the average age of menopause is 51, most women who follow guidelines for healthy diets, maintain an appropriate weight, engage in aerobic and weight-bearing exercise, practice health care prevention and maintenance, employ stress reduction measures, stay intellectually and socially engaged, and are financially secure can anticipate living more than 30 years postmenopausal. For most of that period women can enjoy a quality of life that is physically and psychologically fulfilling and even more creative than earlier in their lives.[67]

What we used to call old age and its accompanying ailments had more to do with ill health than age. The focus of research on aging has been, until recently, on losses of status, societal value, and physical and mental health, emphasizing illness and dying, and loss of friends, family, and economic security. More recent research has demonstrated the factors that contribute to aging well[68,69] but aging is still viewed negatively in the United States where the elderly are often depicted and stereotyped as socially useless and burdens. The exception has been a trend for increasing numbers of grandparents assuming primary child-care responsibilities among some subgroups, especially African American families. In contrast, in many other societies such as Asian and African, the old have been traditionally respected for their wisdom and as keepers and teachers of valued traditions who continue to have significant roles in the society.

There is a long-standing double standard in regard to aging in many societies, including the United States. Women are generally seen as reaching middle age and old age at least 5 years earlier than men.[70] Negative stereotypes about the physical appearance, behavioral attributes, and sexual attractiveness of old women (in contrast to old men) are strongly reinforced by the media. Discrimination based on age is added to that based on sex and compounded for those who are economically deprived and from ethnic minority groups.[71] Increasing numbers of those women (and fewer men) who can afford it attempt to ward off the appearance of aging in our youth-obsessed culture through plastic surgery, Botox, liposuction, and other measures.

Recent research counters societal stereotypes of midlife and old age, finding this time of life often less stressful and highly positive for women (and men). Longitudinal studies and anecdotal reports of college-educated women found a higher sense of self-confidence, power, and generativity in women in their 60s and a lower level of psychological distress than in women in their 20s and 40s.[72] For some women, the midlife, menopausal, postmaternal years may be a time to review their lives and family and career choices and make life changes that increase their sense of well-being in later life.[68,71] Other women who, for various reasons, were unable to make positive changes and life-course corrections were more likely to ruminate and be discontented with their lives.[73] Education and income appear to make a big difference in the quality of life as women age. As more of the cohorts of women who benefited from the societal changes of the second-wave women's movement reach old age, they are more likely to have more positive views and experiences of aging than did their mothers and grandmothers.

SUMMARY AND FUTURE DIRECTIONS

This article focuses on psychosocial aspects of women's adult lives with a particular emphasis on the dramatic and evolving changes that have occurred in both societal and internalized expectations of women's roles and normative life cycle since the second women's movement of the 1960s and beyond. Women's adult life cycle has become increasingly complex and varied as to life choices and timing of career and family. Despite these changes, workplace gender discrimination, sexual harassment, tokenism, and microinequities persist for many women with resultant emotional, physical, economic, and interpersonal sequelae. Role overload, conflict, and strain and other stresses related to efforts to combine career and a family and personal life or to intrapsychic issues may occur. However, research demonstrates that for many women multiple roles are mutually enriching and result in a greater sense of well-being than experienced by women with a single role. Although stress in the workplace was initially viewed as the problem of the individual worker requiring information and stress-management techniques, there is growing recognition that this is a societal issue that would benefit from workplace changes that would better enable workers to integrate work and personal lives, and private and public spheres.

Research on women's work and family roles has changed its emphasis and questions studied from the initial concerns about the possible adverse impacts of women's expanding their traditional roles to include work outside the home, to assumptions that work and family are competing or conflicting roles, to a recognition that work and family are both appropriate, normative. and rewarding aspects of women's adult lives.

For women in midlife and old age, although negative stereotyping of older women and aging in general persists in American society, there is growing recognition of the increased sense of well-being and creativity in the later stages of life experienced by many older women (and men). The tremendous interindividual variability of experiences in midlife and old age is noted to be dependent on many factors, including health, socioeconomic status, ethnicity, and birth cohort.

Physicians, especially those in specialties that focus exclusively or predominantly on women and families, need to be particularly well-informed about the issues discussed in this article both on a personal and a professional level. The issues of retention and leadership pertaining to women physicians in the changing and often dysfunctional culture of medicine has drawn attention to the adverse impact on physicians of both genders, as well as on patient care and trainee education. In the manner of "Physician, heal thyself," women physicians and physicians caring for women need to be attentive to issues affecting women's health and look for opportunities to work toward societal and institutional affirmative changes as a means of helping themselves, as well as the patients they serve.

REFERENCES

1. Gutek BA. Asymmetric changes in men's and women's roles. In: Long BC, Kahn SE, editors. Women, work and coping: a multidisciplinary approach to workplace stress. Montreal (Canada): McGill-Queen's University Press; 1993.
2. Shrier DK. Career and workplace issues. In: Kornstein SG, Clayton AH, editors. Women's mental health: a comprehensive textbook. New York: Guilford Press; 2002. p. 527–41.
3. Shrier DK. Psychosocial aspects of women's lives: work, family, and life cycle issue. Psychiatr Clin North Am 2003;26:741–57.
4. Bateson MC. Composing a life. New York: Penguin Books; 1990.
5. Sheehy G. New passages: mapping your life across time. New York: Random House; 1995.
6. Levinson DJ. The seasons of a woman's life. New York: A Knopf Inc; 1996.
7. Seiden AM. Psychological issues affecting women throughout the life cycle. Psychiatr Clin North Am 1989;12(1):1.
8. Cook EP, Heppner MJ, O'Brien KM. Career development of women of color and white women: assumptions, conceptualization, and interventions from an ecological perspective. Career Development Quarterly 2002;50:291–305.
9. Gilbert LA, Rader J. Current perspectives on women's adult roles: work, family, and life. In: Unger RD, editor. Psychology of women and gender. New York: John Wiley & Sons; 2001. p. 166–7.
10. Nieva VF. Work and family linkages. In: Larwood L, Stromberg AH, Gutek BA, editors, Women and work: an annual review, vol. 1. London: Sage Publications; 1985. p. 176.
11. US Department of Labor. Women in the labor force: a datebook. Washington, DC: Bureau of Labor Statistics; 2006.
12. Woollett A, Marshall H. Motherhood and mothering. In: Unger RK, editor. Handbook of the psychology of women and gender. New York: John Wiley & Sons; 2001. p. 171.
13. Bickel J, Brown AJ, Generation X. Implications for faculty recruitment and development in academic health centers. Acad Med 2005;80(3):205–10.

14. Xie Y, Shauman KA. Women in science: career processes and outcomes. Cambridge (MA): Harvard University Press; 2005.
15. Gutek BA, Done RS. Sexual harassment. In: Unger RK, editor. Psychology of women and gender. New York: John Wiley & Sons; 2001.
16. Shrier DK, editor. Sexual harassment in the workplace and academia: psychiatric issues. Washington, DC: American Psychiatric Press; 1996.
17. Shrier DK, Zucker AN, Mercurio AE, et al. Generation to generation: discrimination and harassment experiences of physician mothers and their physician daughters. J Womens Health 2007;16:882–94.
18. Shrier DK, Shrier LA, Rich M, et al. Pediatricians leading the way: integrating a career and a family/personal life over the life cycle. Pediatrics 2007;117:519–22.
19. Schor JB. The overworked American: the unexpected decline of leisure. New York: Basic Books; 1991.
20. Bond JT, Thompson C, Galinsky E, et al. The national study of the changing workforce. New York: Families and Work Institute; 2002.
21. Ayers L, Cusak M, Crosby F. Combining work and home. Occup Med 1993;8(4): 821–31.
22. Viggiano T. Career management for individual and institutional vitality: a life cycle model for professional development. Boston: Harvard Macy Institute Program for Leaders in Healthcare Education; 2005.
23. Bencko C, Weisberg AC. Mass career customization: aligning the workplace with today's nontraditional workforce. Cambridge (MA): Harvard Business School Press; 2007.
24. US Department of Health and Human Services Office on Women's Health. Beyond parity workbook for action: transforming academic medicine through women's leadership. Bethesda (MD): US Department of Health and Human Services; 2005.
25. Women and medicine: proceedings of the conference chaired by Catherine D. DeAngelis, MD, MPH. Josiah Macy, Jr Foundation; 2007.
26. Hewlett SA, Luce CB, Servon LJ, et al. The Athena factor: reversing the brain drain in science, engineering and technology. Research report from center for work-life policy. New York: Columbia University; 2008.
27. Hewlett SA. Off-ramps and on-ramps. Boston (MA): Harvard Business School Press; 2007.
28. Joshi S, Leichne J, Melanson K, et al. Work-life balance. A case of social responsibility or competitive advantage. Worklifebalance.com, Inc; 2002.
29. Bowman MA, Frank E, Allen DI, editors. Women in medicine: career and life management. 3rd edition. New York: Springer; 2002.
30. Hochschild AR, Machung A. The second shift. New York: The Penguin Group; 2003.
31. National Academy of Sciences, National Academy of Engineering, and Institute of Medicine. Beyond bias and barriers: fulfilling the potential of women in academic science and engineering. Washington, DC: The National Academies Press; 2006.
32. Mason MA, Goulden M. Do babies matter: the effect of family formation on the lifelong careers of academic men and women. Academe 2002;88:212.
33. Unger RK, Crawford M, editors. Women and gender: a feminist psychology. 2nd edition. New York: McGraw-Hill; 1996. p. 446, 463.
34. Conley FK. Walking out on the boys. New York: Farrar, Straus & Giroux; 1998.
35. Bernstein AE, Lenhart SA. The psychodynamic treatment of women. Washington, DC: American Psychiatric Press; 1993. p. 137, 147, 178, 207.

36. Lenhart SA. Physical and mental health aspects of sexual harassment. In: Shrier DK, editor. Sexual harassment in the workplace and academia: psychiatric issues. Washington, DC: American Psychiatric Press; 1996.

37. Lenhart SA, Shrier DK. Potential costs and benefits of sexual harassment litigation. Psychiatr Ann 1996;26(3):132–8.

38. Jensvold MF. Potential for misuse and abuse of psychiatry in workplace sexual harassment. In: Shrier DK, editor. Sexual harassment in the workplace and academia: psychiatric issues. Washington, DC: American Psychiatric Press; 1996.

39. Person ES. Women working: fears of failure, deviance and success. J Am Acad Psychoanal 1982;10:67–84.

40. Stiver I. Work inhibitions in women. Wellesley (MA): The stone center for developmental services and studies. Work in progress, #82(3).

41. Jordan JV, Kaplan AG, Miller JB, et al, editors. Women's growth in connection. New York: Guilford Press; 1991.

42. Fletcher JK. A relational approach to the protean worker. In: Hall DG, editor. The career is dead—long live the career: a relational approach to careers. San Francisco (CA): Jossey-Bass; 1996.

43. Miller JB, Stiver IP. The healing connection: how women form relationships in therapy and in life. Wellesley (MA): The Stone Center; 1997.

44. Grundy E, Henretta JC. Between elderly parents and adult children: a new look at the intergenerational care provided by the 'sandwich generation'. Aging Soc 2006;26(5):707–22.

45. Lebow G, Kane B. Coping with your difficult older parent: stressed-out children. New York: Avon; 1999.

46. Association of American Medical Colleges. Women in US academic medicine. Statistics and benchmarking report, 2006–2007. Washington (DC): AAMC; 2007.

47. Morrissey CS, Schmidt ML. Fixing the system, not the women: an innovative approach to faculty advancement. J Womens Health 2008;17(8):1399–498.

48. Association of American Medical colleges. The changing representation of men and women in academic medicine. AAMC Anal Brief 2005;5(2):1–2.

49. Wright AL, Schwindt LA, Bassford TL, et al. Gender differences in academic advancement: patterns, causes, and potential solutions in one US college of medicine. Acad Med 2003;78(5):500–8.

50. Cropsey KL, Masho SW, Shiang R, et al. Why do faculty leave: reasons for attrition of women and minority faculty from a medical school: four-year results. J Womens Health 2008;17(7):1111–8.

51. Waldman JD, Kelly F, Arora S, et al. The shocking cost of turnover in health care. Health Care Manage Rev 2004;29(1):2–7.

52. Pololi L, Conrad P, Knight S, et al. A study of the relational aspects of the culture of academic medicine. Acad Med 2009;84(1):106–14.

53. Keeton K, Fenner DE, Johnson TR, et al. Predictors of physician career satisfaction, work-life balance, and burnout. Obstet Gynecol 2007;199(4):949–55.

54. McMurray JE, Linzer M, Konrad TR, et al. The work lives of women physicians: results from the physician work life study. The SGIM career satisfaction study group. J Gen Intern Med 2000;15:372–80.

55. Beach MC, Innui TS. Relationship-centered care research network. Relationship-centered care: a constructive reframing. J Gen Intern Med 2006;21(Suppl 1): S3–8.

56. Safran DG, Miller W, Beckman H. Organizational dimensions of relationship-centered care: theory, evidence and practice. J Gen Intern Med 2006; 21(Suppl 1):S9–S15.

57. American Foundation for Suicide Prevention Consensus Statement. Confronting depression and suicide in physicians. JAMA 2003;289(23):3161–6.
58. Frank F, McMurray JE, Linzer M, et al. Career satisfaction of US women physicians: results from the women physicians' health study. Ann Intern Med 1999; 159:1417.
59. Shollen SL, Bland CJ, Finstad DA, et al. Organizational climate and family life: how these factors affect the status of women faculty at one medical school. Acad Med 2009;84(1):87–94.
60. Shrier DK, Brodkin AM, Sondheimer A. Parenting and professionalism: competing and enriching commitments. J Am Med Womens Assn 1993;18(4): 122–4.
61. Scarr S, Eisenberg M. Child care research: issues, perspectives, and results. Annu Rev Psychol 1993;44:613–44.
62. Barnett RC, Rivers C. She works/he works: how two-income families are happier, healthier, and better off. New York: HarperCollins; 1996. p. 166.
63. Gilbert LA. Two careers/one family: the promise of gender equality. London: Sage Publications; 1993.
64. Barnett RC. Toward a review and reconceptualization of the work/family literature. Genet soc Gen Psychol Mongr 1998;124(2):125–82.
65. Bailyn L, Fletcher JK, Kolb D. Unexpected connections: considering employees' personal lives can revitalize your business. Sloan Manage Rev 1997;38(4):11–9.
66. Canetto SS. Older adult women: issues, resources and challenges. In: Unger RD, editor. Handbook of the psychology of women and gender. New York: John Wiley & Sons; 2001.
67. Cohen GD. The creative age: awakening human potential in the second half of life. New York: Avon Books; 2000.
68. National Institute on Aging. Healthy aging: lessons from the Baltimore Longitudinal Study of Aging. National Institute on Aging, National Institutes of Health. Bethesda (MD): U.S. Department of Health & Human Services; 2008.
69. Vaillant GE. Aging well: surprising guideposts to a happier life from the landmark Harvard study of adult development. New York: Little, Brown and Co; 2002.
70. Kite ME, Wagner LS. Attitudes toward older adults. In: Nelson TD, editor. Ageism: stereotyping and prejudice against older persons. Cambridge (MA): MIT Press; 2002. p. 129–61.
71. Unger RK. Midlife and beyond. In: Unger RK, Crawford M, editors. Women and gender: a feminist psychology. 3rd edition. New York: McGraw-Hill; 2003.
72. Zucker AN, Ostrove JM, Stewart AJ. College-educated women's personality development in adulthood: perceptions and age differences. Psychol Aging 2002;17:236–44.
73. Stewart AJ, Vandewater EA. "If I had it to do over again…" Midlife review, midcourse corrections, and women's well-being in later life. J Pers Soc Psychol 1999;76:270–83.

When Depression Complicates Childbearing: Guidelines for Screening and Treatment During Antenatal and Postpartum Obstetric Care

Maria Muzik, MD, MS[a],*, Sheila M. Marcus, MD[b],
Julie E. Heringhausen, BSN[c], Heather Flynn, PhD[a]

KEYWORDS

- Depression • Peripartum • Obstetric care
- Infant outcomes • Medication • Psychotherapy

BACKGROUND AND PREVALENCE

Across the United States, prevalence studies show that 1 in 5 women experience an episode of major depressive disorder (MDD) during their lifetime.[1] The onset of depressive symptoms is seen most often between ages 20 and 40, the prime age range for childbearing.[2] Studies have shown that 10% to 16% of pregnant or postpartum women fulfill the diagnostic criteria for MDD, and even more women

This is an updated version of the article "Depression in childbearing women: when depression complicates pregnancy," which appeared in *Primary Care: Clinics in Office Practice* (Volume 36, Issue 1, March 2009).

[a] Department of Psychiatry, University of Michigan, Rachel Upjohn Building, 4250 Plymouth Road, Ann Arbor, MI 48109, USA
[b] Department of Psychiatry, Child and Adolescent Psychiatry, University of Michigan, Rachel Upjohn Building, 4250 Plymouth Road, Ann Arbor, MI 48109, USA
[c] Medical School, University of Michigan, 1301 Catherine Street, 5124 MS I, Ann Arbor, MI 48109, USA
* Corresponding author.
E-mail address: muzik@med.umich.edu (M. Muzik).

experience subsyndromal depressive symptoms, which frequently are overlooked.[3,4] Because of this correlation with life events, it is important for health care providers to be aware of: (1) the frequency of depression in this population; (2) signs, symptoms, and appropriate screening methods; and (3) the health risks for the mother and growing fetus if depression is undetected or untreated. A study by Marcus and colleagues[5] in 2003 found that of pregnant women screened in an obstetrics setting who reported significant depressive symptoms, 86% were not receiving any form of treatment. Although most women seek some prenatal care during their pregnancy,[5] many women do not seek mental health services because of stigma; thus, antenatal visits to an obstetrician or primary care provider may provide an opportunity for screening and intervention for depression in this high-risk group. However, screening procedures alone have not been found to affect depression outcomes.[6] Because management of a depressed, pregnant, or postpartum woman also includes care of her growing fetus or her breastfeeding infant, treatment may be complicated and requires an informed, multidisciplinary approach, including input from an obstetrician, psychiatrist, and pediatrician, to provide optimal care.[7]

ANTENATAL DEPRESSION
Clinical Features and Risk Factors

The Diagnostic and Statistical Manual of Mental Disorders, Fourth Edition (DSM-IV) defines the diagnosis of depression using the same criteria for men and women, although research shows some variation in female presentation. MDD diagnosis must include existence of depressed or irritable mood or inability to experience pleasure. In addition, 4 of the following symptoms must be present: feelings of guilt, hopelessness, and worthlessness; sleep disturbance (insomnia or hypersomnia); appetite or weight changes; attention or concentration difficulties; decreased energy or unexplainable fatigue; psychomotor agitation or retardation; and, in severe cases, thoughts of suicide.[8] Women may present in a clinic with more seasonal depression or symptoms of atypical depression (eg, hypersomnia, hyperphagia, carbohydrate craving, weight gain, heavy feeling in arms and legs, worse mood in the evenings, and initial insomnia).[8] Anxiety and obsessive worries centering on pregnancy outcomes and fetal safety are common in pregnancy.[9] Many of these symptoms overlap with the physical and mental changes experienced during pregnancy, making them difficult to distinguish, and, therefore, they often are disregarded.[10]

Practitioners caring for pregnant women should be aware of personal and epidemiologic factors that place women most at risk for depression. An important primary risk factor is a previous personal history (particularly during pregnancy or post partum) or a family history of depression.[11] Another common risk factor is a woman's perception of limited social support and presence of social conflict. Recent literature shows that even when women report adequate social support, if they also report interpersonal conflict, then they are at a high risk for depression.[12] Obstetricians and care providers in antenatal clinics routinely address social support for pregnant women and encourage strengthening their support networks. It may be important also to address interpersonal conflict in the clinical interview.[12] Asking questions about feeling let down and unloved, feeling tense from arguing, and the frequency of unpleasant and distressing social interactions may be adequate to screen for social conflict and identify women who would benefit from clinical interventions addressing these interpersonal conflicts.[12] Other risk factors for depression include (1) history of physical, emotional, or sexual abuse; (2) history of (or current) cigarette smoking, alcohol consumption, or substance use; (3) stressors, such as financial or occupational obligations; (4) stressful health concerns or relationships[9]; (5) living alone; and (6) ambivalence about the pregnancy.[13]

SCREENING

In 2002, the US Preventive Services Task Force published findings that a positive answer to either or both of 2 universal depression screening questions was a quick and effective way to screen for depression: (1) "Over the past two weeks, have you ever felt down, depressed, or hopeless?" or (2) "Have you felt little interest or pleasure in doing things?" Affirmative answers initiate a more in-depth screening tool to gather more information toward the diagnosis.[14] The 2 measures used most commonly to screen for depression for adults in ambulatory care are the Beck Depression Inventory (2–3 minutes to complete)[15] and the revised Center for Epidemiologic Studies Depression Scale (5–10 minutes to complete).[16]

The Edinburgh Postnatal Depression Scale (EPDS) is a screening tool used internationally to assess depression during pregnancy and post partum.[17] The EPDS can screen for postpartum depression as early as early as 3 to 5 days after a woman gives birth with a score greater than 9.5.[18] If a woman scores higher than 15 during pregnancy or 13 post partum, then a further assessment is necessary for a diagnosis of depression.[19] Several screening instruments can be used to assess symptom severity and general functioning. One of these is the BASIS-24, a 24-item scale that measures symptoms and general functioning in 6 major areas: depression/functioning, relationships, self-harm, emotional lability, psychosis, and substance abuse.[20] Screening tools do not address the duration of symptoms, degree of impairment, or comorbid psychiatric disorders, including anxiety disorders[21]; thus, if a patient scores beyond the cut-off range for any of these tools, DSM-IV diagnostic criteria should be assessed through further interview.

Regardless of the screening method used, it is important to further question patients who manifest depressive symptoms on screening. An experienced practitioner may discern whether a patient requires more definitive treatment or if an increase in score is caused by a transient psychosocial stressor. Katon and Seeling[22] found that using screening tools in conjunction with "depression caremanagers" may improve the quality of care. Such nurse caremanagers provide education, track adherence with medication and psychotherapy, and support the patients in taking an active role in their illness. Where psychiatrists are available, practices may also benefit from using a collaborative care model with a psychiatric consultant who comanages difficult cases with the primary and antenatal care clinicians during the acute phase of their illness. A recent meta-analysis found that there was a 2-fold increase in medication compliance over 6 months with the collaborative care approach compared with patients following only with primary care, and enhanced functional outcomes were noted in these patients 2 to 5 years later.[23] An obstetric clinic-based study found that antenatal depression screening combined with nurse-delivered feedback and referral did not substantially affect rates of depression treatment use, suggesting the need for additional treatment linkage efforts.[6]

Most women do not follow through with a mental health referral[6] and each woman seems to face unique logistical and psychological barriers to engaging in treatment.[24] Therefore, to provide optimal and effective personalized care, clinicians in obstetrics need to ask women about treatment preferences and individual-specific barriers to follow through.

CONSEQUENCES OF DEPRESSION IN PREGNANCY

Unidentified and untreated depression can have detrimental effects on mother and child. Suicide is the most catastrophic possible outcome of undertreated depression. In addition, depressed women are more likely to participate in unhealthy practices during pregnancy, such as smoking and illicit substance abuse. These women have higher rates of poor nutrition, in part because of lack of appetite, leading to poor weight gain during pregnancy and risking intrauterine growth retardation. Depressed women may be less compliant with prenatal care and feel less invested in the care toward their pregnancy. Finally, women who have depression have increased pain and discomfort during their pregnancies, reporting worse nausea, stomach pain, shortness of breath, gastrointestinal symptoms, heart pounding, and dizziness compared with nondepressed women.[25] Untreated maternal depression in pregnancy has been associated with poor pregnancy and birth outcomes, such as maternal preeclampsia, low birth weight, smaller head circumferences, increased risk for premature delivery, increased surgical delivery interventions, lower Apgar scores, and more admissions to neonatal intensive care units (ICUs).[26–28]

Research suggests that maternal depression leads to alteration in a mother's neuro-endocrine axis and uterine blood flow, which may contribute to premature delivery, low birth weight, and preeclampsia.[29,30] Negative birth outcomes are associated most highly with depression symptoms in the second and third trimesters.[31] Babies of mothers who suffered from depression during their pregnancy have elevated cortisol and catecholamine levels at birth.[32] These infants cry more often and are more difficult to console than babies born to nondepressed mothers.[28] Babies of women at high risk for depression are shown to have more irregular sleep patterns and longer amounts of time in bed before falling asleep.[33] If depression continues into the postpartum period, the risk for long-term effects on a child, such as poor mother-infant attachment, delayed cognitive and linguistic skills, impaired emotional development, and behavioral issues, exist.[34–37] Studies show these babies are fussier, vocalize their needs less, and make fewer positive facial expressions than infants of nondepressed mothers.[38] If a baby is exposed to a depressed maternal environment during early infancy, and the mother has recurrent depressive episodes, the child shows changes in neuroendocrine functioning and more behavior problems at school entry.[39] As these children grow, perhaps because of early exposure or the continued stressful home environment, they are more likely to have emotional instability and conduct disorders, attempt suicide, and require mental health services themselves.[40,41]

TREATMENT OF DEPRESSION DURING PREGNANCY

There are few current medical standards for treatment of women who have depression during pregnancy, in part because ethical constraints preclude randomized controlled trials using pharmacotherapy during gestation. Most women do not seek treatment, but for those who do, many physicians are unsure of how to balance maternal medication needs with risk for exposure to the growing fetus.[42] Because many pregnancies are unplanned and undetected for some time, all women of childbearing age should have their depression managed as if they are or will become pregnant. Primary care providers should engage in preconception planning with all women of childbearing age who have or are at risk for depressive illness. Treatment planning for the use of pharmacotherapy during conception and the first trimester is among the most important decision points for women and their physicians. Obstetricians and other prenatal care providers (eg, midwives and nurses) play a crucial role during this sensitive time period as they are the primary contacts for pregnant women; these professionals can facilitate the detection of depressive symptoms, support the woman's treatment engagement, and provide referral to psychiatry, and they can also support in decision-making about medication intake or engagement in counseling. Intense communication among providers from a multidisciplinary perspective in the context of a collaborative care model is crucial for optimal pregnancy outcomes. Women diagnosed with depression who have been asymptomatic for more than a year may wish to attempt to reduce or discontinue their antidepressants a few months before conception and throughout the pregnancy.[43] However, 1 study found that 60% of women taking antidepressants at the time of their baby's conception had depressive symptoms during the pregnancy.[44] Women should be monitored closely for relapse of depressive symptoms. Of women who discontinued their antidepressants during pregnancy, 68% experienced relapse symptoms compared with 26% of women who continued their medication regimen.[45] If a woman's depression history contains multiple relapses or severe symptoms, including suicide attempts and multiple inpatient psychiatric admissions, it is recommended that she remain on antidepressants for her own safety, regardless of pregnancy status.[43]

Although research studies indicate that no major malformations are associated with antidepressant use during pregnancy, no specific antidepressant has been proven completely safe. All psychotropic medications cross the placenta and enter the amniotic fluid.[46] General guidelines include some straightforward principles: (1) keep the medication regimen simple, (2) use monotherapy, and (3) avoid medication changes during the pregnancy. Use of multiple medications in sequence and medication augmentation strategies all increase the exposure of the fetus.[32] A woman's prior history of pharmacotherapy should be considered when choosing a medication.[32] Although many factors influence pharmacotherapy during pregnancy, drugs with fewer metabolites, drug-drug interactions, more protein binding (preventing placental passage), and lesser teratogenic risk if known should be prioritized when possible.[32]

SPONTANEOUS ABORTION

Research results are mixed when examining rates of antidepressant use and its relationship to spontaneous abortion, and may be confounded by methodological problems (small study samples) or the effects of the illness itself.[47] Although prior work linked bupropion exposure in pregnancy with significant risk for spontaneous abortion,[48] a more recent study using a large sample of 940 women taking various antidepressants (including selective serotonin reuptake inhibitors [SSRIs], bupropion, and mirtazapine) during early pregnancy confirmed a statistically significant higher rate of spontaneous abortions (13% vs 8% in unexposed women) among the exposed women regardless of type of antidepressant used[49]; in this study prior spontaneous abortion was also an independent risk factor for current spontaneous abortion.

TERATOGENICITY

The literature on antidepressant use is growing, particularly regarding the use of SSRIs during pregnancy and possible risk for teratogenicity. Although the popular press creates controversy regarding the safety of SSRIs, research to date does not confirm major congenital malformations.[50] In 2005, GlaxoSmithKline[51] published a report based on a claims database study of 815 infants that showed babies born to mothers who were taking paroxetine during their first trimester had a 1.5- to 2-fold increased risk for congenital heart defects, in particular atrial and ventricular septal defects. Einarson and colleagues[52] more recently demonstrated that the rate of cardiac defects for babies exposed to paroxetine in the first trimester and nonexposed infants was the same (0.7%, not statistically significant) and within the expected cardiac malformation risk range for all pregnancies. At the time of writing, the use of paroxetine remains controversial. Most practitioners avoid its use during pregnancy except for those women who have demonstrated a preferential past positive response to this agent. When paroxetine is used, it is recommended to monitor the fetus with fetal echocardiography.[32]

The National Birth Defects Prevention Study in 2007 found no significant relationship between SSRIs and congenital cardiovascular malformations; however, it did find an association between SSRIs (especially paroxetine during the first trimester) and infants who had anencephaly, craniosynostosis, and omphalocele.[53] Conversely, the Slone Epidemiology Center Birth Defects Study published at approximately the same time noted no increased risk for craniosynostosis, omphalocele, or heart defects with overall SSRI use by pregnant women.[54] This study did find some significant relationships between sertraline and omphalocele and between paroxetine and right ventricular outflow tract obstruction defects.[54] Although these findings indicated some increased risk for specific rare birth defects with specific drug exposure, the overall absolute risk for birth defects with the use of SSRIs is small; therefore, these medications are considered safe for use during pregnancy.[53,54]

NEONATAL ADAPTATION

Studies show that up to 30% of infants exposed to SSRIs in utero during the third trimester are likely to have symptoms of poor neonatal adaptation.[55] These symptoms include short-term self-limited jitteriness, tachycardia, hyperthermia, vomiting, hypoglycemia, irritability, inconsolable crying, abnormal muscle tone, eating difficulties, sleep disturbances, seizures, and respiratory distress,[55] which lead to an overall increased rate of neonatal ICU admissions for these newborns. A recent paper suggested that the neonatal adaptation symptoms clustered in 3 symptom categories based on 3 proposed underlying pathophysiologic mechanisms: serotonergic toxicity (eg, tremor, tachypnea, diaphoresis, and irritability/agitation), antidepressant discontinuation syndrome (eg, hyperthermia, vomiting, increased muscle tonus, and convulsions), and symptoms caused by the immaturity of the newborn's central nervous system (eg, decreased suckling reflex, eating difficulties).[56] Studies assessing neonatal outcomes and complications do not correct for commonly co-occurring risk factors, including maternal smoking or use of alcohol or other substances.[20] Ferreira and colleagues,[57] correcting for these confounding variables, found no increased incidence of preterm labor or neonatal ICU admission for babies exposed to SSRIs or venlafaxine in utero; however, some infants did exhibit neonatal adaptation syndrome symptoms.

Neonatal respiratory problems are commonly associated with prenatal antidepressant exposure.[57–60] Recent studies have reported an increased risk of persistent pulmonary hypertension of the newborn with maternal use of SSRI near term.[59–61] Consequently, many neonatal respiratory complications, ranging from mild tachypnea to a need for respiratory support, could be explained either by the neonate's in utero exposure to antidepressants (ie, consistent with underlying persistent pulmonary hypertension) or by postnatal antidepressant discontinuation syndrome, mainly reported in infants whose mothers had near-term exposure to venlafaxine.[62] More recently, Oberlander and colleagues[63] reported that length of gestational SSRI exposure, rather than timing, increased the risk for neonatal respiratory distress, lower birth weight, and reduced gestational age, even when controlling for maternal illness and medication dose, thus complicating the decision-making process for clinicians when contemplating fetal SSRI exposure. Although some international literature suggests tapering antidepressants in the third trimester to avoid late gestation exposure, most practitioners in the United States avoid this, as it predisposes women to a substantially heightened risk for late pregnancy and postpartum morbidity secondary to depression.[64] As with any decision regarding pharmacotherapy during pregnancy, a consideration toward tapering should be considered on an individual basis, considering the risks for maternal illness versus the risk for neonatal withdrawal symptoms.[20]

The bulk of the literature to date does not reveal increased risk for congenital malformations associated with pregnant women taking tricyclic antidepressants (TCAs),[65] which historically were the medications of choice for treatment of depression but currently are not used extensively. Doses of TCAs may need to be increased as much as 1.6 times the prepregnancy dose in the second half of pregnancy to establish therapeutic levels as a result of increased plasma volumes and metabolism.[66] Case reports have presented babies with TCA exposure experiencing temporary withdrawal symptoms within the first 12 hours of life, including jitteriness, irritability, urinary retention, bowel obstruction, and occasionally seizures.[65,67] Nulman and colleagues[68] found no associations between maternal use of TCAs or fluoxetine during pregnancy and long-term effects on global IQ, language, or behavioral development in preschool children. Further research is needed to examine long-term outcomes for these children.

Limited information is available regarding exposure to atypical antidepressants, such as bupropion, mirtazapine, trazodone, and venlafaxine in utero.[65,69] Like SSRIs and TCAs, venlafaxine has been implicated in cases of neonatal withdrawal.[70]

NONPHARMACOLOGIC TREATMENTS

Psychotherapy also has been studied in the treatment of depression and is considered to be an evidence-based treatment of mood disorders.[71] Interpersonal psychotherapy (IPT) or cognitive behavioral therapy (CBT) in particular are commonly recommended psychotherapeutic treatments for unipolar depression.[72] IPT is useful in addressing interpersonal conflicts, role transitions, and unresolved grief. In addition to improving symptoms, IPT has been shown also to improve social functioning.[71] CBT specifically targets negative thinking and behaviors that maintain depression.[72] Couples counseling may also be indicated in women who have significant strain with their partner.

Women seeking treatment of depression also may benefit from nutrition counseling and regular low-impact exercise.[20,73] Recently, there has been much interest in treating depressed pregnant women with the omega-3 fatty acids eicosapentaenoic acid (EPA) and docosahexaenoic acid (DHA), and there are emerging affirmative data on their safety and benefit.[74] Many providers advise pregnant women who take herbal supplements for their depression to cease during pregnancy, because limited safety data in pregnancy exist. There has also been interest in research on mind-body modalities as treatment options for depression in pregnancy, some of which have been practiced for thousands of years, such as progressive muscle relaxation, yoga, or awareness-enhancing meditation.[75,76] Although much of this research has methodological limitations (eg, lack of randomized controlled trials), there seems to be converging evidence for the efficacy of mind-body modalities during pregnancy used in conjunction with prenatal care. Studies have shown that it is safe and effective for pregnant women who have severe depression to participate in electroconvulsive therapy if they and their provider see this as the best therapy option.[77,78]

POSTPARTUM DEPRESSION
Background, Prevalence, and Clinical Features

Postpartum depression develops in approximately 10% to 20% of women who give birth,[79] with higher percentages in adolescents, mothers of premature infants, and women living in urban areas.[80,81] Women who have low income and limited partner support also are at higher risk.[82,83] Women with 2 or more risk factors are more likely to have stable depressive symptoms across the first 2 years post partum.[84] Postpartum depression often is undetected and commonly underdiagnosed.[85] Many women expect an adjustment period after having a baby and, therefore, may not recognize that the symptoms of depression are out of the ordinary.[85] They may not want to admit they have a problem, they believe they need to prove they are a good mother, or they believe that seeking treatment will result in immediate removal of their child by child protective services. Many women do not seek treatment because of the combination of demanding care of the newborn infant and the lack of energy and motivation that comes with the disease process.[71] Furthermore, after the 6-week postpartum visit, a new mother who received her prenatal care from an obstetrician may not have routine health care scheduled, and she may believe she has nowhere to seek help.[85] If postpartum depression is left untreated, the symptoms last an average of 7 months but can extend into the second year after delivery.[71,85] Depression has a wide impact, influencing all members of families, and can lead to relationship distress, family conflict, or loss of income and, in extreme cases, it can result in placement of children in care outside the home.[86]

The DSM-IV[8] defines postpartum depression with the same symptom criteria as used for depression before or during pregnancy but specifies that it begins within the first 4 weeks after the baby is born. Onset can occur from 24 hours after giving birth to several months later.[85] Many epidemiologic studies define postpartum depression as depressive symptom onset within 3 months post partum and others as within the first year after delivery.[87] Depression symptoms often are accompanied by comorbid anxiety and commonly women have many concerns about their efficacy as a mother or are preoccupied with the health, feeding, and sleeping behaviors of their infants. As in pregnancy, MDD with postpartum onset must have the requisite clinical symptoms present for at least 2 weeks.[8]

Continuum of Affective Symptoms During Post Partum

Postpartum depression must be differentiated from the "baby blues" and postpartum psychosis. The baby blues are reported to occur in up to 70% of women after delivery.[88] These women feel sad, weepy, irritable, anxious, and confused, with increased sensitivity, fatigue, sleep disturbances, and appetite changes.[8] The symptoms usually peak approximately 4 days post partum and abate by day 10.[85,86] Although these symptoms may last only a few hours to days, women who experience the baby blues are at a higher risk for developing postpartum depression. In women who were diagnosed with postpartum depression 6 weeks after delivery, two-thirds had experienced baby blues symptoms.[89] The baby blues, however, almost always resolve within 2 weeks.

Postpartum psychosis occurs less commonly, having an impact on 0.2% of women of childbearing age.[90] Women may experience hallucinations, delusions, unusual behavior, agitation, disorganized thought, and inability to sleep for several nights.[8,86] Often the hallucinations and delusions center on the baby, and immediate intervention is vital to protect the lives of mother and child.[8] Typically this disorder presents within 2 weeks post partum or sooner.[8] Most often, postpartum psychosis is the result of affective psychosis, most commonly bipolar affective disorder.[8] Any woman who has had an episode of postpartum psychosis in a prior pregnancy should be screened carefully for bipolar disorder. Women who have had a prior episode of postpartum psychosis are at a high risk for a subsequent episode, and specific treatment guidelines have been suggested.[91] Some clinicians suggest reintroduction of lithium or other mood stabilizers in late pregnancy or immediately post partum (within the first 24–48 hours of labor) to attenuate the risk for postpartum psychotic relapse. In women who decide against peripartum prophylactic treatment, treating obstetricians and midwives should be vigilant for early signs of postpartum psychotic decompensation, and have low threshold to consult with psychiatry. Postpartum psychosis is considered a psychiatric emergency because of the potential for catastrophic suicide or infanticide.[86]

RISK FACTORS AND EPIDEMIOLOGY

Risk factors for postpartum depression should be identified before or during pregnancy and discussed at length between patient and provider. Many women who develop postpartum depression have had antenatal symptoms of depression.[92] Once a woman experiences postpartum depression, she is at risk for depression relapses with or without additional pregnancies.[93] Research shows that women who have had previous episodes of postpartum depression have a 25% risk for recurrence.[94] Experts debate whether or not the rapid decline in reproductive hormone levels after delivery contributes to depression development. Bloch and colleagues[95] found that when a decline of estradiol and progesterone was simulated in nonpregnant women, 63% of the women who had a history of postpartum depression experienced some changes in mood, whereas the women who did not have a history of postpartum depression did not experience any emotional changes. Thus, women who have a history of postpartum depression may be more sensitive to the systemic decrease in gonadal steroids post delivery. Other risk factors for postpartum depression include past depressive symptoms not related to pregnancy, a family history of depression, and factors that influence depression at any time point, including poor social support, social conflict, and life stressors.[96]

IDENTIFICATION AND SCREENING OF POSTPARTUM DEPRESSION

Health care providers can have difficulty differentiating postpartum depression symptoms from the normative adjustment of a woman to a new infant. Physicians should take into account the circumstances (eg, extreme fatigue, even though a baby may be sleeping through the night) and intensity of the symptoms.[85] Routine postpartum visits and well-infant pediatric visits present an ideal time for depression screening.[97] Although referral to a mental health clinician can be an important part of accurate diagnosis and appropriate treatment intensity, obstetric clinician support and encouragement for referral follow through has been found to be important.[98] Otherwise, physicians can use a screening question, such as "Have you had depressed mood or decreased interest or pleasure in activities most of the day nearly every day for the past 2 weeks?"[8] Affirmative responses should cue a provider to screen for other neurovegetative symptoms, including appetite and sleep changes, hopelessness, and difficulty paying attention. Significant impairment in social or occupational functioning should prompt a psychiatric referral. Suicidality or the risk for harm to an infant requires an assessment for inpatient hospitalization. Concomitant illicit substance abuse likewise merits a prompt evaluation. If EPDS scores are lower than 10 on clinical assessment but a patient still has some depressive symptoms, a reevaluation a few weeks later is recommended.[86] Other disease processes can mimic depression or can occur concomitantly. Patients presenting with symptoms of postpartum depression should routinely be tested for anemia and thyroid function, especially because hypothyroidism and hyperthyroidism occur more frequently post partum and can lead to alterations in mood.[86]

TREATMENT OF POSTPARTUM DEPRESSION

Antidepressant medication and psychotherapy are the foundation of treatment of postpartum depression. SSRIs are medications prescribed most commonly but other agents should be considered with a patient's prior positive treatment response. Because of the high risk for recurrence in women who have a previous history of postpartum depression, 1 study suggests providing prophylactic sertraline to prevent onset of symptoms.[94] Some literature suggests that women who have postpartum depression may be likely to have a more positive response to serotonergic agents, such as SSRIs and venlafaxine, than to TCAs.[99,100] The antidepressant dose may be started at half the recommended amount and increased slowly; postpartum women seem more sensitive to the side effects of these medications. Increased anxious symptoms at initiation of medications is a common concern.[101] Once a steady effective dose is reached, then pharmacotherapy should continue for at least 6 months to prevent a relapse of symptoms.[8] If there is no improvement with antidepressants after 6 weeks of therapy, a psychiatric consultation is appropriate.[86]

Many women are hesitant to take antidepressants while breastfeeding a child. All antidepressants are secreted to some degree into the breast milk; however, ethical concerns prevent large randomized controlled trials in lactating mothers to determine efficacy and safety.[43] Paroxetine and sertraline have been studied in lactating women, and, as with all medications, are secreted into breast milk. Infant serum levels are low to undetectable with these agents, however.[102,103] Fluoxetine has higher rates of secretion into breast milk. Because fluoxetine and its metabolite, norfluoxetine, have long half-lives, they can accumulate in an infant's blood, reaching detectable levels.[104] Case reports link maternal fluoxetine use to colic, prolonged crying, and vomiting, so it is not considered the first-line SSRI for breastfeeding women.[105] If a mother has a positive history of response to fluoxetine, the benefit outweighs the risk and it should be continued while monitoring the child for side effects.

Most lactating infants have no sequelae despite exposure to SSRIs during lactation. Mothers taking any antidepressant should be mindful of their infant's temperament and behavior, especially premature and sick newborns, who may be predisposed to dehydration,[86] and should notify their physician if they notice irritability, difficulty feeding, or disturbed sleep patterns.[43] No adverse effects are noted in infants when breastfeeding mothers take TCAs.[106] Breastfeeding while taking doxepin has been reported to cause severe muscle hypotonia, vomiting, drowsiness, and jaundice in babies, and therefore is not recommended.[107] Small case reports of atypical antidepressants have found no negative effects on infants with maternal use of mirtazapine or trazodone,[108,109] increased risk for drowsiness and lethargy with nefazodone (only 1 case),[110] and increased seizure risk with exposure to bupropion if a baby has a history of seizures.[107,111] Larger studies are needed to explore these effects further. Research on long-term effects of SSRI and TCA exposure through breast milk on children shows no alteration in IQ, language development, or behavior.[107]

For postpartum women who have sleep difficulties, diphenhydramine may be helpful.[112] Lorazepam can be used for women who have profound sleep disruption; it has fewer active metabolites, reduces nighttime anxiety, and enhances sleep. Lorazepam, however, is excreted into breast milk in low concentrations.[113,114] Several studies have observed that in lactating mothers taking lorazepam, there are no adverse effects on infants and no change in the amount of milk consumed. Caution should be taken when prescribing lorazepam during an infant's first few weeks of life because of the immaturity of the hepatic metabolism.[113,114]

Interpersonal therapy (IPT) is ideally suited to postpartum mothers, as almost all women have some concerns regarding role transitions and social support that occur during this important life milestone. IPT specifically targets effective elicitation of social support, adjustment to role changes, and unresolved grief that may contribute to distress around motherhood. Likewise, CBT has been shown to reduce depressive symptoms[115] by targeting unrealistic expectations that some women may have, such as the need to be a "perfect" mother, or a sense of shame at not being overjoyed with their infant during the immediate postpartum period. In addition, CBT encourages engagement in activities that are pleasurable and rewarding for the woman. Both psychotherapies have been shown to reduce or eliminate depression during an acute phase of treatment (up to approximately 16 weeks).[71] Pilot studies are currently exploring the efficacy of the treatment provided by telephone, to allow women to receive treatment without leaving their home.[116] Many women, especially those who have lactation concerns with pharmacotherapy, may be more comfortable beginning with IPT or CBT.[71] A recent qualitative study found that concerns and knowledge about antidepressant medications preclude treatment use among perinatal women.[24] In addition, behavioral strategies, such as adjusting the sleep schedule (having each member of the caring dyad share some of the nighttime responsibilities) and using the support of other family members to assist with nighttime feedings, may enhance a woman's ability to sleep at night.[117]

More recent work suggests that treating postpartum depression alone may not be sufficient in protecting children against long-term poor outcomes, and that dyadically based postpartum therapy interventions may be more beneficial for improving outcomes for infants of depressed mothers.[35] These relationship-based treatments may be short or long term, rooted in psychodynamic and attachment theories,[118,119] and are sometimes combined with skill-based techniques targeting relaxation and coping.[120,121] These dyadic relationship-based psychotherapies seem to affect parenting and child outcomes positively despite mixed improvement of depression in the mothers.[122,123]

Debate exists about the prospect of hormone therapy for postpartum depression. One study evaluated the effects of transdermal 17β-estradiol versus placebo and found a significant decrease in depression scores in the estradiol group.[124] Half of the women receiving estradiol, however, were also taking antidepressants, so the effect of hormone therapy alone is unclear. In addition, the hypercoagulable state of postpartum women may limit the clinical usefulness of estrogen treatments. Prophylactic progesterone (norethisterone enanthate) post partum compared with placebo demonstrated an increased risk for depressive symptoms in the treatment group.[125] More research is needed to explore hormonal treatment possibilities further.

SUMMARY

Obstetric care providers need to be aware that depression in women during their childbearing years is common. Routine depression screening, particularly at prenatal care visits, coupled with the use of physician collaborators to assist in connecting women with care, is paramount. During prenatal interviews, providers should be aware of risk factors for depression, including previous history of depression and interpersonal conflict. Links have been made between depression during pregnancy and poor pregnancy outcomes, such as preeclampsia, insufficient weight gain, decreased compliance with prenatal care, and premature labor. The literature suggests that overall the risks of SSRIs are small during pregnancy relative to the risk for undertreatment of depression. If depression continues post partum, there is an increased risk for poor mother-infant attachment, delayed cognitive and linguistic skills, impaired emotional development, and behavioral issues. Longer term, these children are more likely to have emotional instability or conduct disorders and to require mental health services. To prevent these outcomes, postpartum depression screening with the EPDS or simple screening questions should be a priority for post-partum follow-up visits. Antidepressant treatments, IPT, adjunctive behavioral treatment, and involving family in the supportive care of postpartum women often are helpful strategies. More research is needed to determine the long-term and developmental effects in children exposed to antidepressants during pregnancy and lactation.

REFERENCES

1. Kessler RC, Zhao S, Blazer DG, et al. Prevalence, correlates, and course of minor depression and major depression in the National Comorbidity Survey. J Affect Disord 1997;45:19.
2. Weissman MM, Olfson M. Depression in women: implications for health care research. Science 1995;269:799.
3. Brown MA, Solchany JE. Two overlooked mood disorders in women: subsyndromal depression and prenatal depression. Nurs Clin North Am 2004;39:83.
4. Gotlib IH, Whiffen VE, Mount JH, et al. Prevalence rates and demographic characteristics associated with depression in pregnancy and the postpartum. J Consult Clin Psychol 1989;57:269.
5. Marcus SM, Flynn HA, Blow FC, et al. Depressive symptoms among pregnant women screened in obstetrics settings. J Womens Health (Larchmt) 2003;12:373.
6. Flynn HA, O'Mahen H, Massey L, et al. The impact of a brief obstetrics clinic-based intervention on treatment use for perinatal depression. J Womens Health 2006;15:1195.
7. ACOG educational bulletin. Seizure disorders in pregnancy. Number 231, December 1996. Committee on Educational Bulletins of the American College of Obstetricians and Gynecologists. Int J Gynaecol Obstet 1997;56:279.
8. American Psychiatric Association. Diagnostic and statistical manual of mental disorders. 4th edition. Washington, DC: American Psychiatric Association; 1994.
9. Ross L, McLean L. Anxiety disorders during pregnancy and the postpartum period: a systematic review. J Clin Psychiatry 2006;67:1285.
10. Kumar R, Robson KM. A prospective study of emotional disorders in childbearing women. Br J Psychiatry 1984;144:35.
11. Altshuler LL, Cohen LS, Moline ML, et al. Treatment of depression in women: a summary of the expert consensus guidelines. J Psychiatr Pract 2001;7(3):185.
12. Westdahl C, Milan S, Magriples U, et al. Social support and social conflict as predictors of prenatal depression. Obstet Gynecol 2007;110:134.
13. Altshuler LL, Hendrick V, Cohen LS. Course of mood and anxiety disorders during pregnancy and the postpartum period. J Clin Psychiatry 1998;59(Suppl 2):29.
14. USPSTF. Screening for depression: recommendations and rationale. Ann Intern Med 2002;136:760.
15. Feinman JA, Cardillo D, Palmer J, et al. Development of a model for the detection and treatment of depression in primary care. Psychiatr Q 2000;71:59.

16. Radloff LS. The CES-D scale: a self-report depression scale for research in the general population. Appl Psychol Meas 1977;1:385.
17. Cox JL, Holden JM, Sagovsky R. Detection of postnatal depression. Development of the 10-item Edinburgh Postnatal Depression Scale. Br J Psychiatry 1987;150:782.
18. Jardri R, Pelta J, Maron M, et al. Predictive validation study of the Edinburgh Postnatal Depression Scale in the first week after delivery and risk analysis for postnatal depression. J Affect Disord 2006;93:169.
19. Matthey S, Henshaw C, Elliott S, et al. Variability in use of cut-off scores and formats on the Edinburgh Postnatal Depression Scale: implications for clinical and research practice. Arch Womens Ment Health 2006;9:309.
20. Ross AS, Hall RW, Frost K, et al. Antenatal & neonatal guidelines, education & learning system. J Ark Med Soc 2006;102:328.
21. Muzik M, Klier CM, Rosenblum KL, et al. Are commonly used self-report inventories suitable for screening postpartum depression and anxiety disorders? Acta Psychiatr Scand 2000;102:71.
22. Katon WJ, Seelig M. Population-based care of depression: team care approaches to improving outcomes. J Occup Environ Med 2008;50:459.
23. Gilbody S, Bower P, Fletcher J, et al. Collaborative care for depression: a cumulative meta-analysis and review of longer-term outcomes. Arch Intern Med 2006; 166:2314.
24. Flynn HA, Henshaw E, O'Mahen HA. et al. Patient perspectives on improving the depression referral processes in obstetrics settings: a qualitative study. General Hospital Psychiatry, in press.
25. Zuckerman B, Amaro H, Bauchner H, et al. Depressive symptoms during pregnancy: relationship to poor health behaviors. Am J Obstet Gynecol 1989;160:1107.
26. Chung TK, Lau TK, Yip AS, et al. Antepartum depressive symptomatology is associated with adverse obstetric and neonatal outcomes. Psychosom Med 2001;63:830.
27. Wadhwa PD, Sandman CA, Porto M, et al. The association between prenatal stress and infant birth weight and gestational age at birth: a prospective investigation. Am J Obstet Gynecol 1993;169:858.
28. Zuckerman B, Bauchner H, Parker S, et al. Maternal depressive symptoms during pregnancy, and newborn irritability. J Dev Behav Pediatr 1990;11:190–4.
29. Teixeira JM, Fisk NM, Glover V. Association between maternal anxiety in pregnancy and increased uterine artery resistance index: cohort based study. BMJ 1999;318:153.
30. Wadhwa PD, Dunkel-Schetter C, Chicz-DeMet A, et al. Prenatal psychosocial factors and the neuroendocrine axis in human pregnancy. Psychosom Med 1996;58:432.
31. Hoffman S, Hatch MC. Depressive symptomatology during pregnancy: evidence for an association with decreased fetal growth in pregnancies of lower social class women. Health Psychol 2000;19:535.
32. ACOG Committee on Practice Bulletins–Obstetrics. ACOG Practice Bulletin. Clinical management guidelines for obstetrician-gynecologists number 92. Use of psychiatric medications during pregnancy and lactation. Obstet Gynecol 2008;111(4):1001–20.
33. Heringhausen J, Marcus S, Muzik M, et al. Neonatal sleep patterns and relationship to maternal depression. In: Poster Presentation American Academy of Child & Adolescent Psychiatry Annual Meeting. Chicago, October 28–November 2, 2008.

34. Coghill SR, Caplan HL, Alexandra H, et al. Impact of maternal postnatal depression on cognitive development of young children. Br Med J 1986; 292:1165.
35. Forman DR, O'Hara MW, Stuart S, et al. Effective treatment for postpartum depression is not sufficient to improve the developing mother-child relationship. Dev Psychopathol 2007;19:585.
36. Alpern L, Lyons-Ruth K. Preschool children at social risk. Chronicity and timing of maternal depressive symptoms and child behavior at school and at home. Dev Psychopathol 1993;5:371.
37. Bifulco A, Figueiredo B, Guedeney N, et al. Maternal attachment style and depression associated with childbirth: preliminary results from a European and US cross-cultural study. Br J Psychiatry 2004;184:31.
38. Field T. Infants of depressed mothers. Infant Behav Dev 1995;18:1.
39. Essex MJ, Klein MH, Cho E, et al. Maternal stress beginning in infancy may sensitize children to later stress exposure: effects on cortisol and behavior. Biol Psychiatry 2001;52:776.
40. Lyons-Ruth K, Wolfe R, Lyubchik A. Depression and the parenting of young children: making the case for early preventive mental health services. Harv Rev Psychiatry 2000;8:148.
41. Weissman MM, Prusoff BA, Gammon GD, et al. Psychopathology in the children (ages 6–18) of depressed and normal parents. J Am Acad Child Psychiatry 1984;23:78.
42. Einarson A, Miropolsky V, Varma B, et al. Determinates of physicians' decision-making regarding the prescribing of antidepressant medication during pregnancy. In: Fifteenth International Conference of the Organization of Teratology Information Services (OTIS). Scottsdale (AZ), June 22, 2008
43. Gonsalves L, Schuermeyer I. Treating depression in pregnancy: practical suggestions. Cleve Clin J Med 2006;73:1098.
44. Hostetter A, Stowe ZN, Strader JRJ, et al. Dose of selective serotonin uptake inhibitors across pregnancy: clinical implications. Depress Anxiety 2000;11:51.
45. Cohen LS, Altshuler LL, Harlow BL, et al. Relapse of major depression during pregnancy in women who maintain or discontinue antidepressant treatment. JAMA 2006;295:499.
46. Hostetter A, Richie JC, Stowe ZN. Amniotic fluid and umbilical cord blood concentrations of antidepressants in 3 women. Biol Psychiatry 2000;48:1032.
47. Hemels ME, Einarson A, Koren G, et al. Antidepressant use during pregnancy and the rates of spontaneous abortions: a meta-analysis. Ann Pharmacother 2005;39:803.
48. Chun-Fai-Chan B, Koren G, Fayez I, et al. Pregnancy outcome of women exposed to bupropion during pregnancy: a prospective comparative study. Am J Obstet Gynecol 2005;192:932.
49. Einarson A, Choi J, Einarson T, et al. Rates of spontaneous and therapeutic abortions following use of antidepressants in pregnancy: results from a large prospective database. J Obstet Gynaecol Can 2009;31:452.
50. Einarson A. Risks/safety of psychotropic medication use during pregnancy. Can J Clin Pharmacol 2009;16:58.
51. GlaxoSmithKline. Available at: http://www.gsk.com/media/paroxetine_pregnancy.htm. Accessed October 18, 2009.
52. Einarson A, Pistelli A, DeSantis M, et al. Evaluation of the risk of congenital cardiovascular defects associated with use of paroxetine during pregnancy. Am J Psychiatry 2008;165:749.

53. Alwan S, Reefhuis J, Rasmussen SA, et al. Use of selective serotonin-reuptake inhibitors in pregnancy and the risk of birth defects. N Engl J Med 2007;356:2684.
54. Louik C, Lin AE, Werler MM, et al. First-trimester use of selective serotonin-reuptake inhibitors and the risk of birth defects. N Engl J Med 2007;356:2675.
55. Koren G, Matsui D, Einarson A, et al. Is maternal use of selective serotonin reuptake inhibitors in the third trimester of pregnancy harmful to neonates? CMAJ 2005;172:1457.
56. Boucher N, Bairam A, Beaulac-Baillargeon L. A new look at the neonate's clinical presentation after in utero exposure to antidepressants in late pregnancy. J Clin Psychopharmacol 2008;28.
57. Ferreira E, Carceller AM, Agogue C, et al. Effects of selective serotonin reuptake inhibitors and venlafaxine during pregnancy in term and preterm neonates. Pediatrics 2007;119:52.
58. Moses-Kolko EL, Bogen D, Perel J, et al. Neonatal signs after late in utero exposure to serotonin reuptake inhibitors: literature review and implications for clinical applications. JAMA 2005;293:2372.
59. Chambers CD, Johnson KA, Dick LM, et al. Birth outcomes in pregnant women taking fluoxetine. N Engl J Med 1996;335:1010.
60. Kallen B, Olausson PO. Maternal use of selective serotonin re-uptake inhibitors and persistent pulmonary hypertension of the newborn. Pharmacoepidemiol Drug Saf 2008;17:801.
61. Chambers CD, Hernandez-Diaz S, Van Marter LJ, et al. Selective serotonin-reuptake inhibitors and risk of persistent pulmonary hypertension of the newborn. N Engl J Med 2006;354:579.
62. Boucher N, Koren G, Beaulac-Baillargeon L. Maternal use of venlafaxine near term: correlation between neonatal effects and plasma concentrations. Ther Drug Monit 2009;31:404.
63. Oberlander TF, Warburton W, Misre S, et al. Effects of timing and duration of gestational exposure to serotonin reuptake inhibitor antidepressants: population-based study. Br J Psychiatry 2008;192:338.
64. Einarson A, Selby P, Koren G, et al. Abrupt discontinuation of psychotropic drugs during pregnancy: dilemmas and guidelines. Am J Psychiatry 2001;26:44.
65. Altshuler LL, Cohen LS, Szuba MP, et al. Pharmacologic management of psychiatric illness during pregnancy: dilemmas and guidelines. Am J Psychiatry 1996;153:592.
66. Sharma V. A cautionary note on the use of antidepressants in postpartum depression. Bipolar Disord 2006;8:411.
67. Schimmell MS, Katz EZ, Shaag Y, et al. Toxic neonatal effects following maternal clomipramine therapy. J Toxicol Clin Toxicol 1991;29:479.
68. Nulman I, Rovet J, Stewart DE, et al. Neurodevelopment of children exposed in utero to antidepressant drugs. N Engl J Med 1997;336:258.
69. Einarson TR, Einarson A. Newer antidepressants in pregnancy and rates of major malformations: a meta-analysis of prospective comparative studies. Pharmacoepidemiol Drug Saf 2005;14:823.
70. Way CM. Safety of newer antidepressants in pregnancy. Pharmacotherapy 2007;27:546.
71. O'Hara MW, Stuart S, Gorman LL, et al. Efficacy of interpersonal psychotherapy for postpartum depression. Arch Gen Psychiatry 2000;57:1039.
72. Bhatia SC, Bhatia SK. Depression in women: diagnostic and treatment considerations. Am Fam Physician 1999;60:225.

73. Daley AJ, Macarthur C, WInter H, et al. The role of exercise in treating post-partum depression: a review of the literature. J Midwifery Womens Health 2007;52:56.

74. Freeman MP, Hibbeln JR, Wisner KL, et al. Omega-3 fatty acids: evidence basis for treatment and future research in psychiatry. J Clin Psychiatry 1954;67:2006.

75. Beddoe AE, Lee KA. Mind-body interventions during pregnancy. J Obstet Gynecol Neonatal Nurs 2008;37:165.

76. Beddoe AE, Yang CP, Kennedy HP, et al. The effects of mindfulness-based yoga during pregnancy on maternal psychological and physical distress. J Obstet Gynecol Neonatal Nurs 2009;38:310.

77. Anderson EL, Reti IM. ECT in pregnancy: a review of the literature from 1941 to 2007. Psychosom Med 2009;71:235.

78. Miller LJ. Use of electroconvulsive therapy during pregnancy. Hosp Community Psychiatry 1994;45:444.

79. Steiner M. Perinatal mood disorders: position paper. Psychopharmacol Bull 1998;34:301.

80. Hobfoll SE, Ritter C, Lavin J, et al. Depression prevalence and incidence among inner-city pregnant and postpartum women. J Consult Clin Psychol 1995;63:445.

81. Logsdon MC, Usui W. Psychosocial predictors of postpartum depression in diverse groups of women. West J Nurs Res 2001;23:563.

82. Secco ML, Profit S, Kennedy E, et al. Factors affecting postpartum depressive symptoms of adolescent mothers. J Obstet Gynecol Neonatal Nurs 2007;36:47.

83. Shanok AF, Miller L. Depression and treatment with inner-city pregnant and parenting teens. Arch Womens Ment Health 2007;10:199.

84. Klier CM, Rosenblum KL, Zeller M, et al. A multi-risk approach to predicting chronicity of postpartum depression symptoms. Depress Anxiety 2008;25:718.

85. Epperson CN. Post-partum major depression: detection and treatment. Am Fam Physician 1999;59:2247.

86. Wisner KL, Parry BL, Piontek CM, et al. Clinical practice. Postpartum depression. N Engl J Med 2002;347:194.

87. Kendell R, Chalmers JC, Platz C. Epidemiology of puerpereal psychoses. Br J Psychiatry 1987;150:662.

88. O'Hara MW, Swain AM. Rates and risk of post-partum depression–a meta-analysis. Int Rev Psychiatry 1996;8:37.

89. Hannah P, Adams D, Lee A, et al. Links between early post-partum mood and post-natal depression. Br J Psychiatry 1992;160:777.

90. Harlow BL, Vitonis AF, Sparen P, et al. Incidence of hospitalization for post-partum psychotic and bipolar episodes in women with and without prior pre-pregnancy or prenatal psychiatric hospitalizations. Arch Gen Psychiatry 2007;64:42.

91. Cohen LS. Treatment of bipolar disorder during pregnancy. J Clin Psychiatry 2007;68(Suppl 9):4.

92. Milgrom J, Gemmill AW, Bilszta JL, et al. Antenatal risk factors for post-natal depression: a large prospective study. J Affect Disord 2008;108:147.

93. Cooper PJ, Murray L. Course and recurrence of post-natal depression. Evidence for the specificity of the diagnostic concept. Br J Psychiatry 1995;166:191.

94. Wisner KL, Perel J, Peindl KS, et al. Prevention of recurrent post-partum depression: a randomized clinical trial. J Clin Psychiatry 2001;62:82.

95. Bloch M, Schmidt PJ, Danaseau M, et al. Effects of gonadal steroids in women with a history of post-partum depression. Am J Psychiatry 2000;157:924.

96. Wisner KL, Stowe ZN. Psychobiology of post-partum mood disorders. Semin Reprod Endocrinol 1997;15:77.
97. Gjerdingen DK, Yawn BP. Post-partum depression screening: importance, methods, barriers, and recommendations for practice. J Am Board Fam Med 2007;20:280.
98. Flynn HA, Blow FC, Marcus SM. Rates and predictors of depression treatment among pregnant women in hospital-affiliated obstetrics practices. Gen Hosp Psychiatry 2006;28:289.
99. Cohen LS, Viguera AC, Bouffard SM, et al. Venlaflaxine in the treatment of post-partum depression. J Clin Psychiatry 2001;62:592.
100. Wisner KL, Peindl KS, Gigliotti TV, et al. Tricyclics vs. SSRIs for post-partum depression. Arch Womens Ment Health 1999;1:189.
101. Wisner KL, Perel J, Peindl KS, et al. Effects of the post-partum period on nortrip-tyline pharmacokinetics. Psychopharmacol Bull 1997;33:243.
102. Stowe ZN, Owens MJ, Landry JC, et al. Sertraline and desmethylsertraline in human breast milk and nursing infants. Am J Psychiatry 1997;154:1255.
103. Spigset O, Carleborg L, Norstrom A, et al. Peroxetine level in breast milk. J Clin Psychiatry 1996;57:39.
104. Kristensen JH, Ilett KF, Hackett LP, et al. Distribution and excretion of fluoxetine and norfluoxetine in human milk. Br J Clin Pharmacol 1999;48:521.
105. Lester BM, Cucca J, Andreozzi L, et al. Possible association between fluoxetine hydrochloride and colic in an infant. J Am Acad Child Adolesc Psychiatry 1993; 32:1253.
106. Yoshida K, Smith B, Craggs M, et al. Investigation of pharmacokinetics and of possible adverse effects in infants exposed to tricyclic antidepressants in breast-milk. J Affect Disord 1997;43:225.
107. Hale TW. Drug therapy and breast-feeding: anti-depressants, anti-psychotics, anti-manics, and sedatives. Neo Reviews 2004;5:E451.
108. Kristensen JH, Ilett KF, Rampono J, et al. Transfer of the anti-depressant mirta-zapine into breast milk. Br J Clin Pharmacol 2007;63:322.
109. Verbeeck RK, Ross SG, McKenna EA, et al. Excretion of trazodone in breast milk. Br J Clin Pharmacol 1986;22:367.
110. Yapp P, Ilett KF, Kristensen JH, et al. Drowsiness and poor feeding in a breast-fed infant: association with nefazodone and its metabolites. Ann Pharmacother 2000;34:1269.
111. Chaudron LH, Schoenecker CJ. Bupropion and breastfeeding: a case of a possible infant seizure. J Clin Psychiatry 2004;65:881.
112. Ringdahl EN, Pereira SL, Delzell JE, et al. Treatment of primary insomnia. J Am Board Fam Pract 2004;17:212.
113. Summerfield RJ, Nielsen MS. Excretion of lorazepam into breast milk. Br J Anaesth 1985;57:1042.
114. Johnstone MJ. The effect of lorazepam on neonatal feeding behaviour at term. Pharmatherapeutica 1982;3:259.
115. Milgrom J, Negri LM, Gemmill AW, et al. A randomized controlled trial of psychological interventions for post-natal depression. Br J Clin Psychol 2005; 44:529.
116. Flynn HA, Henshaw E, O'Mahen H, et al. Personalizing CBT for perinatal depres-sion: results of a qualitative study on improving intervention engagement and effectiveness. Ann Arbor (MI): Team UofMDoPP; 2008.
117. Gay CL, Lee KA, Lee SY, et al. Sleep patterns and fatigue in new mothers and fathers. Biol Res Nurs 2004;5:311.

118. Cohen NJ, Muir E, Lojkasek M, et al. Watch, wait, and wonder: testing the effectiveness of a new approach to mother-infant psychotherapy. Infant Ment Health J 1999;20:429.
119. Fraiberg S, Edelson E, Shapiro V. Ghosts in the nursery. A psychoanalytic approach to the problems of impaired infant-mother relationships. In: Fraiberg L, editor. Selected writings of Selma Fraiberg. Columbus (OH): Ohio State University Press; 1987. p. 100–36.
120. Field T, Grizzle N, Scafidi F, et al. Massage therapy for infants of depressed mothers. Infant Behav Dev 1996;19:107.
121. Field T, Pickens J, Prodromidis M, et al. Targeting adolescent mothers with depressive symptoms for early intervention. Adolescence 2000;35:381.
122. Cicchetti D, Cohen D, editors. Attachment and developmental psychopathology. (Developmental psychopathology). New Jersey: John Wiley & Sons; 2006. p. 207–26.
123. Clark R, Tluczek A, Wenzel A. Psychotherapy for postpartum depression: a preliminary report. Am J Orthopsychiatry 2003;73:441.
124. Gregoire AJ, Kumar R, Everitt B, et al. Transdermal oestrogen for treatment of severe post-natal depression. Lancet 1996;347:930.
125. Lawrie TA, Hofmeyr GJ, De Jager M, et al. A double-blind randomised placebo controlled trial post-natal norethisterone enanthate: the effect on post-natal depression and serum hormones. Br J Obstet Gynaecol 1998;105:1082.

Update and Critique of Natural Remedies as Antidepressant Treatments

David Mischoulon, MD, PhD[a,b,*]

KEYWORDS

- Omega-3 • St John's wort • Hypericum
- S-Adenosyl methionine • SAMe • Eicosapentaenoic
- Docosahexaenoic • Depression

Natural or "alternative" remedies have been routinely used in Asia and Europe for centuries,[1] and the popularity of these medications in the United States and worldwide has accelerated dramatically over the past decade. Increasing numbers of patients now are asking their doctors whether they might benefit from natural treatments, and many patients see a variety of practitioners in addition to physicians, including herbalists, naturopaths, and other healers. Because natural remedies are readily available over the counter, many individuals are choosing to self-medicate without professional supervision.

The National Institutes of Health has recognized that up to 25% of people in the United States seek and obtain alternative treatments,[2] and Eisenberg and colleagues[3]

The author has received research support from the following companies: Schwabe, NordicNaturals, Amarin (Laxdale Ltd), Lichtwer, Cederroth, SwissMedica, Ganeden, and Bristol-Meyers-Squibb (BMS). He has received honoraria from BMS, Pfizer, Pamlab, Virbac, NordicNaturals, and Reed Medical Education/MGH Psychiatry Academy (commercial entities supporting the MGH Psychiatry Academy are listed on the Academy's Web site http://www.mghcme.org). He has received royalty income from Back Bay Scientific. This publication was made possible in part by grant number 5K23AT001129-05 from the National Center for Complementary and Alternative Medicine. Its contents are solely the responsibility of the author and do not necessarily represent the official views of the National Center for Complementary and Alternative Medicine, National Institutes of Health.

This is an updated version of the article "Update and Critique of Natural Remedies as Antidepressant Treatments", which appeared in *Psychiatric Clinics of North America* (Volume 30, Issue 1, March 2007).

[a] Depression Clinical and Research Program, Department of Psychiatry, Massachusetts General Hospital, 50 Staniford Street, Suite 401, Boston, MA 02114, USA

[b] Harvard Medical School, 25 Shattuck Street, Boston, MA 02115, USA

* Depression Clinical and Research Program, Department of Psychiatry, Massachusetts General Hospital, 50 Staniford Street, Suite 401, Boston, MA 02114.

E-mail address: dmischoulon@partners.org

Obstet Gynecol Clin N Am 36 (2009) 789–807
doi:10.1016/j.ogc.2009.10.005
0889-8545/09/$ – see front matter © 2009 Elsevier Inc. All rights reserved.

found that 33% of patients at Boston's Beth Israel Medical Center use some form of complementary and alternative medicine. In 1990 there were more visits to alternative treatment practitioners nationwide than to primary care physicians.[3] The World Health Organization reported that that more than 70% of the world's population uses nonconventional medicine.[4] Growing numbers of academic investigators are performing clinical and basic research on these agents, and medical schools and residency training programs are starting to include complementary and alternative medicine in their curricula. Most physicians, however, still feel relatively unequipped to advise patients who ask about alternative treatments, and many practitioners remain highly skeptical of their potential value.

The benefits and liabilities of herbal remedies and other natural treatments still are largely unclear. Medical research has historically overlooked this area, and nutraceutical companies do not routinely fund studies on these medications.[5] Perhaps the most unfortunate—and dangerous—public misconception about these alternative medications is the belief that, just because something is "natural," it is automatically safe. Although historically the relatively few reports of serious adverse effects from these medications have been a large part of their appeal,[1] there increasingly have been cases of individuals who have had toxic reactions from these agents, whether or not they exceeded the recommended dosage.[1,6] Likewise, there are limited data regarding the safety and efficacy of combining alternative medications with conventional ones, but reports of adverse interactions have begun to emerge for some substances.

Natural medications, with the exception of homeopathic remedies, generally are not regulated by the US Food and Drug Administration (FDA).[5,7] Consequently, optimal doses for these medications are poorly established, as are the active ingredients, contraindications, drug-drug interactions, and potential toxicities. Another consequence of the lack of regulation is that preparations made by different companies vary with regard to form, quality, or purity of the medication, and hence in effectiveness.

Although natural medications are available for most physical and medical problems, there are relatively fewer ones for psychiatric disorders; these treatments are mainly limited to mood and anxiety symptoms and senescent cognitive decline. This article reviews 3 of the best-studied natural medications for mood disorders, St John's wort (hypericum), S-adenosyl methionine (SAMe), and the omega-3 fatty acids eicosapentaenoic acid (EPA) and docosahexaenoic acid (DHA).

ST JOHN'S WORT

Hypericum is an extract of the flower of St John's wort (*Hypericum perforatum* L.) that has been used for the treatment of depression for centuries.[1] Physicians in Europe have long considered hypericum effective for treating mild to moderate depression. In the past decade, interest in St John's wort has increased dramatically in the United States and worldwide, and today it is one of the biggest-selling natural remedies on the market.

Mechanisms of Action

The mechanism of action of hypericum is not fully understood. The extract from St John's wort contains polycyclic phenols, hypericin and pseudohypericin, which are among the presumed active components; other compounds include flavonoids (hyperoside, quercetin, isoquercitrin, rutin), kaempferol, luteolin, biapigenin, and hyperforin.[8–10] Hypericin, believed to be one of the main active components in hypericum, decreases serotonin receptor density.[11] Because hypericin does not cross the blood-brain barrier, one proposed mechanism of action for hypericin is the inhibition of monocyte cytokine production of interleukin-6 and interleukin-1β, resulting in a decrease in corticotrophin-releasing hormone and thus dampening production of cortisol.[12] Hypericin also may inhibit reuptake of serotonin, norepinephrine, and dopamine,[11] and may thus result in reduced expression of beta adrenoreceptors and increased density of serotonin (5-HT2A and 5-HT1A) receptors.[13] Hypericin also may have affinity for γ-aminobutyric acid receptors.

More recent investigations have implicated hyperforin as a possible active ingredient.[14] Laakmann and colleagues[15] performed a randomized, double-blind, placebo-controlled 6-week study of 2 different extracts of hypericum on 147 patients. The 2 extracts contained 0.5% and 5% hyperforin, respectively. Patients who received the hypericum extract with 5% hyperforin showed greater improvement in mean Hamilton Depression Scale (HAM-D) scores than the group receiving the 0.5% hyperforin extract, and the latter group showed only slightly greater improvement than the placebo group.

Various mechanisms of antidepressant action for hyperforin have been proposed, including serotonin reuptake inhibition and norepinephrine and acetylcholine reuptake inhibition. Some studies suggest inhibition of serotonin, dopamine, norepinephrine, γ-aminobutyric acid, and L-glutamate,[16] although serotonergic mechanisms probably are most important. Other mechanisms have been proposed also, including reduced expression of cortical β-adrenoceptors and 5-HT2 receptors, and synaptosomal release similar to that caused by reserpine.[14]

Other components of hypericum, including the flavonoids, are irreversible monoamine oxidase-A inhibitors, but the concentration of these compounds in the extract are so small that they are unlikely to be involved in the antidepressant mechanism.[17]

Most commercially available St John's wort preparations are standardized either to hypericin or hyperforin. Because there are several different preparations of the medication, the amount of other active ingredients may vary with different preparations, and there are no published head-to-head trials with different brands of hypericum.

Efficacy

In general, hypericum has been reported to have efficacy greater than placebo and equal to active controls. There are approximately 35 to 40 published trials, including 26 placebo-controlled studies and 14 with a standard antidepressant as the active comparator.[18] Most studies have been conducted in Europe, usually with patients already in clinical care in general practice settings.[1] Results in such studies may be more predictive of effectiveness and acceptability in clinical practice but may differ widely from results in a controlled research setting. For example, the European studies generally report little about the methods of recruitment, whether consecutive patients were recruited, and what, if any, exclusion criteria were applied. Patient groups in many European studies of hypericum were not limited to major depression and included other diagnoses.[1,14]

In clinical trials hypericum has been compared with low doses of both imipramine and maprotiline.[19-22] Doses of imipramine and maprotiline used in European clinical practice tend to be lower than those considered adequate by psychopharmacologists in the United States. In these clinical trials, the typical dose of imipramine or maprotiline is 75 mg/d. Despite the inadequate doses of active controls, the response rates in these trials seemed comparable to those in studies that use higher doses of tricyclic antidepressant agents (TCAs) (eg, imipramine >150 mg/d). The lack of a placebo control makes it difficult to interpret the results, but hypericum seemed to be at least as effective as low doses of imipramine and maprotiline. In these studies, response rates for hypericum ranged from 35.3% to 81.8%, and response for TCAs ranged from 41.2% to 77.8%.

A meta-analysis by Nierenberg[23] examined 4 studies comprising a heterogeneous group of depressive conditions, in which hypericum, 300 mg 3 times a day, was judged to be effective in 79 of 120 subjects (65.8%), whereas placebo was considered effective in only 36 of 125 subjects (28.8%; $\chi^2 = 32.24$; $P<.0001$). The placebo response rate seemed comparable to that observed in many outpatient studies of antidepressants conducted in the United States.

A meta-analysis by Linde and colleagues[24] examined 15 trials comparing hypericum with placebo and 8 trials comparing hypericum with TCAs in 1757 patients who had mild to moderate depression. In 6 trials that used single preparations of hypericum (containing only St John's wort), hypericum yielded greater response rates than placebo (55.1% for hypericum vs 22.3% for placebo) and comparable response rates to tricyclic antidepressants (63.9% for hypericum vs 58.5% for tricyclic antidepressants). In 2 trials that used combination preparations of hypericum (containing St John's wort and other herbal medications such as Kava), hypericum was found to be more effective than TCAs (67.7% vs 50%). A meta-analysis by Voltz[25] suggested that hypericum may not be effective for acute treatment of severely depressed patients.

In the 2000s, approximately 10 notable studies by North American, European, and South American investigators have been published. Many of these studies are distinguished by their large-scale, randomized, double-blind design or by comparing St John's wort with newer antidepressants, particularly the selective serotonin reuptake inhibitors (SSRIs), as well as with placebo.

In a 6-week trial with 375 patients, Lecrubier and colleagues[26] found that St John's wort, 900 mg/d, was significantly more effective than placebo, especially in patients who had higher baseline HAM-D scores. In an 8-week trial with 200 depressed subjects, Shelton and colleagues[27] found that St John's wort, 900 to 1200 mg/d, was no more effective than placebo in the full intent-to-treat analysis, although among completers the remission rates were significantly higher with St John's wort than with placebo.

Brenner and colleagues[28] compared St John's wort, 900 mg/d, with sertraline, 75 mg/d, in 30 depressed subjects for 6 weeks. St John's wort yielded a 47% response rate and sertraline a 40% response rate. The difference was not statistically significant. Gastpar and colleagues[29] also compared St John's wort, 612 mg/d, with sertraline, 50 mg/d, in 241 depressed subjects for 12 weeks, with 161 subjects receiving an additional 12 weeks of treatment for a total treatment period of 6 months. By the first 12 weeks, hypericum was found to yield a response rate comparable to sertraline, and this response was maintained in subjects who continued for the full 6 months. van Gurp and colleagues[30] compared St John's wort, 900 to 1800 mg/d, with sertraline, 50 to 100 mg/d, in 12 community-based primary care offices. Eighty-seven depressed subjects were treated for 12 weeks. No significant differences in mean HAM-D scores were found, and St John's wort resulted in significantly fewer adverse events.

Schrader[31] compared St John's wort, 500 mg/d, with fluoxetine, 20 mg/d, for 6 weeks in 240 depressed subjects. St John's wort yielded a 60% response rate and fluoxetine a 40% response rate. Results barely reached significance in favor of St John's wort. The investigators noted that St John's wort had a more favorable adverse effects profile. Only 8% of subjects receiving St John's wort reported adverse events compared with 23% receiving fluoxetine. Behnke and colleagues[32] compared St John's wort with fluoxetine in 70 mildly to moderately depressed subjects for 6 weeks. This study found HAM-D score decreases of 50% for St John's wort and 58% for fluoxetine, with the efficacy of St John's wort approximately 80% that of fluoxetine on the HAM-D and the von Zerssen Depression scales.

The Hypericum Depression Study Group[33] compared St John's wort at doses of 900 to 1500 mg/d versus sertraline, 50 to 100 mg/d, or placebo for 8 weeks in 340 depressed subjects. St John's wort and sertraline both yielded a response rate of approximately 24%; the response rate for placebo was 32%. This report, along with that of Shelton and colleagues,[27] resulted in a great deal of media attention during 2002, and St John's wort sales worldwide dropped temporarily in the immediate aftermath.[5]

Fava and colleagues[34] at the Massachusetts General Hospital (MGH) conducted a study similar to that of the Hypericum Group, comparing St John's wort, 900 mg/d, with fluoxetine, 20 mg/d, versus placebo for 12 weeks. The study was powered for 180 subjects, but the sponsor closed the study prematurely because of the media hysteria over the previously mentioned negative studies, which were published while the MGH study was in progress. Consequently, only 135 subjects were recruited. The results showed a trend toward significance for St John's wort against placebo with regard to decrease in HAM-D scores, and a significant advantage for St John's wort against fluoxetine. Remission rates were 38% for St John's wort, 30% for fluoxetine, and 21% for placebo, but these differences did not reach significance. In view of the placebo response rate, which was consistent with the literature, the investigators concluded that the observed results were "real" and suggested that if the full complement of 180 subjects had been recruited, both St John's wort and fluoxetine would have beaten placebo by a statistically significant margin.

Moreno and colleagues[35] compared hypericum, 900 mg/d, with fluoxetine, 20 mg/d, or placebo in 72 depressed subjects. After 8 weeks, the investigators found that hypericum yielded a remission rate of 12%, significantly lower than that of fluoxetine (34.6%) and placebo (45%).

How should these recent studies be interpreted in the context of the previous literature? A recent Cochrane review declared similar response rates overall for St John's wort, SSRIs, and TCAs, but cautioned about the "inconsistent and confusing" nature of the data.[18] In comparisons between St John's wort and placebo, the results tended to favor St John's wort but more so in cases for which there was not a strict diagnosis of major depressive disorder. Trials with strictly diagnosed depression according to the *Diagnostic and Statistical Manual of Mental Disorders*, 4th edition (DSM-IV) criteria showed less robust results.[18] More studies are necessary to clarify some of the questions about efficacy that the aforementioned studies have raised.

Safety and Tolerability

In the past few years, increasing numbers of adverse drug-drug interactions between St John's wort and other medications have been reported in the literature. These interactions are thought to occur largely through the liver enzyme CYP-450-3A4, and have resulted in decreased activity of several drugs, including warfarin, cyclosporin, oral contraceptives, theophylline, phenprocoumon, digoxin, indinavir, and irinotecan.[36–40] Extreme caution, therefore, is required with human immunodeficiency virus–positive patients who take protease inhibitors, cancer patients receiving chemotherapy, and transplant recipients who take immunosuppressive drugs. It also is recommended that St John's wort not be combined with SSRIs, because anecdotes of "serotonin syndrome" have been reported, presumably related to the monoamine oxidase inhibitor activity of St John's wort.[41]

When St John's wort is used as monotherapy, adverse events are relatively uncommon and mild.[42] Patients have complained of dry mouth, dizziness, constipation, other gastrointestinal symptoms, and confusion.[1-42] Woelk and colleagues[43] followed 3250 patients treated with hypericum by 633 physicians in routine clinical practice, and found that only 2.4% of patients mentioned side effects of gastrointestinal symptoms and allergic reactions. Only 1.5% of patients stopped taking the drug because of these side effects. So far, there seem to be no published reports assessing the effects of a hypericum overdose.

Phototoxicity has long been associated with hypericum in grazing animals and has been reported, albeit rarely, in humans.[44] Brockmoller and colleagues[45] found that doses of hypericum as high as 1800 mg caused minor increases in sensitivity to UV light in humans but no phototoxicity. Siegers and colleagues[46] have recommended that patients who take an overdose of hypericum should be isolated from UV radiation for 7 days, but this caution may not necessarily apply to patients receiving regular doses. As a general precaution, the author and colleagues recommend that patients who take St John's wort use sunscreen and other protection when spending large amounts of time in the sun.

At least 17 cases of psychosis resulting from St John's wort have been reported, of which 12 comprised mania or hypomania.[47] Bipolar patients therefore should be advised to use St John's wort only with a concurrent mood stabilizer.

Recommendations and Special Considerations for Women Who are Pregnant or Breastfeeding

Hypericum has been shown to be more effective than placebo and equal to low-dose TCAs in most controlled trials, but has had less impressive results against the SSRIs and placebo in the more recent studies, perhaps in part because of the recruitment of more severely or chronically depressed patient samples.[14]

Recommended doses of St John's wort based on the literature fall between 900 mg/d and 1800 mg/d, usually divided on a twice- or thrice-daily basis. St John's wort seems to have a relatively benign side effect profile although, given the risk of interactions, care needs to be taken with patients taking multiple medications. Likewise, in view of the risk of cycling, caution should be exercised in patients who have bipolar disorder.

The literature as a whole suggests that St John's wort may be less effective in cases of more severe or more chronic depression, and people who have milder forms of depression therefore may be the best candidates for St John's wort. A collaborative study of St John's wort for minor depression at MGH, the University of Pittsburgh Medical Center, and Cedars-Sinai Medical Center has recently been completed, and data analysis is currently underway. Hypericum needs to be studied further in depressed subjects who have rigorously diagnosed DSM-IV major depression, using placebo and active controls for acute treatment periods of at least 8 to 12 weeks. Longer-term continuation treatment also merits investigation, and systematic tracking of side effects needs to be further developed.

Little is known about toxic effects that hypericum may have during pregnancy and breastfeeding. A systematic literature review[48] found that in utero exposure to St John's wort in animals may be associated with low birth weight but led to no adverse effects on cognitive development; breastfeeding while on St John's wort was associated with colic and drowsiness or lethargy.[48] Given the cytochrome-P450 induction of St John's wort, concerns were raised over its potential interference with other medications administered during pregnancy or lactation.[48] One small prospective study found no significant differences in fetal malformations in women exposed to St John's wort during pregnancy, compared with pregnant women on other antidepressants and pregnant women with no teratogen exposure.[49] Studies examining hyperforin and hypericin levels in breast milk have suggested safety for children and mothers,[50,51] and one small prospective study suggests no increase in adverse events in children exposed to St John's wort in mother's milk, though cases of lethargy and drowsiness were reported.[52] The data, however, are scant and long-term studies of safety are required.[53] In the absence of safety data, it is recommended that women who are pregnant or intend to become pregnant avoid St John's wort.

S-ADENOSYL METHIONINE

S-Adenosyl methionine (SAMe) (**Box 1**) is a methyl donor in the brain, involved in the pathways for synthesis of hormones, neurotransmitters, nucleic acids, proteins, and phospholipids.[54] Of particular interest is its activity as an intermediate in the synthesis of norepinephrine, dopamine, and serotonin,[54] which suggests its potential role in mood regulation. Widely prescribed in Europe for decades, SAMe gained popularity in the United States following its release as an over-the-counter dietary supplement in 1998 to 1999. It is considered a potential treatment for major depression as well as for several other medical conditions.[54]

Mechanisms of Action

SAMe is synthesized from the amino acid L-methionine through the one-carbon cycle, a metabolic pathway involving the vitamins folate and B12.[54] Deficiencies of both these vitamins have long been associated with depression. For example, 10% to 30% of depressed patients may have low folate, and these patients may respond less well to antidepressants.[55] Administration of folate augmentation to partial responders to antidepressants has yielded encouraging results.[56,57] Vitamin B12 is converted to methylcobalamin, which also is involved in the synthesis of various central nervous system neurotransmitters. B12 deficiency may result in an earlier age of onset of depression.[58] The final pathway of these vitamin deficiencies may be reduced SAMe, leading to diminished synthesis of vital neurotransmitters. The replenishment of folate and B12 may in turn result in increased SAMe and neurotransmitter synthesis. Indeed, low SAMe levels have been found in the cerebrospinal fluid of depressed individuals,[59] and higher plasma SAMe levels have been associated with improvement in depressive symptoms.[60] The enzyme methionine adenosine transferase, necessary for the manufacture of SAMe, has decreased activity in depressed schizophrenic patients but increased activity in manic patients.[61–63] If correction of B-vitamin deficiencies can increase SAMe levels and hence alleviate depressive symptoms, it is reasonable to postulate that direct administration of SAMe also could reverse a depressed state.

Box 1
S-Adenosyl methionine

$$NH_2\text{-}CH\text{-}CH_2\text{-}CH_2\text{-}S\text{-}Adenosyl$$
$$O=C\cdot OH \qquad CH_3$$

This derivative of the amino acid methionine functions by donating a methyl (-CH3) group in a variety of metabolic reactions, including the synthesis of neurotransmitters.

Efficacy

There are approximately 45 published randomized clinical trials of SAMe for treatment of depression, of which at least 8 used an active comparator.[54,64–66] SAMe demonstrated superiority to placebo in 6 of 8 placebo-controlled studies with sample sizes ranging from 40 to 100 individuals, and equivalency to placebo in the other 2 studies.[54,65,66] In 6 of 8 comparison studies with TCAs, SAMe was equivalent in efficacy to TCAs and was more effective than imipramine in one study.[54,65,66] Doses of SAMe in these studies ranged from 200 to 1600 mg/d administered orally, intramuscularly, or intravenously.[54,65,66]

Overall, trials of oral SAMe suggest efficacy comparable to TCAs and superiority to placebo at doses between 200 and 1600 mg/d.[64–66] Although some early studies yielded equivocal results because of problems with dissolution and stability of early oral SAMe preparations,[54,65,66] current oral SAMe preparations are tosylated and are more stable, and thus are more suitable for research use. As yet there are no published reports comparing SAMe with newer antidepressants such as SSRIs, but such studies are in progress.

SAMe may have a relatively faster onset of action than conventional antidepressants.[54,65,66] In one study, some patients improved within a few days, and most did so within 2 weeks.[67] Likewise, 2 studies showed that the combination of SAMe and a low-dose TCA resulted in earlier onset of action than a TCA alone.[68,69]

A recent study by Alpert and colleagues[70] examined the efficacy of SAMe as an adjunctive treatment for partial and nonresponders to SSRIs. Thirty subjects who had residual depression despite SSRI or venlafaxine treatment received a 6-week course of SAMe, 800 to 1600 mg. Response and remission rates with SAMe augmentation were 50% and 43%, respectively, and the treatment was well tolerated. The results suggest a possible role for SAMe as an augmenting agent in cases of partial or no response to SSRIs. A placebo-controlled follow-up augmentation study comparing SAMe against placebo in SSRI nonresponders has recently been completed by the authors' group, and analysis of these findings is in progress.

Other reports suggest that SAMe is effective for dementia-related cognitive deficits, depression in patients who have Parkinson disease or other medical illness, psychological distress during the puerperium, and opioid and alcohol detoxification.[66]

Safety and Tolerability

SAMe is well tolerated and relatively free of adverse effects. There is no apparent hepatotoxicity or anticholinergic effects. Side effects include mild insomnia, lack of appetite, constipation, nausea, dry mouth, sweating, dizziness, and nervousness.[54] Cases of increased anxiety, mania, or hypomania in bipolar depression have been reported,[54,71,72] and therefore care must be taken with patients who have a history of bipolar disorder. These patients should be advised not to take SAMe unless they are receiving a concurrent mood stabilizer. So far, there seem to be no significant drug-drug interactions between SAMe and FDA-registered drugs.

Recommendations and Special Considerations for Women who are Pregnant or Breastfeeding

There is encouraging evidence that SAMe is effective for treatment of major depression, both as monotherapy and as an adjunct to FDA-approved antidepressants. Some studies have suggested a faster onset of action for SAMe than for conventional antidepressants, and it may accelerate the effect of conventional antidepressants when combined. SAMe seems to be well tolerated, with a relatively benign side effect profile. SAMe may be especially good for patients who are sensitive to antidepressant-related side effects, particularly the elderly and those who have medical comorbidity. There is no apparent toxicity, except for risk of cycling in patients who have bipolar depression. Recommended doses range from 400 to 1600 mg/d,[54,65,66] although in clinical practice the author and colleagues have observed some individuals who require at least 3000 mg/d for alleviation of depression. More research is needed to determine optimal SAMe doses, and head-to-head comparisons with newer antidepressants should help clarify the place of SAMe in the psychopharmacologic armamentarium.

SAMe is relatively expensive, with prices ranging from $0.75 to $1.25 for a 400-mg tablet. Because insurance plans do not cover over-the-counter supplements, the out-of-pocket cost can be prohibitive to many patients, particularly those who may require higher doses. Careful shoppers who search the Internet may be able to purchase SAMe at more accessible prices, but they should verify the reputation of the seller. With increasing numbers of manufacturers and competition in the marketplace, it is hoped that the price of SAMe will drop in the foreseeable future.

As with St John's wort, there is a lack of data regarding safety during pregnancy and lactation. Some studies have found that pregnancy may result in impaired methylation and lower levels of SAMe,[73] suggesting a potential benefit from SAMe administration in pregnant women. SAMe supplementation in pregnant women with intrahepatic cholestasis has been associated with beneficial effects.[74] Although SAMe seems to be a mostly safe over-the-counter agent (ie, a chemical that humans already manufacture, with no drug-drug interactions, and minimal and mild adverse effects), consideration for SAMe administration in selected cases may be reasonable.[53] However, given the limited data the pregnant woman is likely better off avoiding SAMe, particularly when considering that there are many registered antidepressants with proven track records for safety and efficacy during pregnancy.

OMEGA-3 FATTY ACIDS

During the past century, intake of omega-3 fatty acids in the Western diet has decreased dramatically, while intake of processed foods rich in omega-6–containing vegetable oils has increased. This dietary shift has resulted in a higher physiologic ratio of omega-6:omega-3 fatty acids in Western countries compared with countries with higher fish and omega-3 consumption.[75–79] The modern Western diet and the additional stresses of twenty-first century life have been postulated to create a baseline proinflammatory state in humans that may contribute to cardiovascular disease and also may play a role in the development of mood disorders.[80] Administration of omega-3 supplements may potentially reverse this proinflammatory state by correcting the omega-6:omega-3 ratio, thus providing beneficial cardiovascular and mood-related effects. Several recent treatment studies have yielded encouraging, albeit preliminary, evidence of clinical efficacy for omega-3 fatty acids as mood-enhancing agents. The 2 omega-3 fatty acids thought to be relevant to psychiatry are EPA and DHA (**Box 2**), both of which are found primarily in fish oil. Investigations into their efficacy have examined EPA and DHA separately and in combination with each other.

Mechanisms of Action

How might the omega-3 fatty acids exert their mood-enhancing effect? Proposed mechanisms for the amelioration of depression include an effect on membrane-bound receptors and enzymes involved in the regulation of neurotransmitter signaling, as well as regulation of calcium ion influx through calcium channels.[80] Hamazaki and

---

Box 2
Docosahexaenoic acid and eicosapentaenoic acid

Docosahexaenoic acid

$CH_3-CH_2-CH=CH-CH_2-CH=CH-CH_2-CH=CH-CH_2-CH=CH-CH_2-CH=$
$CH-CH_2-CH=CH-CH_2-CH_2-COOH$

Docosahexaenoic acid (22:6, n-3) has a 22-carbon chain and 6 double bonds. The leftmost carbon is termed the "omega" carbon, and the first double bond occurs on the third carbon from the left, hence the term "omega-3."

Eicosapentaenoic acid

$CH_3-CH_2-CH=CH-CH_2-CH=CH-CH_2-CH=CH-CH_2-CH=CH-CH_2-CH=$
$CH-CH_2-CH_2-CH_2-COOH$

Eicosapentaenoic acid (20:5, n-3) has a 20-carbon chain and 5 double bonds. The first double bond occurs on the third carbon from the left.

---

colleagues[81] found that administration of a combination of EPA and DHA to healthy subjects resulted in a lowering of plasma norepinephrine levels compared with placebo, and the investigators proposed that omega-3s could exert their effect by interaction with the catecholamines. Omega-3 fatty acids also may inhibit secretion of inflammatory cytokines, thus leading to decreased corticosteroid release from the adrenal gland and dampening of mood-altering effects associated with cortisol.[80,82] For example, EPA inhibits the synthesis of prostaglandin E2, thus dampening the synthesis of *p*-glycoprotein, the latter of which may be involved in antidepressant resistance.[82] In this regard, EPA resembles amitriptyline, which also inhibits *p*-glycoprotein and is generally considered useful for resistant depression.

Efficacy

Approximately 20 controlled trials and a few open studies with EPA or DHA suggest that supplementation with omega-3 fatty acids at doses about 5 or more times the standard dietary intake in the United States may yield antidepressant or mood-stabilizing effects. Various meta-analyses of depression studies with omega-3[83–86] generally support the efficacy of omega-3, but are limited by mixed samples of augmentation and monotherapy studies, small sample sizes, inclusion of bipolar subjects, and different preparations and doses of omega-3, ranging from 1 to 10 g/d.

Peet and Horrobin[87] conducted a randomized, placebo-controlled, dose-finding study of ethyl-eicosapentaenoate (ethyl-EPA) as adjunctive therapy for 70 adults who had persistent depression despite treatment with a standard antidepressant. Subjects who received 1 g/d EPA for 12 weeks showed significantly higher response rates (53%) than subjects receiving placebo (29%), with notable improvement of depressed mood, anxiety, sleep disturbance, libido, and suicidality. The 2 g/d group showed little evidence for a drug:placebo difference, and the 4 g/d group showed a nonsignificant trend toward improvement. These results suggest that there may be an optimal dose of omega-3 that humans require for maximum benefit, and it is possible that an overcorrection of the omega-6:omega-3 ratio with higher omega-3 doses may limit the antidepressant effect of EPA.

Su and colleagues[88] conducted an 8-week, double-blind, placebo-controlled trial comparing adjunctive omega-3 (6.6 g/d) with placebo in 28 depressed patients. Patients in the omega-3 group had a significant decrease in HAM-D scores compared with placebo. In a sample of 20 subjects who had major depressive disorder and were receiving antidepressant therapy, Nemets and colleagues[89] found a statistically significant benefit of adjunctive EPA, 1 g/d, and a clinically important difference in the mean reduction of the 24-item HAM-D scale by the study end point at week 4 compared with placebo (12.4 vs 1.6). Frangou and colleagues[90] treated 75 depressed subjects with ethyl-EPA at 1 g/d, 2 g/d, or placebo for 12 weeks. EPA outperformed placebo significantly in both EPA treatment arms, based on HAM-D scores; the higher dose of EPA seemed to confer no added benefit compared with 1 g/d. A recent randomized controlled study by the authors' group examined EPA monotherapy for depression, and found an advantage for EPA compared with placebo, though the study was limited by a smaller than projected sample size.[91]

A small study by Silvers[92] suggested that 8 g of "fish oil" was not more effective than 8 g of "olive oil," but this underpowered study was limited by problems with attrition, dosage, and choice of rating scales. Regarding DHA, one placebo-controlled study with 36 subjects showed lack of efficacy of DHA monotherapy, 2 g/d, for depression.[93] A 3-armed dose-finding study of DHA monotherapy[94] demonstrated greater efficacy for DHA doses of 1 g/d compared with 2 g/d and 4 g/d, which, similarly to the study of EPA by Peet and Horrobin, suggests a therapeutic window for DHA as well as EPA.

Freeman and colleagues[95] performed a dose-finding trial of omega-3 in 16 women who had postpartum depression. Subjects received 0.5 g/d, 1.4 g/d, or 2.8 g/d. HAM-D scores and the Edinburgh Post Natal Depression Scale both decreased by approximately 50% for all groups, and there seemed to be no dose-response effect. Marangell and colleagues[96] found no preventive effect of postpartum depression with open omega-3 mix (EPA and DHA), 2960 mg/d, in a small sample of pregnant women. A prospective large-scale study[97] found no association between fish intake or n-3 intake and risk of postpartum depression.

Omega-3 fatty acids may have efficacy for bipolar as well as unipolar mood disorders. Using high doses of an omega-3 fatty acid mix (6.2 g EPA plus 3.4 g DHA) versus placebo over a 4-month period, Stoll and colleagues[98] found that among 30 patients who had bipolar I or II disorder, a Kaplan-Meier survival analysis revealed a significantly longer duration of remission for those receiving adjunctive omega-3 fatty acid mix versus placebo along with their current mood-stabilizing regimen.

Keck and colleagues[99] were unable to replicate the results of Stoll and colleagues in a larger-scale study. In their double-blind, placebo-controlled trial of adjunctive EPA, 6 g/d, for 4 months in patients who had bipolar depression (n = 57) or rapid cycling (n = 59), EPA did not separate from placebo. Systematic reviews of bipolar studies suggested that most of the observed benefit in bipolar subjects is with regard to depressive rather than manic symptoms.[100,101]

Osher and colleagues[102] treated 12 bipolar I depressed subjects with open adjunctive EPA, 1.5 to 2 g/d, for up to 6 months. Ten patients completed at least 1 month of follow-up, and 8 achieved a 50% or greater reduction in HAM-D scores. No cycling occurred with any patients. Further investigation is needed to determine whether bipolar disorder actually requires higher doses of omega-3 fatty acids than unipolar illness, and to unravel the respective contributions of EPA and DHA.

The relationship between omega-3 fatty acid treatment and a range of other psychiatric syndromes also has been studied to a lesser extent; the resulting data are equivocal. Conditions investigated include borderline personality disorder, schizophrenia, attention-deficit disorder, and obsessive-compulsive disorder.[103–110] These investigations tend to consist of smaller patient samples, and their conflicting results reflect this limitation.

Safety and Tolerability

The omega-3s have been shown to be very safe. Most complaints of side effects such as gastrointestinal upset and fishy aftertaste tend to occur with higher doses (>5 g/d) and with less pure preparations. At the more typical doses of 1 g/d with highly purified omega-3 preparations, these adverse effects are less common. There is a documented risk of bleeding, which seems to be minimal, particularly with doses less than 3 g/d. Individuals taking anticoagulants such as warfarin need to take care, and should not use omega-3s without physician supervision.[83] Given a few documented cases of cycling in bipolar patients,[83] omega-3s should be used with care in this population and preferably with a concomitant mood stabilizer.

Recommendations and Special Considerations for Women who are Pregnant or Breastfeeding

The data supporting the use of omega-3 fatty acids for depression are encouraging, particularly with regard to EPA. Low doses of omega-3 fatty acids may be an effective and well-tolerated monotherapy or adjunctive therapy for depressed adults. A recent review by Freeman and colleagues[83] recommends that depressed individuals may safely use approximately 1 g/d of an EPA-DHA mixture but should not substitute omega-3s for conventional antidepressants at this time. Likewise, individuals who take more than 3 g/d of omega-3 should do so under a physician's supervision.[83]

Most studies thus far have used omega-3s as adjunctive agents; given their apparent safety and tolerability, their effectiveness as monotherapy should be investigated further. Likewise, the issue of whether EPA or DHA is more effective in the treatment of depression remains to be clarified. Finally, the mechanism of action of the omega-3s, particularly their interplay with the immune system, merits further investigation. Studies addressing these questions are currently underway at the MGH and Cedars-Sinai Medical Center. It is hoped that these and other future investigations will clarify some of the lingering unanswered questions about this exciting and potentially valuable treatment.

The omega-3 fatty acids may be particularly well suited for treatment of specific patient populations (eg, pregnant or lactating women) for whom antidepressants must be used with caution,[111] for elderly people who may not tolerate side effects of conventional antidepressant agents, and for those who have medical comorbidity, particularly cardiovascular disease and possibly autoimmune conditions, for which there may be dual benefits. That said, it remains difficult to recommend omega-3s as a first-line antidepressant during pregnancy, in view of the well-documented safety and efficacy of the tricyclic antidepressants and the SSRIs. Various lines of investigation have demonstrated benefit from omega-3s to expectant mothers in whom fish intake is often restricted during pregnancy, and to unborn children and infants, particularly with regard to neural development[112,113] and allergy prevention.[114] However, what the safe upper limit of omega-3 supplements may be in pregnancy is not known.[113] Pregnant women who are depressed and are considering omega-3 therapy should first discuss the matter with their physician, and consider a consultation with a psychiatrist who is well versed in the use of natural products.

SUMMARY

Natural medications such as St John's wort, SAMe, and omega-3 fatty acids eventually may prove to be valuable additions to the pharmacologic armamentarium, both as monotherapy and as adjunctive therapy for mood disorders. Current research data are compelling, from a standpoint of both efficacy and safety, but before clinicians can recommend these as first-line treatments, more well-designed controlled studies in large patient populations are needed. During the past decade, the National Institutes of Health, the National Institute for Mental Health, and the National Center for

Complementary and Alternative Medicine have widened their support for research on the efficacy and safety of alternative treatments, and increasing numbers of academic institutions are undertaking large-scale, multicenter studies on the natural medications reviewed here as well as on others. These studies should help answer some of the yet unsettled questions about natural medications.

Physicians who are considering recommending natural antidepressants to their patients should emphasize that these treatments are relatively unproven and that it remains to be seen whether they would be appropriate or preferable to the conventional psychotropic agents.[115,116] In the absence of more conclusive data, the best candidates for alternative treatments may be patients for whom a delay in adequate treatment would not be devastating (eg, the mildly symptomatic patient who has a strong interest in natural remedies). Other good candidates may include patients who have been unresponsive to conventional antidepressants or particularly intolerant of side effects; these patients, however, often are the most difficult to treat, and alternative agents seem best suited for the mildly ill.[116] Care should be taken with patients who are taking multiple medications, in view of adverse drug-drug interactions that have emerged with increased use of alternative treatments. Pregnant women are probably safer using registered antidepressants, though current knowledge suggests that the omega-3 fatty acids and SAMe should eventually be proven safe in pregnancy. St John's wort, in view of its documented interactions and presence of myriad plant-derived chemicals of unknown significance, will require more rigorous safety testing before it can be recommended in pregnancy. Finally, as with all psychotropic agents, natural medications should be used preferably under the supervision of a physician.

REFERENCES

1. Schulz V, Hansel R, Tyler VE. Rational phytotherapy: a physician's guide to herbal medicine. 4th edition. Berlin: Springer; 2001. 78–86.
2. National Institutes of Health Office of Alternative Medicine 1997. Clinical practice guidelines in complementary and alternative medicine. An analysis of opportunities and obstacles. Practice and Policy Guidelines Panel. Arch Fam Med 1997;6: 149–54.
3. Eisenberg DM, Kessler RC, Foster C, et al. Unconventional medicine in the United States: prevalence, costs, and patterns of use. N Engl J Med 1993; 328:246–52.
4. Krippner S. A cross cultural comparison of four healing models. Altern Ther Health Med 1995;1:21–9.
5. Mischoulon D. Nutraceuticals in psychiatry, part 1: social, technical, economic, and political perspectives. Contemporary Psychiatry 2004;2(11):1–6.
6. Mischoulon D. Nutraceuticals in psychiatry, part 2: review of six popular psychotropics. Contemporary Psychiatry 2004;3(1):1–8.
7. National Institutes of Health Office of Alternative Medicine. Alternative medicine: expanding medical horizons. Rockville (MD): National Institutes of Health Office of Alternative Medicine; 1992.
8. Muller-Kuhrt L, Boesel R. Analysis of hypericins in hypericum extract. Nervenheilkunde 1993;12:359–61.
9. Staffeldt B, Kerb R, Brockmoller J, et al. Pharmacokinetics of hypericin and pseudohypericin after oral intake of the *Hypericum perforatum* extract LI 160 in healthy volunteers. Nervenheilkunde 1993;12:331–8.
10. Wagner H, Bladt S. Pharmaceutical quality of hypericum extracts. Nervenheilkunde 1993;12:362–6.

11. Müller W, Rossol R. Effects of hypericum extract on the expression of serotonin receptors. Nervenheilkunde 1993;12:357–8.

12. Thiele B, Ploch M, Brink I. Modulation of cytokine expression by hypericum extract. Nervenheilkunde 1993;12:353–6.

13. Teufel-Mayer R, Gleitz J. Effects of long-term administration of hypericum extracts on the affinity and density of the central serotonergic 5-HT1 A and 5-HT2 A receptors. Pharmacopsychiatry 1997;30(Suppl 2):113–6.

14. Nierenberg AA, Lund HG, Mischoulon D. St John's wort: a critical evaluation of the evidence for antidepressant effects. In: Mischoulon D, Rosenbaum J, editors. Natural medications for psychiatric disorders: considering the alternatives. 2nd edition. Philadelphia: Lippincott Williams & Wilkins; 2008. p. 27–38.

15. Laakmann G, Schule C, Baghai T, et al. St John's wort in mild to moderate depression: the relevance of hyperforin for the clinical efficacy. Pharmacopsychiatry 1998;31(Suppl 1):54–9.

16. Orth HC, Rentel C, Schmidt PC. Isolation, purity analysis and stability of hyperforin as a standard material from *Hypericum perforatum* L. J Pharm Pharmacol 1999;51(2):193–200.

17. Bladt S, Wagner H. MAO inhibition by fractions and constituents of hypericum extract. Nervenheilkunde 1993;12:349–52.

18. Linde K, Mulrow CD, Berner M, et al. St John's wort for depression. Cochrane Database Syst Rev 2005;(2):CD000448.

19. Vorbach EU, Hubner WD, Arnoldt KH. Effectiveness and tolerance of the hypericum extract LI 160 in comparison with imipramine. Randomized double blind study with 135 out-patients. Nervenheilkunde 1993;12:290–6 Also in J Geriatr Psychiatry Neurol 1994;7(Suppl 1):S19–23.

20. Harrer G, Hubner WD, Podzuweit H. Effectiveness and tolerance of the hypericum preparation LI 160 compared to maprotiline. Multicentre double-blind study with 102 outpatients. Nervenheilkunde 1993;12:297–301.

21. Martinez B, Kasper S, Ruhrmann B, et al. Hypericum in the treatment of seasonal affective disorders. Nervenheilkunde 1993;12:302–7.

22. Wheatley D. LI 160, an extract of St John's wort, versus amitriptyline in mildly to moderately depressed outpatients—a controlled 6-week clinical trial. Pharmacopsychiatry 1997;30(Suppl 2):77–80.

23. Nierenberg AA. St John's wort: a putative over-the-counter herbal antidepressant. J Depress Disord Index & Reviews 1998;III:16–7.

24. Linde K, Ramirez G, Mulrow CD, et al. St John's wort for depression—an overview and meta-analysis of randomized clinical trials. Br Med J 1996;313:253–8.

25. Volz HP. Controlled clinical trials of hypericum extracts in depressed patients—an overview. Pharmacopsychiatry 1997;30(Suppl 2):72–6.

26. Lecrubier Y, Clerc G, Didi R, et al. Efficacy of St John's wort extract WS 5570 in major depression: a double-blind, placebo-controlled trial. Am J Psychiatry 2002;159(8):1361–6.

27. Shelton RC, Keller MB, Gelenberg A, et al. Effectiveness of St John's wort in major depression: a randomized controlled trial. JAMA 2001;285(15):1978–86.

28. Brenner R, Azbel V, Madhusoodanan S, et al. Comparison of an extract of hypericum (LI 160) and sertraline in the treatment of depression: a double-blind, randomized pilot study. Clin Ther 2000;22(4):411–9.

29. Gastpar M, Singer A, Zeller K. Efficacy and tolerability of hypericum extract STW3 in long-term treatment with a once-daily dosage in comparison with sertraline. Pharmacopsychiatry 2005;38(2):78–86.

30. van Gurp G, Meterissian GB, Haiek LN, et al. St John's wort or sertraline? Randomized controlled trial in primary care. Can Fam Physician 2002;48: 905–12.
31. Schrader E. Equivalence of St John's wort extract (Ze 117) and fluoxetine: a randomized, controlled study in mild-moderate depression. Int Clin Psychopharmacol 2000;15(2):61–8.
32. Behnke K, Jensen GS, Graubaum HJ, et al. *Hypericum perforatum* versus fluoxetine in the treatment of mild to moderate depression. Adv Ther 2002;19(1): 43–52.
33. Hypericum Depression Trial Study Group. Effect of *Hypericum perforatum* (St John's wort) in major depressive disorder: a randomized controlled trial. JAMA 2002;287:1807–14.
34. Fava M, Alpert J, Nierenberg AA, et al. A double-blind, randomized trial of St John's wort, fluoxetine, and placebo in major depressive disorder. J Clin Psychopharmacol 2005;25(5):441–7.
35. Moreno RA, Teng CT, Almeida KM, et al. *Hypericum perforatum* versus fluoxetine in the treatment of mild to moderate depression: a randomized double-blind trial in a Brazilian sample. Rev Bras Psiquiatr 2006;28(1):29–32.
36. Baede-van Dijk PA, van Galen E, Lekkerkerker JF. [Drug interactions of *Hypericum perforatum* (St John's wort) are potentially hazardous]. Ned Tijdschr Geneeskd 2000;144(17):811–2 [in Dutch].
37. Miller LG. Herbal medicinals: selected clinical considerations focusing on known or potential drug-herb interactions. Arch Intern Med 1998;158:2200–11.
38. Moore LB, Goodwin B, Jones SA, et al. St John's wort induces hepatic drug metabolism through activation of the pregnane X receptor. Proc Natl Acad Sci U S A 2000;97(13):7500–2.
39. Miller JL. Interaction between indinavir and St John's wort reported. Am J Health Syst Pharm 2000;57(7):625–6.
40. Piscitelli SC, Burstein AH, Chaitt D, et al. Indinavir concentrations and St John's wort. Lancet 2000;355(9203):547–8.
41. Hu Z, Yang X, Ho PC, et al. Herb-drug interactions: a literature review. Drugs 2005;65(9):1239–82.
42. Schulz V. Safety of St John's wort extract compared to synthetic antidepressants. Phytomedicine 2006;13(3):199–204.
43. Woelk H, Burkhard G, Grunwald J. Evaluation of the benefits and risks of the hypericum extract LI 160 based on a drug monitoring study with 3250 patients. Nervenheilkunde 1993;12:308–13.
44. Beattie PE, Dawe RS, Traynor NJ, et al. Can St John's wort (hypericin) ingestion enhance the erythemal response during high-dose ultraviolet A1 therapy? Br J Dermatol 2005;153(6):1187–91.
45. Brockmoller J, Reum T, Bauer S, et al. Hypericin and pseudohypericin: pharmacokinetics and effects on photosensitivity in humans. Pharmacopsychiatry 1997; 30(Suppl 2):94–101.
46. Siegers CP, Biel S, Wilhelm KP. Phototoxicity caused by hypericum. Nervenheilkunde 1993;12:320–2.
47. Stevinson C, Ernst E. Can St John's wort trigger psychoses? Int J Clin Pharmacol Ther 2004;42(9):473–80.
48. Dugoua JJ, Mills E, Perri D, et al. Safety and efficacy of St John's wort (hypericum) during pregnancy and lactation. Can J Clin Pharmacol 2006;13(3): e268–76.

49. Moretti ME, Maxson A, Hanna F, et al. Evaluating the safety of St John's wort in human pregnancy. Reprod Toxicol 2009;28(1):96–9.

50. Klier CM, Schäfer MR, Schmid-Siegel B, et al. John's wort (*Hypericum perforatum*)—is it safe during breastfeeding? Pharmacopsychiatry 2002;35(1): 29–30.

51. Klier CM, Schmid-Siegel B, Schäfer MR, et al. St John's wort (*Hypericum perforatum*) and breastfeeding: plasma and breast milk concentrations of hyperforin for 5 mothers and 2 infants. J Clin Psychiatry 2006;67(2):305–9.

52. Lee A, Minhas R, Matsuda N, et al. The safety of St John's wort (*Hypericum perforatum*) during breastfeeding. J Clin Psychiatry 2003;64(8):966–8.

53. Freeman MP. Complementary and alternative medicine for perinatal depression. J Affect Disord 2009;112(1–3):1–10.

54. Spillmann M, Fava M. *S*-adenosyl-methionine (ademethionine) in psychiatric disorders. CNS Drugs 1996;6:416–25.

55. Alpert JE, Mischoulon D, Nierenberg AA, et al. Nutrition and depression: focus on folate. Nutrition 2000;16:544–6.

56. Coppen A, Bailey J. Enhancement of the antidepressant action of fluoxetine by folic acid: a randomised, placebo controlled trial. J Affect Disord 2000;60: 121–30.

57. Alpert JE, Mischoulon D, Rubenstein GEF, et al. Folinic acid (leucovorin) as an adjunctive treatment for SSRI-refractory depression. Ann Clin Psychiatry 2002; 14:33–8.

58. Fava M, Borus JS, Alpert JE, et al. Folate, B12, and homocysteine in major depressive disorder. Am J Psychiatry 1997;154:426–8.

59. Bottiglieri T, Godfrey P, Flynn T, et al. Cerebrospinal fluid *S*-adenosylmethionine in depression and dementia: effects of treatment with parenteral and oral *S*-adenosylmethionine. J Neurol Neurosurg Psychiatr 1990;53:1096–8.

60. Bell KM, Potkin SG, Carreon D, et al. *S*-adenosylmethionine blood levels in major depression: changes with drug treatment. Acta Neurol Scand Suppl 1994;154: 15–8.

61. Bottiglieri T, Chary TK, Laundy M, et al. Transmethylation in depression. Ala J Med Sci 1988;25:296–301.

62. Matthysse S, Baldessarini RJ. *S*-adenosylmethionine and catechol-*O*-methyl-transferase in schizophrenia. Am J Psychiatry 1972;128:1310–2.

63. Tolbert LC. MAT kinetics in affective disorders and schizophrenia. An account. Ala J Med Sci 1988;25:291–6.

64. Bressa GM. *S*-Adenosyl-L-methionine (SAMe) as antidepressant: meta-analysis of clinical studies. Acta Neurol Scand 1994;154(Suppl):7–14.

65. Papakostas GI, Alpert JE, Fava M. *S*-Adenosyl methionine in depression: a comprehensive review of the literature. Curr Psychiatry Rep 2003;5:460–6.

66. Mischoulon D, Fava M. Role of *S*-adenosyl-L-methionine in the treatment of depression: a review of the evidence. Am J Clin Nutr 2002;76(Suppl 5): 1158S–61S.

67. Fava M, Giannelli A, Rapisarda V, et al. Rapidity of onset of the antidepressant effect of parenteral *S*-adenosyl-L-methionine. Psychiatry Res 1995;56:295–7.

68. Alvarez E, Udina C, Guillamat R. Shortening of latency period in depressed patients treated with SAMe and other antidepressant drugs. Cell Biol Rev 1987;S1:103–10.

69. Berlanga C, Ortega-Soto HA, Ontiveros M, et al. Efficacy of *S*-adenosyl-L-methionine in speeding the onset of action of imipramine. Psychiatry Res 1992;44: 257–62.

70. Alpert JE, Papakostas G, Mischoulon D, et al. S-adenosyl-L-methionine (SAMe) as an adjunct for resistant major depressive disorder: an open trial following partial or nonresponse to selective serotonin reuptake inhibitors or venlafaxine. J Clin Psychopharmacol 2004;24(6):661–4.

71. Carney MWP, Chary TNK, Bottiglieri T. Switch mechanism in affective illness and oral S-adenosylmethionine (SAM). Br J Psychiatry 1987;150:724–5.

72. Carney MW, Martin R, Bottiglieri T, et al. Switch mechanism in affective illness and S-adenosylmethionine. Lancet 1983;1:820–1.

73. Guerra-Shinohara EM, Morita OE, Peres S, et al. Low ratio of S-adenosylmethionine to S-adenosylhomocysteine is associated with vitamin deficiency in Brazilian pregnant women and newborns. Am J Clin Nutr 2004;80(5):1312–21.

74. Frezza M, Surrenti C, Manzillo G, et al. Oral S-adenosylmethionine in the symptomatic treatment of intrahepatic cholestasis. A double-blind, placebo-controlled study. Gastroenterology 1990;99(1):211–5.

75. Adams PB, Lawson S, Sanigorski A, et al. Arachidonic acid to eicosapentaenoic acid ration in blood correlates positively with clinical symptoms of depression. Lipids 1996;31:157–61.

76. Hibbeln JR, Salem N. Dietary polyunsaturated fatty acids and depression: when cholesterol does not satisfy. Am J Clin Nutr 1995;62:1–9.

77. The changing rate of major depression: cross national comparisons. Cross-National Collaborative Group. JAMA 1992;268:3098–105.

78. Hibbeln JR. Fish consumption and major depression [letter]. Lancet 1998;351:1213.

79. Hibbeln JR. Long-chain polyunsaturated fatty acids in depression and related conditions. In: Peet M, Glen I, Horrobin DF, editors. Phospholipid spectrum disorder in psychiatry. Carnforth (UK): Marius Press; 1999. p. 195–210.

80. Stoll AL. Omega-3 fatty acids in mood disorders: a review of neurobiological and clinical actions. In: Mischoulon D, Rosenbaum J, editors. Natural medications for psychiatric disorders: considering the alternatives. Philadelphia: Lippincott Williams & Wilkins; 2008. p. 39–67.

81. Hamazaki K, Itomura M, Huan M, et al. Effect of omega-3 fatty acid-containing phospholipids on blood catecholamine concentrations in healthy volunteers: a randomized, placebo-controlled, double-blind trial. Nutrition 2005;21(6):705–10.

82. Murck H, Song C, Horrobin DF, et al. Ethyl-eicosapentaenoate and dexamethasone resistance in therapy-refractory depression. Int J Neuropsychopharmacol 2004;7(3):341–9.

83. Freeman MP, Hibbeln JR, Wisner KL, et al. Omega-3 fatty acids: evidence basis for treatment and future research in psychiatry. J Clin Psychiatry 2006;67:1954–67.

84. Appleton KM, Hayward RC, Gunnell D, et al. Effects of n-3 long-chain polyunsaturated fatty acids on depressed mood: systematic review of published trials. Am J Clin Nutr 2006;84(6):1308–16.

85. Lin PY, Su KP. A meta-analytic review of double-blind, placebo-controlled trials of antidepressant efficacy of omega-3 fatty acids. J Clin Psychiatry 2007;68(7):1056–61.

86. Rogers PJ, Appleton KM, Kessler D, et al. No effect of n-3 long-chain polyunsaturated fatty acid (EPA and DHA) supplementation on depressed mood and cognitive function: a randomised controlled trial. Br J Nutr 2008;99(2):421–31.

87. Peet M, Horrobin DF. A dose-ranging study of the effects of ethyl-eicosapentaenoate in patients with ongoing depression despite apparently adequate treatment with standard drugs. Arch Gen Psychiatry 2002;59(10):913–9.

88. Su KP, Huang SY, Chiu CC, et al. Omega-3 fatty acids in major depressive disorder. A preliminary double-blind, placebo-controlled trial. Eur Neuropsychopharmacol 2003;13(4):267–71.

89. Nemets B, Stahl ZM, Belmaker RH. Addition of omega-3 fatty acid to maintenance medication treatment for recurrent unipolar depressive disorder. Am J Psychiatry 2002;159:477–9.

90. Frangou S, Lewis M, McCrone P. Efficacy of ethyl-eicosapentaenoic acid in bipolar depression: randomised double-blind placebo-controlled study. Br J Psychiatry 2006;188:46–50.

91. Mischoulon D, Papakostas GI, Dording CM, et al. A double-blind randomized controlled trial of ethyl-eicosapentaenoate (EPA-E) for major depressive disorder. J Clin Psychiatry 2009 [Epub ahead of print].

92. Silvers KM, Woolley CC, Hamilton FC, et al. Randomized double-blind placebo-controlled trial of fish oil in the treatment of depression. Prostaglandins Leukot Essent Fatty Acids 2005;72:211–8.

93. Marangell LB, Martinez JM, Zboyan HA, et al. A double-blind, placebo-controlled study of the omega-3 fatty acid docosahexaenoic acid in the treatment of major depression. Am J Psychiatry 2003;160(5):996–8.

94. Mischoulon D, Best-Popescu C, Laposata M, et al. A double-blind dose-finding pilot study of docosahexaenoic acid (DHA) for major depressive disorder. Eur Neuropsychopharmacol 2008;18:639–45.

95. Freeman MP, Hibbeln JR, Wisner KL, et al. Randomized dose-ranging pilot trial of omega-3 fatty acids for postpartum depression. Acta Psychiatr Scand 2006; 113(1):31–5.

96. Marangell LB, Martinez JM, Zboyan HA, et al. Omega-3 fatty acids for the prevention of postpartum depression: negative data from a preliminary, open-label pilot study. Depress Anxiety 2004;19(1):20–3.

97. Strøm M, Mortensen EL, Halldorsson TI, et al. Fish and long-chain n-3 polyunsaturated fatty acid intakes during pregnancy and risk of postpartum depression: a prospective study based on a large national birth cohort. Am J Clin Nutr 2009; 90(1):149–55.

98. Stoll AL, Severus EW, Freeman MP, et al. Omega3 fatty acids in bipolar disorder: a preliminary double-blind, placebo-controlled trial. Arch Gen Psychiatry 1999; 56:407–12.

99. Keck PE, Mintz J, McElroy SL, et al. Double-blind, randomized, placebo-controlled trials of ethyl-eicosapentanoate in the treatment of bipolar depression and rapid cycling bipolar disorder. Biol Psychiatry 2006;60:1020–2.

100. Parker G, Gibson NA, Brotchie H, et al. Omega-3 fatty acids and mood disorders. Am J Psychiatry 2006;163(6):969–78.

101. Montgomery P, Richardson AJ. Omega-3 fatty acids for bipolar disorder. Cochrane Database Syst Rev 2008;(2):CD005169.

102. Osher Y, Bersudsky Y, Belmaker RH. Omega-3 eicosapentaenoic acid in bipolar depression: report of a small open-label study. J Clin Psychiatry 2005;66(6):726–9.

103. Zanarini MC, Frankenburg FR. Omega-3 fatty acid treatment of women with borderline personality disorder: a double-blind, placebo-controlled pilot study. Am J Psychiatry 2003;160:167–9.

104. Mellor JE, Laugharne JDE, Peet M. Omega-3 fatty acid supplementation in schizophrenic patients. Hum Psychopharmacol 1996;11:39–46.

105. Vaddadi KS, Courtney T, Gilleard CJ, et al. A double-blind trial of essential fatty acid supplementation in patients with tardive dyskinesia. Psychiatry Res 1989; 27:313–23.

106. Emsley R, Myburgh C, Oosthuizen P, et al. Randomized, placebo-controlled study of ethyl-eicosapentaenoic acid as supplemental treatment in schizophrenia. Am J Psychiatry 2002;159:1596–8.

107. Fenton WS, Dickerson F, Boronow J, et al. A placebo-controlled trial of omega-3 fatty acid (ethyl eicosapentaenoic acid) supplementation for residual symptoms and cognitive impairment in schizophrenia. Am J Psychiatry 2001;158:2071–4.

108. Maidment ID. Are fish oils an effective therapy in mental illness—an analysis of the data. Acta Psychiatr Scand 2000;102:3–11.

109. Fux M, Benjamin J, Nemets B. A placebo-controlled cross-over trial of adjunctive EPA in OCD. J Psychiatr Res 2004;38(3):323–5.

110. Peet M, Brind J, Ramchand CN, et al. Two double-blind placebo-controlled pilot studies of eicosapentaenoic acid in the treatment of schizophrenia. Schizophr Res 2001;49(3):243–51.

111. Chiu C-C, Huang S-Y, Shen WW, et al. Omega-3 fatty acids for depression in pregnancy [letter]. Am J Psychiatry 2003;160:385.

112. Greenberg JA, Bell SJ, Ausdal WV. Omega-3 fatty acid supplementation during pregnancy. Rev Obstet Gynecol 2008;1(4):162–9.

113. Innis SM. Omega-3 fatty acids and neural development to 2 years of age: do we know enough for dietary recommendations? J Pediatr Gastroenterol Nutr 2009; 48(Suppl 1):S16–24.

114. Furuhjelm C, Warstedt K, Larsson J, et al. Fish oil supplementation in pregnancy and lactation may decrease the risk of infant allergy. Acta Paediatr 2009;98: 1461–7.

115. Eisenberg DM. Advising patients who seek alternative medical therapies. Ann Intern Med 1997;127(1):61–9.

116. Mischoulon D, Rosenbaum JF. The use of natural medications in psychiatry: a commentary. Harv Rev Psychiatry 1999;6:279–83.

Sleep, Hormones, and Memory

Jan Born, PhD[a],*, Ullrich Wagner, PhD[b]

KEYWORDS

• Hormones • Hypothalamo-pituitary-adrenal-system • Memory
• Sleep

Although knowledge about the mechanisms of sleep is rapidly growing, its function remains elusive. A common view is that sleep, which is an organismic state free of any stress, serves primarily to recover the organism from the stress of the wake phase. However, whereas the restorative function of sleep is intuitively comprehended at the subjective level, it is difficult to define any recovery function of sleep in physiologic terms.[1] If sleep recovered the body from stress would the release of stress hormones not be expected to be at a minimum at morning awakening? However, the release of cortisol reaches a circadian peak at that time. Considering the function of sleep from a physiologic perspective requires concepts more specifically related to the neuronal and metabolic processes that are orchestrated by the brain in a sleep-specific way. This article follows the hypothesis that a primary function of sleep pertains to the consolidation of memory. In recent years, this view has received substantial support from a rapidly growing number of experiments performed in various species and at different levels of behavioral, cellular, and molecular analysis.[2–7]

Memory formation can be divided into 3 fundamental subprocesses (**Fig. 1**). First, the information to be stored is taken up, that is, encoded into a cellular network to establish a preliminary memory trace. Second, retention of the newly encoded traces requires some kind of consolidation, that is, strengthening of the new traces, because these are initially labile and subject to processes of decay and forgetting. Consolidation counteracts forgetting, which occurs because of the decay of the fresh trace or because of retroactive interference from subsequently encoded material. Third, once stored, the information can be retrieved, and typically a test of retrieval is used to confirm existence of a memory because the memory trace cannot be directly measured. Encoding and retrieval of information are processes that occur mainly during wakefulness when the organism has to cope acutely with a great diversity of stressors. In contrast, the

Supported by the Deutsche Forschungsgemeinschaft SFB 654 – Plasticity and Sleep.

This is an updated version of the article "Sleep, hormones, and memory," which appeared in *Sleep Medicine Clinics* (Volume 2, Issue 2, June 2007).

[a] Department of Neuroendocrinology, University of Lübeck, Haus 23a, Ratzeburger Allee 160, 23538 Lübeck, Germany

[b] School of Psychology, Bangor University, Brigantia Building, Penrallt Road, Bangor, Gwynedd LL57 2AS, UK

* Corresponding author.

E-mail address: born@kfg.uni-luebeck.de (J. Born).

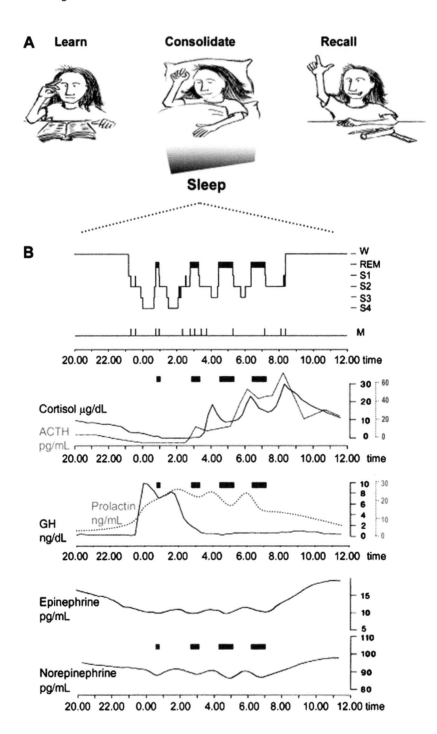

consolidation of newly acquired memories takes place preferentially during sleep, when the challenge by acute stressors is minimal. It is supposed that processes of consolidation are shifted to the sleep phase, because relying on the same cellular networks as those used for the acute processing of stressors, these processes of consolidation would interfere with proper encoding and retrieval operations during wakefulness.

Memory formation is conceptualized as a general biological function that pertains not only to the neurobehavioral system but also to memory in other systems that adapt to stressors in the long term, like the immune system, which learns how to respond to specific antigens. This article discusses evidence (mainly from studies that have been performed in humans in the authors' laboratory) suggesting that the sleep-specific regulation of endocrine activity subserves the consolidation of memories. Although a few studies support the notion that neuroendocrine activity during sleep enhances immunologic memory formation also,[8–10] this article is restricted to neurobehavioral memory.

THE UNIQUE NEUROENDOCRINE REGULATION OF SLEEP

Sleep consists of the cyclic occurrence of non-rapid eye movement (non-REM) sleep and REM sleep, with the deepest stages of non-REM sleep (stages 3 and 4) termed slow wave sleep (SWS). Sleep is entrained to the circadian rhythm and external zeit-gebers such that in humans sleep normally occurs during nighttime. Because of the coupling to a circadian oscillator, nocturnal sleep in humans can be roughly divided into an early and a late part distinctly differing in sleep architecture. During early sleep, SWS is predominant, whereas the other core sleep stage (REM sleep) occurs only in marginal amounts. During late sleep this relationship is reversed: REM sleep predominates whereas the amount of SWS is greatly reduced.

The dynamics of sleep architecture are paralleled by distinct temporal patterns of endocrine activity embracing almost all hormonal systems. Sleep can be associated with 3 types of hormonal patterns: (1) a uniform change in hormonal release throughout the night, (2) a differential change during early and late sleep, and (3) a pattern strictly bound to the non-REM–REM sleep cycle (see **Fig. 1**). For example, release of melatonin is generally increased during nocturnal sleep, whereas release of epinephrine and norepinephrine is reduced.[11,12] Early SWS-dominated sleep is associated with distinctly increased somatotropic secretory activity but suppressed hypothalamo-pituitary-adrenal (HPA) activity, whereas during late REM-rich sleep, this relationship is reversed.[1,13] Finally, there is a general synchronization of endocrine activity to the non-REM–REM sleep cycle such that secretory activity prevails during periods of non-REM sleep, whereas activity is suppressed during REM sleep. This synchronization holds for hormonal release regulated via the hypothalamo-pituitary system and for the sympatho-adrenal system.[12,14–16]

Fig. 1. (*A*) Memory formation comprises 3 subprocesses: (1) "learning," which refers to the encoding of information into a neuronal memory trace, (2) "consolidation" of the fresh memory trace for long-term storage, and (3) "recall" of the memories. Learning and recall of memories take place effectively only during wakefulness, whereas memories are consolidated optimally only during sleep. (*B*) Individual nocturnal sleep profile and associated blood concentrations of ACTH, cortisol, GH, prolactin, epinephrine, and norepinephrine. Note, minimum levels of ACTH and cortisol in the presence of high GH levels during early sleep rich in SWS (S3 and S4), whereas during late REM-rich sleep this pattern is reversed. Epinephrine and norepinephrine concentrations are generally decreased during sleep. Release of all hormones is downregulated during REM sleep (*black bars*, copied also to the panels below).

The neuroendocrine architecture of sleep evolves from an interaction between circadian oscillators and the systems that regulate sleep. The strength of the influence differs for the 2 factors depending on the type of hormone. In some cases, the nocturnal change in hormonal release reflects mainly a circadian rhythm in the absence of any direct influence of sleep. Melatonin concentrations, for example, peak around midnight whether sleep occurs during nighttime or is shifted acutely to daytime hours.[11,17]

In other cases, circadian oscillators and sleep exert influences on hormonal release that can be in the same or opposite directions. Release of thyrotropin (thyroid stimulating hormone [TSH]) is a robust marker of the circadian clock, showing a distinct surge during early night.[11] Regular nocturnal sleep reduces the surge, indicating opposing influences of sleep and circadian oscillators on TSH release during this time.

In contrast to the release of TSH, activity of the HPA system is influenced synergistically by circadian oscillators and sleep. Plasma concentrations of corticotropin (adrenocorticotropic hormone [ACTH]) and cortisol show a stable 24-hour pattern with maximum concentrations around the time of morning awakening and nadir concentrations during the early hours of nocturnal sleep. This pattern changes only marginally during conditions of continuous 24 hours of wakefulness, which has led some researchers to exclude (erroneously) any influence of sleep on HPA secretory activity. In fact, sleep actively and synergistically adds to the inhibition of ACTH and cortisol release during early sleep and also to the activation of the HPA system during late sleep. The former effect can be unmasked by stimulating pituitary-adrenal activity during sleep through secretagogues like corticotropin-releasing hormone (CRH) or vasopressin.[18–20] The secretory response to the releasing hormones when injected during SWS in early sleep is distinctly reduced in comparison with the response to these substances injected at the same dose and the same time of night while the subject is awake (**Fig. 2**). This inhibitory action of SWS during early sleep on the release of ACTH and cortisol is most likely mediated via the secretion of a release-inhibiting factor during this period, although the specific molecule remains to be characterized.

CRH administration during late sleep in these studies did not increase ACTH and cortisol secretory responses when compared with responses in waking subjects at the same time of the night. Nevertheless, late sleep seems to contribute to the morning increase in HPA activity by disinhibiting the system, as indicated by findings from another study.[21] In this study, subjects were aroused after a 3-hour period of early nocturnal sleep and then stayed awake. Arousing the subject induces a transient increase in ACTH and cortisol concentrations.[22,23] However, during the succeeding wake period, HPA secretory activity as indicated by ACTH and cortisol release was significantly lower than during the corresponding time interval of the control condition during which subjects continued sleeping. Because the pituitary-adrenal secretory response to intravenous CRH was not affected by late sleep, the disinhibition during this sleep interval is likely mediated via a mechanism acting at the hypothalamic or a supraordinate level of the HPA system.

Somatotropic activity represents a well-documented example of hormonal regulation with predominant dependence on sleep. Release of growth hormone (GH) peaks during early sleep in close temporal association with the first periods of SWS.[24,25] Sleep during daytime is likewise associated with increased GH release, but the nocturnal GH surge can be prevented by keeping the subject awake. Like GH, secretion of prolactin seems to be particularly linked to SWS and the associated slow wave electroencephalogram activity.[26] Although less clear, there is evidence that plasma catecholamine concentrations are likewise subject to a primary regulation by sleep.

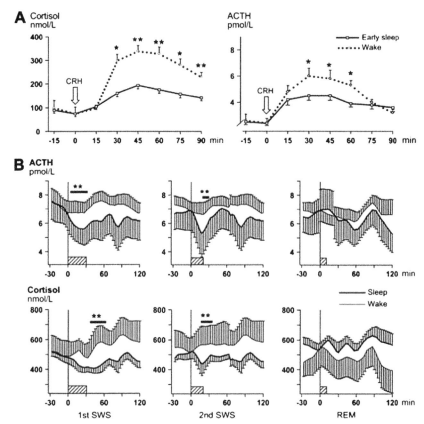

Fig. 2. (*A*) Mean (±SEM) plasma concentration of cortisol and ACTH before (−15 to 0 minutes) and after (15 to 90 minutes) bolus injection of CRH (50 μg) during early nocturnal sleep, mostly during SWS (*solid lines*) and at the same time of night while subjects stayed awake (*dotted lines*) (n = 14). (*B*) Mean (±SEM) plasma concentration of cortisol and ACTH during continuous infusion of CRH (30 μg/h, preceded by a bolus of 30 μg CRH). Concentrations during sleep (*thick lines*) between 30 minutes before and 2 hours after the first nocturnal period of SWS (*left*), second period of SWS (*middle*), and first epoch of REM sleep (*right*) were compared with levels during corresponding time intervals of a condition of continuous wakefulness (*thin lines*). For the comparison, hormone concentrations were averaged time-locked to the individual onset of the 3 different sleep epochs and to the respective time points of the wake condition (and adjusted to a common preonset baseline). Hatched horizontal bars indicate average length of the respective sleep epoch. Asterisks indicate significant (*P*<.05) differences between effects of the sleep and wake condition. (*Data from* Bierwolf C, Struve K, Marshall L, et al. Slow wave sleep drives inhibition of pituitary-adrenal secretion in humans. J Neuroendocrinol 1997;9(6):479–84; and Späth-Schwalbe E, Uthgenannt D, Voget G, et al. Corticotropin-releasing hormone-induced adrenocorticotropin and cortisol secretion depends on sleep and wakefulness. J Clin Endocrinol Metab 1993;77:1170–73.)

Sleep, and particularly REM sleep, reduces blood concentrations of norepinephrine and epinephrine.[12,16] In general, however, a clear-cut dissociation of circadian and sleep-related mechanisms in the regulation of hormonal release, especially in the sympatho-adrenal and the HPA systems, is methodologically difficult because of possible confounding variables like motor activity, body position, light exposure, and food intake that interact with circadian and sleep-related mechanisms of hormonal regulation.

SLEEP ENHANCES THE CONSOLIDATION OF MEMORIES

An enhancing effect of sleep on memory consolidation has been demonstrated for major types of neuropsychologically distinct memories (declarative, emotional, and procedural memories). Declarative memory refers to the explicit memories for facts and events, and experimentally is often tested using paired associate learning tasks (like the learning of lists of word pairs). Encoding and, initially, retrieval of these memories relies essentially on the hippocampus.[27] However, with time retrieval becomes independent of the hippocampus, presumably because of a gradual transfer of these memories to other mainly neocortical networks.[28] Emotional memory is known to rely essentially on the amygdala.[29,30] It is often assessed by the "emotional enhancement," that is, the extent to which the memory for an emotional stimulus (eg, words with aversive meaning) is superior to the memory for a comparable but neutral stimulus (eg, neutral nonarousing words). The emotional enhancement reflects primarily a modulating influence of the amygdala on hippocampal memory function.[31,32] Procedural memory refers to the memory for sensory and motor skills that are acquired gradually by repeated practice. It does not require hippocampal or amygdalar function, but among others relies strongly on striatocortical circuitry.[33] In studies of sleep-dependent memory formation, procedural memory has often been assessed by the finger-tapping task, which requires the subject to tap as fast and as accurately as possible a certain sequence of finger taps (on a keyboard).[34]

A frequently used design in studies on sleep-associated memory consolidation compares recall after a retention period filled with nocturnal sleep (with learning in the evening before, and recall in the morning after) with recall after a retention period filled with daytime wakefulness (with learning in the morning and recall in the evening of the day). However, this approach confounds circadian phase with effects of sleep. To keep circadian phase constant, other studies compared retention periods across nocturnal periods of sleep versus wakefulness. With this approach, impaired recall after the nocturnal vigil may reflect fatigue hampering processes of retrieval rather than inferior consolidation during the wake phase. The deprivation of sleep is known to induce a multitude of cognitive impairments that cannot be taken to infer, in reverse, the function of normal sleep. To avoid confounds of sleep deprivation, designs were used in more recent studies in which subjects either slept or remained awake the first night after learning, and recall was not tested until after a second night, which enabled recovery sleep before retrieval testing. Also, retention was compared for shorter periods of sleep and wakefulness to keep deprivation effects in the wake condition minimal.

Employing such designs, recent studies confirmed earlier findings that sleep after learning, in comparison with wakefulness, enhances retention not only of declarative memory for various materials (eg, word pairs, spatial locations),[35–40] but also of emotional memories,[41,42] and procedural memories for visual discrimination and motor skills.[3,34,43,44] For procedural memory tasks a robust gain in performance is observed at a later retrieval testing, the size of which has been shown to depend critically on the presence of sleep after initial training. This gain in performance suggests a latent offline processing of memory representations during sleep that not only stabilizes but enhances skill in the absence of any further practice. A gain in performance at later retrieval testing that depends on sleep has been likewise shown for the hippocampus-dependent declarative memory system.[38,45] These studies showed that sleep supports the gain of explicit (ie, conscious) knowledge about rules and invariant features of stimulus materials that had been acquired implicitly (ie, unconsciously) before sleep. In combination, these findings of performance gains at retrieval testing indicate that sleep does not only passively strengthen memories but that memory consolidation during sleep is an active process that reshapes the newly encoded memory representation and thereby can induce, depending on the type of task, a gain of procedural skill or explicit knowledge. A sleep-specific reorganization of newly encoded memory representations has been confirmed by studies using functional magnetic resonance imaging (fMRI) of the brain. If sleep, compared with wakefulness, followed initial acquisition, later retrieval of declarative memories (of a virtual maze) involved less hippocampal activity but increased striatal activity,[46] later retrieval of emotional memories involved less amygdalar but increased prefrontal and hippocampal activity,[47] and later retrieval of procedural memories (for finger-tapping skill) involved less activity in cortical motor areas but increased activity in regions of the basal ganglia.[48]

SLEEP STAGES AND MEMORY CONSOLIDATION

Traditionally, REM sleep has been considered more important for memory consolidation because this sleep stage is linked to dreams and obvious cognitive processing. However, investigations using selective REM sleep deprivation were not conclusive,[7,35] partly because the repeated arousal from REM sleep imposes a strong stress on subjects, which contaminates later recall performance. To avoid the adverse effects of REM sleep deprivation procedures, Ekstrand's group[49,50] developed an effective approach that compares effects of 3- to 4-hour retention intervals filled with early SWS-rich sleep with those of 3- to 4-hour retention intervals filled with late sleep in which REM sleep is predominant (**Fig. 3**). Effects of early and late sleep are additionally contrasted with those of wake retention intervals during corresponding nighttimes. This approach revealed that retention of hippocampus-dependent declarative memory benefits particularly, but not exclusively, from SWS-dominated early nocturnal sleep, whereas memories not relying on the hippocampus, that is, amygdala-dependent emotional memories and also procedural memories improve particularly, but not exclusively from REM sleep during the late night.[35,36,41] The time spent in lighter non-REM sleep stage 1 and 2, and time awake was closely comparable between the early and late periods of retention sleep in these experiments, which excludes a primary role of these stages for the differential effects of early versus late sleep on memory consolidation.

   A central hypothesis is that the consolidation during sleep relies on a covert reactivation during sleep of the neuronal networks that were used for encoding the new memories during prior wakefulness.[7,28,51] Consistent with this hypothesis, in rats, hippocampal neuron assemblies implicated in encoding of spatial information during maze learning become reactivated in the same temporal order during succeeding SWS.[52] Neuroimaging studies in healthy humans revealed signs of reactivation during sleep after learning, which for declarative tasks (virtual maze learning) occurred in hippocampal regions during SWS, whereas for procedural tasks neural reactivations concentrated on the cuneus and striatal regions during REM sleep.[53–55] Brain stimulation in humans that enhanced the slow oscillations characterizing SWS was found to enhance selectively the retention of declarative memories.[56]

   There are reports that indicate a benefit of procedural memory also from SWS and, vice versa, a benefit from REM sleep for aspects of declarative memory.[43,57] In part this reflects the nature of the experimental tasks, which do not exclusively activate

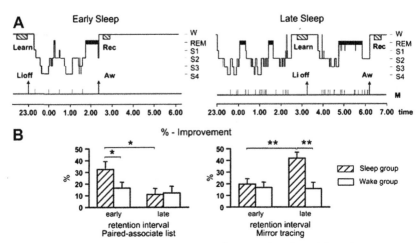

Fig. 3. (*A*) Experimental design to study the influence of early and late sleep on memory consolidation, illustrated by individual sleep profiles. Early sleep: Subjects learned the tasks to a criterion at 10:15 PM. Lights were turned off at 11:00 PM to enable a 3-hour period of early retention sleep. Recall was tested approximately 30 minutes after awakening (Aw). Late sleep: Subjects slept during the first 3 hours of the night to reduce propensity for SWS. They learned the tasks to the criterion at approximately 2:30 AM. Thereafter, lights were turned off to enable a 3-hour period of late retention sleep. Recall was tested approximately 30 minutes after awakening. In additional wake control conditions, subjects remained awake during the corresponding retention periods between learning and recall testing. Note, predominance of SWS during early sleep, and of REM sleep during late sleep. (*B*) Mean improvement (±SEM) in retrieval performance after early and late sleep (*hatched bars*) and respective wake control conditions (*empty bars*) for a declarative (paired-associate word list) and a procedural (mirror-tracing) memory task. There is a double dissociation between memory system and time of night. Whereas declarative memory benefits from early, SWS-rich sleep, procedural memory is enhanced after late, REM sleep-rich. *P*<.05, *P*<.01 for comparisons between conditions. (*Data from* Plihal W, Born J. Effects of early and late nocturnal sleep on declarative and procedural memory. J Cog Neurosci 1997;9:534–47.)

either one of the systems.[58,59] If, accordingly, memory performance reflects an interaction of memory systems, sleep-associated memory consolidation is best described in the "sequential hypothesis"[60] posing that SWS and REM sleep act on different aspects of memory, that is, declarative versus emotional and procedural aspects, respectively, with the sequence of SWS and REM sleep phases producing the final memory enhancement.[61]

HORMONAL EFFECTS ON SLEEP-ASSOCIATED MEMORY CONSOLIDATION

Apart from the differential distribution of SWS and REM sleep, early and late nocturnal sleep are also characterized by strikingly differing patterns of neuroendocrine activity. As mentioned previously, SWS-rich early nocturnal sleep supports the inhibition of HPA activity and, in conjunction with circadian oscillators, helps establish minimum cortisol concentrations during this time (see **Fig. 1**). Concurrently, somatotropic hormonal activity and the release of GH reach a maximum. This pattern is reversed during REM-rich sleep. To what extent does activity of these neuroendocrine axes contribute to the differential pattern of memory consolidation during early and late sleep? This question is tempting, particularly with respect to the consolidation of declarative and emotional memories, as these memory systems strongly rely on hippocampal and amygdalar function (two regions well known to express at high density receptors for a great variety of hormones, including cortisol and GH).[62–65] In an ongoing series of experiments in humans the authors have been aiming to characterize the role of neuroendocrine regulation for sleep-associated memory consolidation.

In an initial study targeting the HPA system, cortisol plasma concentrations were raised selectively during a 3-hour period of early SWS-rich retention sleep by intravenously infusing this hormone while subjects slept (**Fig. 4**).[66] Before retention sleep (ie, 10:15–11 PM), subjects learned to a criterion a declarative word-pair associate learning task and a procedural mirror-tracing task. Postlearning infusion of cortisol, in one of the experimental nights, and of placebo in a control night, started at 11:00 PM when

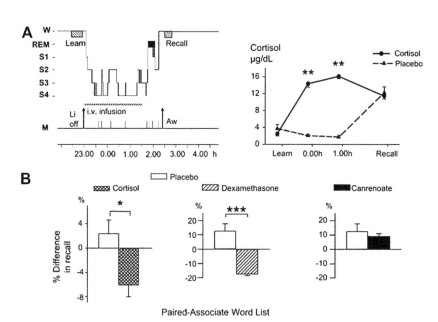

Fig. 4. (A) Left: Experimental design for studying the influence of cortisol on memory consolidation during early nocturnal sleep, illustrated by an individual sleep profile. Before sleep, subjects learned to a criterion memory tasks. Lights were turned off at 11 PM to enable a 3-hour period of SWS-rich early sleep. Recall was tested 15 to 30 minutes after awakening. Infusion of cortisol (versus placebo) started at 11 PM and was discontinued after 2.5 hours. Right: Mean (±SEM) plasma cortisol concentrations during the placebo (*dashed line*) and cortisol conditions (*solid line*). Note, plasma cortisol concentrations in the cortisol condition were enhanced only during the period of retention sleep, but were the same as in the placebo condition at recall testing. (B) Effects of administration of cortisol, dexamethasone, and canrenoate (versus placebo) on retention of declarative memories for word pairs during a period of early SWS-rich sleep. Mean (±SEM) retention is expressed by the number of recalled word pairs at retrieval testing after sleep, with performance at the criterion trial during learning before sleep set to 100%. $P<.01$, $P<.001$. (*Data from* Plihal W, Born J. Memory consolidation in human sleep depends on inhibition of glucocorticoid release. Neuroreport 1999;10(13):2741–7; and Plihal W, Pietrowsky R, Born J. Dexamethasone blocks sleep induced improvement of declarative memory. Psychoneuroendocrinology 1999;24(3): 313–31.)

lights were turned off to enable the 3-hour period of sleep, which was followed by retrieval testing 15 minutes later. The dose of cortisol was low, starting at a rate of 16 mg/h during the first 15 minutes and of 4 mg/h during the remaining time, which induced cortisol concentrations in plasma of about 16 μg/dL during retention sleep, that is, a level comparable with that observed naturally during the early morning hours or during mild stress (see **Fig. 4**). Infusions were discontinued after 2.5 hours, so that plasma cortisol concentrations differed between the placebo and cortisol conditions only during the period of retention sleep, but were practically identical during learning before sleep and retrieval testing after sleep.

The main outcome of this study was that cortisol distinctly impaired the consolidation of declarative memories for the word pairs. Learning performance before sleep was closely comparable between the placebo and cortisol condition. However, striking differences developed at retrieval testing after sleep. After infusion of placebo, the subjects' recall of the word pairs was improved on average by + 2.4% ± 2.2% (with reference to performance at learning), whereas following infusion of cortisol, subjects had forgotten a significant number of word pairs learned before sleep, with this impairment averaging − 6.1% ± 1.8% (P<.01). Although improving across sleep, retrieval of mirror-tracing skills (speed and error rate during tracing figures trained before sleep) was not influenced by cortisol, indicating that the hormone selectively impaired hippocampus-dependent declarative memory function, leaving procedural memory unaffected. The absence of changes in SWS during cortisol infusion provides further but indirect evidence for an action of cortisol on hippocampal function, as this region does not participate in the generation of SWS.

Recent studies have indicated an impairing effect of glucocorticoids specifically on retrieval.[67,68] However, this effect cannot satisfactorily explain the impaired recall of word-pairs after cortisol infusion during sleep, because cortisol infusion in this sleep study was stopped almost 1 hour before retrieval testing and plasma cortisol concentrations measured at retrieval, like those at learning before sleep, were practically identical for the placebo and cortisol conditions. A delayed action of cortisol on retrieval operations is also unlikely in light of the rapid temporal dynamics of the effects on retrieval in previous studies, suggesting a nongenomic mediation of the effect.[69]

MINERALOCORTICOID RECEPTORS VERSUS GLUCOCORTICOID RECEPTORS

Cortisol acts on the brain via 2 different receptors: high-affinity mineralocorticoid receptors (MR) and low-affinity glucocorticoid receptors (GR).[62] Because of the distinctly higher affinity, 70% to 90% of MR are continuously occupied even at nadir cortisol concentrations during early nocturnal sleep. Whereas GR are widely expressed throughout the brain, expression of MR is particularly high in limbic regions, including the hippocampus and the amygdala. Findings conclude that the impairing effect of cortisol on declarative memory consolidation is mediated via predominant activation of GR.

Plihal and colleagues[70] compared effects of dexamethasone (DEX; 2 mg) and placebo on memory consolidation during sleep. DEX is a synthetic glucocorticoid preferentially binding GR. Because of its slow pharmacodynamics, DEX was administered orally 7 hours before periods of retention sleep that covered 3-hour periods of SWS-rich early, 3-hour periods of REM-rich late nocturnal sleep, and corresponding periods of wakefulness. The memory tasks were the same as in the study by Plihal and Born,[66] testing effects of cortisol (ie, word-pair associate learning and mirror tracing). Like cortisol, DEX did not affect the time in SWS during early retention sleep, but distinctly impaired retention of word pairs (see **Fig. 4**). During late retention sleep, DEX reduced the amount of REM sleep but did not affect consolidation of word-pair memories. Further, DEX did not affect memory for mirror-tracing skill during early or late retention sleep, although late REM-rich sleep was, as expected, associated with a superior gain of mirror-tracing skill. Because DEX did not change learning of word pairs before retention sleep, a confounding influence on encoding of memories can be excluded. Also, a primary impairing effect of DEX on retrieval processes could be ruled out in this study, because in this case the impairing effect of DEX on declarative word recall would be expected to occur independently of the timing of retention sleep; however, DEX impaired recall of word pairs selectively after early but not late retention sleep. Brain uptake of DEX might be slower than of cortisol,[71] but its half-life (in blood) is distinctly longer. Hence, administering DEX several hours before testing in these experiments probably allowed accumulation of substantial amounts of substance in the brain. In combination, these data support the notion that enhanced glucocorticoid activity during early sleep impairs the consolidation of newly acquired hippocampus-dependent memories via prevailing activation of brain GR.

In addition to GR, MR also contribute to hippocampal memory consolidation during sleep, as indicated by a recent study[72] investigating effects of metyrapone, a blocker of cortisol synthesis. Metyrapone was given in the evening after subjects had learned texts that were either neutral or emotionally aversive. Compared with the effects of placebo, metyrapone distinctly reduced cortisol levels already during early SWS-rich sleep to values less than half of those during the placebo condition (**Fig. 5**). The suppression persisted throughout the night but had vanished at retrieval testing at 11:00 AM. Notably, in conjunction with distinctly reduced SWS during early sleep, metyrapone impaired retention of the neutral texts, representing a purely hippocampus-dependent memory. REM sleep during the late night remained unchanged, but emotional memory formation, as reflected by the superior recall of the aversive compared with the neutral texts, was supported by metyrapone.

The combined suppression of SWS and consolidation of neutral texts likely reflect insufficient MR activation following metyrapone.[73] As mentioned, during early nocturnal sleep cortisol concentrations reach a minimum, which is associated with preferential binding of high-affinity MR (70%–90%), whereas occupation of low-affinity GR is marginal. Hence, a further, greater than 50% reduction of cortisol concentrations during this time, as observed after metyrapone, primarily reduces MR rather than GR occupation. An involvement of GR is unlikely also because reduced GR activation would be expected to improve rather than impair memory consolidation (as discussed earlier). The view of MR hypoactivation decreasing memory consolidation is also consistent with several studies reporting an impairing effect of metyrapone on declarative memory function in humans during wakefulness.[74,75]

The conclusion of reduced MR occupation after metyrapone to impair declarative memory consolidation during sleep stands in contrast with findings from experiments investigating the effect of canrenoate, which failed to impair sleep-associated declarative memory consolidation.[66] However, selectively blocking MR by administration of the MR antagonist canrenoate (with unchanged cortisol release) shifts the balance between MR and GR activation toward absolute dominance of GR activity, which is a highly artificial condition. Thus, in conjunction with the absolute occupation of MR, the ratio between MR and GR coexpressed in the same hippocampal neurons might be effective in regulating declarative memory consolidation.[76]

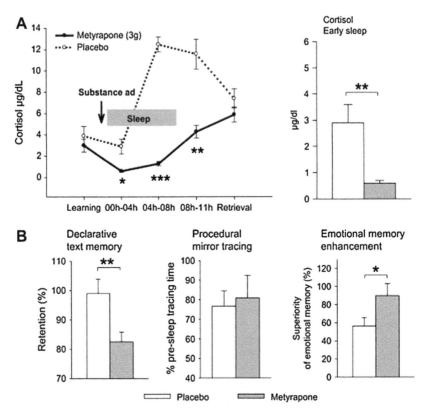

Fig. 5. (A) Left: Mean (±SEM) plasma cortisol concentrations following oral administration of the cortisol synthesis inhibitor metyrapone (3 g, *solid line*) and placebo (*dotted line*) before an 8-hour period of nocturnal retention sleep (*shaded area*). Memory tasks (mirror tracing, neutral and emotional texts) were learned before sleep. Retrieval was tested at 11 AM the next day. Right: Average plasma cortisol concentrations during the early 3-hour period of sleep following metyrapone and placebo. (B) Metyrapone impaired retention of declarative memories for neutral texts (*left*), did not alter consolidation of procedural memories for mirror-tracing skill assessed by speed of tracing (*middle*), and increased emotional memory formation as determined by the percent enhancement in recall of aversive in comparison with neutral texts (*right*) (n = 14), P<.05, P<.01. (*Data from* Wagner U, Degirmenci M, Drosopoulos S, et al. Effects of cortisol suppression on sleep-associated consolidation of neutral and emotional memory. Biol Psychiatry 2005;58:885–93.)

THE LATE SLEEP INCREASE IN CORTISOL

Aside from nadir cortisol concentrations during early sleep, the role of the increase in cortisol during late sleep for memory consolidation has been investigated. Late sleep dominated by REM sleep supports consolidation particularly of emotional and procedural memories. Increasing activation of GR during a period of late REM-rich sleep by administration of DEX did not affect consolidation of procedural mirror-tracing skill, although DEX reduced significantly the time in REM sleep.[70] This negative finding is in line with several other reports suggesting that procedural memory function relying on corticostriatal circuitry is generally less sensitive to effects of corticosteroids.[77]

However, there is evidence that the increase in cortisol concentration during late sleep affects processing of emotional memories depending on amygdalar function (see **Fig. 5**).[72] In this study, mentioned earlier, administration of metyrapone diminished the naturally enhanced cortisol concentrations during late sleep to levels comparable with those normally observed during early sleep. Metyrapone augmented the "emotional enhancement," as determined after sleep by the relative increase in memory for aversive texts in comparison with the memory for neutral texts, both acquired before sleep. Apparently, the late-night increase in cortisol does not facilitate but rather dampens amygdala-dependent emotional processing during REM sleep, thereby possibly preventing overconsolidation of emotional memories. This effect is mediated via GR, as the late-night increase in cortisol activates preferentially this type of corticosteroid receptors.[62] Moreover, the effect of cortisol suppression is presumably directly on limbic processing of emotional representations with only an indirect influence on brain stem centers generating REM sleep, because REM sleep per se remained unchanged by metyrapone.

These findings of a facilitating role of low cortisol levels for amygdala-dependent emotional memory consolidation seem to be at variance with findings in humans and animals indicating a supportive effect of glucocorticoids on emotional memory.[75,78–80] However, none of these studies referred to memory consolidation during sleep, which as an offline mode of processing characterized by downregulated sensory inputs, relies on mechanisms basically different from those serving memory function during wakefulness.[3,7]

SOMATOTROPIC ACTIVITY

First attempts have been made to unravel contributions of the SWS-associated surge in somatotropic activity to memory consolidation. Gais and colleagues[81] blocked GH secretion by intravenously infusing somatostatin in healthy young subjects during the first 3 hours of sleep containing mainly SWS. Declarative and procedural memory consolidation was tested across this period, using a word-pair learning task and a mirror-tracing task, respectively. Although GH was effectively suppressed, memory performance and sleep remained unaffected by GH suppression.

This result was unexpected in light of diverse evidence, indicating that GH does improve memory function; GH enhances memory performance in GH-deficient and elderly patients[82] and was found in rats to prevent the loss of neurons in the hippocampus,[83] to modulate N-methyl-D-aspartate (NMDA) receptor transcription[84] and to enhance long-term memory for one-trial avoidance conditioning.[85] One explanation for GH suppression to remain ineffective is that the function of GH is related to memory function in general and to the maintenance of memory systems, rather than to the acute processing of specific memory contents during sleep.

Alternatively, effects on memory may derive from brain-borne but not from circulating GH. GH is synthesized in the hippocampus, although it is unknown if hippocampal GH is regulated by sleep.[86] Gais and colleagues[81] used somatostatin to suppress peripheral GH. Because somatostatin does not pass the blood-brain barrier and, hence, is not centrally active,[87] the findings do not rule out contributions to declarative memory consolidation of hippocampal sources of GH or of its releasing hormone, GHRH. Also, effects of GHRH and GH on hippocampal memory processing might develop slowly and only some time after somatotropic activity has ceased during sleep. Retrieval testing shortly after the 3-hour period of early retention sleep in those experiments might have been too early to reveal any impairing effects of GH suppression.

Whereas some knowledge has been accumulated about possible effects of circulating hormones like GH and cortisol on sleep-associated memory consolidation, it is unclear to what extent such effects involve hypothalamic releasing and inhibiting factors of the somatotropic and HPA systems, respectively, which reach brain regions relevant to memory processing via collateral pathways. There are also numerous other hormones, including prolactin and adrenal release of catecholamines, that are regulated by sleep and likely involved in memory consolidation during sleep. Norepinephrine is one candidate whose regulation could critically affect hippocampal and amygdalar memory processing during sleep.[88] During SWS, activity of norepinephrine is between the levels observed during wakefulness and REM sleep, in which catecholamine release reaches a minimum.[89] Phasic increases in norepinephrine activity during SWS may represent conditions favorable for synaptic plastic processes presumed to underlie the formation of long-term memories in neocortical networks.[90] Effects of such signals on memory consolidation during sleep might be entirely different from those observed on awake memory function.[91] Investigations of hormonal effects on memory consolidation during sleep are scarce, despite sleep being an ideal brain state for studying the consolidation process.

A MODEL OF HORMONAL INFLUENCES ON MEMORY CONSOLIDATION DURING SLEEP

As mentioned earlier, the central hypothesis in this field of research is that memory consolidation during sleep relies on covert reactivation of the neuronal networks that were used for encoding the information during prior wakefulness.[7,28,51,92] Signs of reactivation after declarative learning were identified mainly during SWS in hippocampal circuitry but also in neocortex. A causative role of reactivation during SWS for consolidation of hippocampus-dependent memories has been recently demonstrated by Rasch and colleagues,[93] who cued memories by presentation of odor during sleep.

Based on the evidence for reactivations as a basic mechanism of memory consolidation during sleep, the consolidation of hippocampus-dependent memories has been conceptualized in the framework of a dialog between neocortex and hippocampus, which also allows for integrating hormonal effects (**Fig. 6**).[7,35,51,94] According to this model, at learning (during wakefulness) information to be stored is encoded into neocortical and hippocampal networks with the hippocampus serving as an intermediate buffer that quickly encodes the information but holds it only temporarily. During subsequent periods of SWS the newly encoded representations are repeatedly reactivated in the hippocampus, which stimulates a transfer of the information from hippocampal to neocortical networks where the information is stored for the long term. Hippocampal memory reactivation is driven by the (<1 Hz) slow oscillations that dominate SWS and exert in parallel a grouping influence on thalamo-cortical spindle activity (10–15 Hz), which presumably facilitates neuronal plastic processes within neocortical networks by stimulating calcium-dependent intracellular mechanisms.[95] Thereby, slow oscillations enable that feedback inputs from these structures (ie, thalamo-cortical spindle activity and hippocampo-cortical memory transfer) arrive at the same time within neocortical networks, with the co-occurrence of these inputs eventually facilitating the formation of long-term memories within neocortical networks.

Hormones exert an impact mainly on the hippocampus to modulate declarative memory consolidation, which expresses at high density a great variety of receptors for the major hormones that are regulated by sleep, including those of the HPA and the somatotropic systems. Cortisol affects hippocampal reactivation and hippocampo-neocortical memory transfer by fine-tuning local neuronal excitability and synaptic

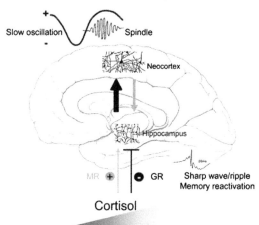

Model of Declarative Memory Consolidation

Fig. 6. Model of hippocampus-dependent declarative memory consolidation during sleep. During wakefulness information is encoded into neocortical networks and parts of it in hippocampal networks (*gray arrow*). During SWS, newly encoded information in the hippocampus is repeatedly reactivated. Reactivations are accompanied by hippocampal sharp wave-ripple activity. They are driven by slow oscillations that originate in neocortical networks (preferentially in those that were used for encoding) and synchronize hippocampal memory reactivation with the occurrence of spindle activity in thalamo-cortical circuitry. Hippocampal reactivation stimulates a transfer of the newly encoded information back to neocortical networks (*thick black arrow*). The hippocampal input arriving in synchrony with spindle input at neocortical circuitry can induce long-term plastic changes selectively at those synapses previously used for encoding, thereby forming a long-term memory of the information in neocortical networks. High concentrations of cortisol inhibit hippocampal memory reactivation and transfer to neocortex via activation of GR. Likewise, memory reactivation and transfer is suppressed in the hippocampus with insufficient occupation of MR.

potentiation via activation of MR and GR.[76] GR activation was found to inhibit glucose transport into hippocampal neurons and glia cells, to suppress hippocampal glutamatergic neurotransmission and excitatory output from CA1 neurons of the hippocampus.[62,96,97] Predominant activation of GR suppressed long-term potentiation (LTP) and primed burst potentiation in hippocampal cells, but stimulated long-term synaptic depression and depotentiation.[98–100] Blockade of GR prolonged maintenance of LTP in hippocampal dentate gyrus.[101,102] The available data indicate that enhanced GR activation globally suppresses excitatory neurotransmission and the induction and maintenance of LTP within hippocampal circuitry (ie, conditions that likely counteract effective reactivation and transfer of memories to neocortical regions during sleep). In contrast, activation of MR has been found to change membrane properties of pyramidal CA1 neurons toward enhanced excitability[103] and to prolong hippocampal LTP.[101] Blockade of MR suppressed the ability to induce LTP in dentate gyrus.[98,102] These data suggest that sufficient activation of high-affinity MR in hippocampal circuitry is a prerequisite for proper reactivation and transfer of memory during SWS.

It is not clear whether similar mechanisms hold for the glucocorticoid-induced suppression of emotional memory consolidation during REM-rich sleep. There is evidence from human imaging studies of increased amygdalar activation during

REM sleep[104] consistent with reactivation of emotional memories during sleep. Sleep-dependent consolidation of emotional memories seems to be associated with a transfer and shift of representations toward increased involvement of prefrontal cortex and hippocampus, but reduced amygdalar involvement.[47] Cortisol might suppress the putative processes of memory reactivation and transfer occurring in the amygdala during REM sleep in the same way as hippocampal memory processing during SWS, although the underlying effects of corticosteroids on neuronal excitability in the amygdala are still obscure.[105] Alternatively, the corticosteroid effect on emotional memory consolidation might be secondary to an influence on hippocampal networks interacting with amygdalar networks during memory reactivation.[31,106,107] According to this view, like activation during wakefulness, reactivation of the basolateral amygdala during REM sleep following an emotional experience feed into hippocampal networks to enhance respective memory representations. This emotional enhancement of hippocampal memories is counteracted by GR activation because of elevated levels of cortisol during REM sleep. As hippocampal portions of the representation per se are enhanced during SWS (at nadir cortisol concentration), the modulation of cortisol during SWS-rich early and REM-rich sleep would contribute to preferential strengthening of declarative aspects of the memory but reducing its affective valence.

The authors propose that neuroendocrine regulation influences memory consolidation during sleep primarily by an action on memory reactivation occurring in the hippocampus and amygdala during SWS and REM sleep, respectively. This view has been substantiated with respect to HPA activity, but needs further validation and has to be extended to other hormones that are tightly regulated by sleep.

REFERENCES

1. Born J, Fehm HL. Hypothalamus-pituitary-adrenal activity during human sleep: a coordinating role for the limbic hippocampal system. Exp Clin Endocrinol Diabetes 1998;106(3):153–63.
2. Maquet P. The role of sleep in learning and memory. Science 2001;294:1048–52.
3. Stickgold R. Sleep-dependent memory consolidation. Nature 2005;437:1272–8.
4. Cirelli C. A molecular window on sleep: changes in gene expression between sleep and wakefulness. Neuroscientist 2005;11(1):63–74.
5. Tononi G, Cirelli C. Sleep function and synaptic homeostasis. Sleep Med Rev 2006;10(1):49–62.
6. Frank MG, Benington JH. The role of sleep in memory consolidation and brain plasticity: dream or reality? Neuroscientist 2006;12(6):477–88.
7. Born J, Rasch B, Gais S. Sleep to remember. Neuroscientist 2006;12(5):410–24.
8. Lange T, Perras B, Fehm HL, et al. Sleep enhances the human antibody response to hepatitis A vaccination. Psychosom Med 2003;65(5):831–5.
9. Lange T, Dimitrov S, Fehm HL, et al. Shift of monocyte function toward cellular immunity during sleep. Arch Intern Med 2006;166(16):1695–700.
10. Dimitrov S, Lange T, Nohroudi K, et al. Number and function of circulating human antigen presenting cells regulated by sleep. Sleep 2007;30(4):401–11.
11. Goichot B, Weibel L, Chapotot F, et al. Effect of the shift of the sleep-wake cycle on three robust endocrine markers of the circadian clock. Am J Phys 1998;275(2 Pt 1):E243–8.
12. Dodt C, Breckling U, Derad I, et al. Plasma epinephrine and norepinephrine concentrations of healthy humans associated with nighttime sleep and morning arousal. Hypertension 1997;30(1 Pt 1):71–6.

13. Steiger A. Sleep and the hypothalamo-pituitary-adrenocortical system. Sleep Med Rev 2002;6(2):125–38.
14. Born J, Kern W, Bieber K, et al. Night-time plasma cortisol secretion is associated with specific sleep stages. Biol Psychiatry 1986;21(14):1415–24.
15. Follenius M, Brandenberger G, Simon C, et al. REM sleep in humans begins during decreased secretory activity of the anterior pituitary. Sleep 1988;11(6): 546–55.
16. Lechin F, Pardey-Maldonado B, van der DB, et al. Circulating neurotransmitters during the different wake-sleep stages in normal subjects. Psychoneuroendocrinology 2004;29(5):669–85.
17. Benhaberou-Brun D, Lambert C, Dumont M. Association between melatonin secretion and daytime sleep complaints in night nurses. Sleep 1999;22(7): 877–85.
18. Bierwolf C, Struve K, Marshall L, et al. Slow wave sleep drives inhibition of pituitary-adrenal secretion in humans. J Neuroendocrinol 1997;9(6):479–84.
19. Späth-Schwalbe E, Uthgenannt D, Voget G, et al. Corticotropin-releasing hormone-induced adrenocorticotropin and cortisol secretion depends on sleep and wakefulness. J Clin Endocrinol Metab 1993;77:1170–3.
20. Späth-Schwalbe E, Uthgenannt D, Korting N, et al. Sleep and wakefulness affect the responsiveness of the pituitary-adrenocortical axis to arginine vasopressin in humans. Neuroendocrinology 1994;60(5):544–8.
21. Späth-Schwalbe E, Gofferje M, Kern W, et al. Sleep disruption alters nocturnal ACTH and cortisol secretory patterns. Biol Psychiatry 1991;29(6): 575–84.
22. Born J, Hansen K, Marshall L, et al. Timing the end of nocturnal sleep. Nature 1999;397(6714):29–30.
23. Wilhelm I, Born J, Kudielka BM, et al. Is the cortisol awakening rise a response to awakening? Psychoneuroendocrinology 2007;32(4):358–66.
24. Born J, Muth S, Fehm HL. The significance of sleep onset and slow wave sleep for nocturnal release of growth hormone (GH) and cortisol. Psychoneuroendocrinology 1988;13(3):233–43.
25. Pietrowsky R, Meyrer R, Kern W, et al. Effects of diurnal sleep on secretion of cortisol, luteinizing hormone, and growth hormone in man. J Clin Endocrinol Metab 1994;78(3):683–7.
26. Spiegel K, Luthringer R, Follenius M, et al. Temporal relationship between prolactin secretion and slow-wave electroencephalic activity during sleep. Sleep 1995;18(7):543–8.
27. Squire LR. Memory and the hippocampus: a synthesis from findings with rats, monkeys, and humans. Psychol Rev 1992;99(2):195–231.
28. Sutherland GR, McNaughton B. Memory trace reactivation in hippocampal and neocortical neuronal ensembles. Curr Opin Neurobiol 2000;10(2):180–6.
29. Le Doux JE. Emotion circuits in the brain. Annu Rev Neurosci 2000;23:155–84.
30. McGaugh JL. The amygdala modulates the consolidation of memories of emotionally arousing experiences. Annu Rev Neurosci 2004;27:1–28.
31. Phelps EA. Human emotion and memory: interactions of the amygdala and hippocampal complex. Curr Opin Neurobiol 2004;14(2):198–202.
32. Dolcos F, LaBar KS, Cabeza R. Interaction between the amygdala and the medial temporal lobe memory system predicts better memory for emotional events. Neuron 2004;42(5):855–63.
33. Doyon J, Benali H. Reorganization and plasticity in the adult brain during learning of motor skills. Curr Opin Neurobiol 2005;15(2):161–7.

34. Walker MP, Brakefield T, Hobson JA, et al. Dissociable stages of human memory consolidation and reconsolidation. Nature 2003;425(6958):616–20.
35. Gais S, Born J. Declarative memory consolidation: mechanisms acting during human sleep. Learn Mem 2004;11(6):679–85.
36. Plihal W, Born J. Effects of early and late nocturnal sleep on declarative and procedural memory. J Cogn Neurosci 1997;9:534–47.
37. Drosopoulos S, Wagner U, Born J. Sleep enhances explicit recollection in recognition memory. Learn Mem 2005;12(1):44–51.
38. Fischer S, Drosopoulos S, Tsen J, et al. Implicit learning—explicit knowing: a role for sleep in memory system interaction. J Cogn Neurosci 2006;18:311–9.
39. Gais S, Lucas B, Born J. Sleep after learning aids memory recall. Learn Mem 2006;13(3):259–62.
40. Ellenbogen JM, Hulbert JC, Stickgold R, et al. Interfering with theories of sleep and memory: sleep, declarative memory, and associative interference. Curr Biol 2006;16(13):1290–4.
41. Wagner U, Gais S, Born J. Emotional memory formation is enhanced across sleep intervals with high amounts of rapid eye movement sleep. Learn Mem 2001;8(2):112–9.
42. Hu P, Stylos-Allan M, Walker MP. Sleep facilitates consolidation of emotional declarative memory. Psychol Sci 2006;17(10):891–8.
43. Gais S, Plihal W, Wagner U, et al. Early sleep triggers memory for early visual discrimination skills. Nat Neurosci 2000;3(12):1335–9.
44. Fischer S, Hallschmid M, Elsner AL, et al. Sleep forms memory for finger skills. Proc Natl Acad Sci U S A 2002;99(18):11987–91.
45. Wagner U, Gais S, Haider H, et al. Sleep inspires insight. Nature 2004; 427(6972):352–5.
46. Orban P, Rauchs G, Balteau E, et al. Sleep after spatial learning promotes covert reorganization of brain activity. Proc Natl Acad Sci U S A 2006;103:7124–9.
47. Sterpenich V, Albouy G, Boly M, et al. Sleep-related hippocampo-cortical interplay during emotional memory recollection. PLoS Biol 2007;5(11):e282.
48. Fischer S, Nitschke MF, Melchert UH, et al. Motor memory consolidation in sleep shapes more effective neuronal representations. J Neurosci 2005;25(49): 11248–55.
49. Fowler MJ, Sullivan MJ, Ekstrand BR. Sleep and memory. Science 1973;179(70): 302–4.
50. Ekstrand BR, Barrett TR, West JN, et al. The effect of sleep on human long-term memory. In: Drucker-Colin RR, McGaugh JL, editors. Neurobiology of sleep and memory. New York: Academic Press; 1977. p. 419–38.
51. Buzsáki G. Memory consolidation during sleep: a neurophysiological perspective. J Sleep Res 1998;7(Suppl 1):17–23.
52. Wilson MA, McNaughton BL. Reactivation of hippocampal ensemble memories during sleep. Science 1994;265(5172):676–9.
53. Peigneux P, Laureys S, Fuchs S, et al. Learned material content and acquisition level modulate cerebral reactivation during posttraining rapid-eye-movements sleep. Neuroimage 2003;20(1):125–34.
54. Peigneux P, Laureys S, Fuchs S, et al. Are spatial memories strengthened in the human hippocampus during slow wave sleep? Neuron 2004;44(3):535–45.
55. Maquet P, Laureys S, Peigneux P, et al. Experience-dependent changes in cerebral activation during human REM sleep. Nat Neurosci 2000;3(8):831–6.
56. Marshall L, Helgadottir H, Molle M, et al. Boosting slow oscillations during sleep potentiates memory. Nature 2006;444(7119):610–3.

57. Rauchs G, Bertran F, Guillery-Girard B, et al. Consolidation of strictly episodic memories mainly requires rapid eye movement sleep. Sleep 2004;27(3): 395–401.
58. Poldrack RA, Rodriguez P. Sequence learning: what's the hippocampus to do? Neuron 2003;37(6):891–3.
59. Poldrack RA, Rodriguez P. How do memory systems interact? Evidence from human classification learning. Neurobiol Learn Mem 2004;82(3):324–32.
60. Giuditta A, Ambrosini MV, Montagnese P, et al. The sequential hypothesis of the function of sleep. Behav Brain Res 1995;69(1–2):157–66.
61. Stickgold R, Whidbee D, Schirmer B, et al. Visual discrimination task improvement: a multi-step process occurring during sleep. J Cogn Neurosci 2000; 12(2):246–54.
62. De Kloet ER, Vreugdenhil E, Oitzl MS, et al. Brain corticosteroid receptor balance in health and disease. Endocr Rev 1998;19(3):269–301.
63. Joels M, De Kloet ER. Mineralocorticoid and glucocorticoid receptors in the brain. Implications for ion permeability and transmitter systems. Prog Neurobiol 1994;43(1):1–36.
64. Nyberg F. Growth hormone in the brain: characteristics of specific brain targets for the hormone and their functional significance. Front Neuroendocrinol 2000; 21:330–48.
65. Schneider HJ, Pagotto U, Stalla GK. Central effects of the somatotropic system. Eur J Endocrinol 2003;149(5):377–92.
66. Plihal W, Born J. Memory consolidation in human sleep depends on inhibition of glucocorticoid release. Neuroreport 1999;10(13):2741–7.
67. DeQuervain DJ, Roozendaal B, McGaugh JL. Stress and glucocorticoids impair retrieval of long-term spatial memory. Nature 1998;394(6695): 787–90.
68. DeQuervain DJ, Roozendaal B, Nitsch RM, et al. Acute cortisone administration impairs retrieval of long-term declarative memory in humans. Nat Neurosci 2000; 3(4):313–4.
69. De Kloet ER, Reul JM. Feedback action and tonic influence of corticosteroids on brain function: a concept arising from the heterogeneity of brain receptor systems. Psychoneuroendocrinology 1987;12(2):83–105.
70. Plihal W, Pietrowsky R, Born J. Dexamethasone blocks sleep induced improvement of declarative memory. Psychoneuroendocrinology 1999;24(3):313–31.
71. Meijer OC, Karssen AM, De Kloet ER. Cell- and tissue-specific effects of corticosteroids in relation to glucocorticoid resistance: examples from the brain. J Endocrinol 2003;178(1):13–8.
72. Wagner U, Degirmenci M, Drosopoulos S, et al. Effects of cortisol suppression on sleep-associated consolidation of neutral and emotional memory. Biol Psychiatry 2005;58:885–93.
73. Neylan TC, Lenoci M, Maglione ML, et al. Delta sleep response to metyrapone in post-traumatic stress disorder. Neuropsychopharmacology 2003;28:1666–76.
74. Lupien SJ, Wilkinson CW, Briere S, et al. The modulatory effects of corticosteroids on cognition: studies in young human populations. Psychoneuroendocrinology 2002;27(3):401–16.
75. Maheu FS, Joober R, Beaulieu S, et al. Differential effects of adrenergic and corticosteroid hormonal systems on human short- and long-term declarative memory for emotionally arousing material. Behav Neurosci 2004;118(2):420–8.
76. Joels M, Hesen W, De Kloet ER. Long-term control of neuronal excitability by corticosteroid hormones. J Steroid Biochem Mol Biol 1995;53(1–6):315–23.

77. Kirschbaum C, Wolf OT, May M, et al. Stress- and treatment-induced elevations of cortisol levels associated with impaired declarative memory in healthy adults. Life Sci 1996;58(17):1475–83.

78. Abercrombie HC, Kalin NH, Thurow ME, et al. Cortisol variation in humans affects memory for emotionally laden and neutral information. Behav Neurosci 2003;117(3):505–16.

79. Buchanan TW, Lovallo WR. Enhanced memory for emotional material following stress-level cortisol treatment in humans. Psychoneuroendocrinology 2001;26: 307–17.

80. Roozendaal B. 1999 Curt P. Richter award. Glucocorticoids and the regulation of memory consolidation. Psychoneuroendocrinology 2000;25(3):213–38.

81. Gais S, Hüllemann P, Hallschmid M, et al. Sleep-dependent surges in growth hormone do not contribute to sleep-dependent memory consolidation. Psychoneuroendocrinology 2006;31(6):786–91.

82. van Dam PS, Aleman A, de Vries WR, et al. Growth hormone, insulin-like growth factor I and cognitive function in adults. Growth Horm IGF Res 2000;10(Suppl B):S69–73.

83. Azcoitia I, Perez-Martin M, Salazar V, et al. Growth hormone prevents neuronal loss in the aged rat hippocampus. Neurobiol Aging 2005;26(5):697–703.

84. LeGreves M, Steensland P, LeGreves P, et al. Growth hormone induces age-dependent alteration in the expression of hippocampal growth hormone receptor and N-methyl-D-aspartate receptor subunits gene transcripts in male rats. Proc Natl Acad Sci U S A 2002;99(10):7119–23.

85. Schneider-Rivas S, Rivas-Arancibia S, Vazquez-Pereyra F, et al. Modulation of long-term memory and extinction responses induced by growth hormone (GH) and growth hormone releasing hormone (GHRH) in rats. Life Sci 1995;56(22): L433–41.

86. Donahue CP, Kosik KS, Shors TJ. Growth hormone is produced within the hippocampus where it responds to age, sex, and stress. Proc Natl Acad Sci U S A 2006;103(15):6031–6.

87. Meisenberg G, Simmons WH. Minireview. Peptides and the blood-brain barrier. Life Sci 1983;32(23):2611–23.

88. McGaugh JL, Roozendaal B. Role of adrenal stress hormones in forming lasting memories in the brain. Curr Opin Neurobiol 2002;12(2):205–10.

89. Hobson JA, Pace-Schott EF. The cognitive neuroscience of sleep: neuronal systems, consciousness and learning. Nat Rev Neurosci 2002;3(9):679–93.

90. Cirelli C, Tononi G. Differential expression of plasticity-related genes in waking and sleep and their regulation by the noradrenergic system. J Neurosci 2000; 20:9187–94.

91. Rasch BH, Born J, Gais S. Combined blockade of cholinergic receptors shifts the brain from stimulus encoding to memory consolidation. J Cogn Neurosci 2006;18:793–802.

92. Ji D, Wilson MA. Coordinated memory replay in the visual cortex and hippocampus during sleep. Nat Neurosci 2007;10(1):100–7.

93. Rasch B, Büchel C, Gais S, et al. Odor cues during slow-wave sleep prompt declarative memory consolidation. Science 2007;315(5817):1426–9.

94. Buzsáki G. The hippocampo-neocortical dialogue. Cereb Cortex 1996;6(2): 81–92.

95. Sejnowski TJ, Destexhe A. Why do we sleep? Brain Res 2000;886(1–2):208–23.

96. De Kloet ER, Joels M, Holsboer F. Stress and the brain: from adaptation to disease. Nat Rev Neurosci 2005;6(6):463–75.

97. Horner HC, Packan DR, Sapolsky RM. Glucocorticoids inhibit glucose transport in cultured hippocampal neurons and glia. Neuroendocrinology 1990;52(1): 57–64.

98. Pavlides C, Ogawa S, Kimura A, et al. Role of adrenal steroid mineralocorticoid and glucocorticoid receptors in long-term potentiation in the CA1 field of hippocampal slices. Brain Res 1996;738(2):229–35.

99. Pavlides C, McEwen BS. Effects of mineralocorticoid and glucocorticoid receptors on long-term potentiation in the CA3 hippocampal field. Brain Res 1999; 851:204–14.

100. Alfarez DN, Wiegert O, Joels M, et al. Corticosterone and stress reduce synaptic potentiation in mouse hippocampal slices with mild stimulation. Neuroscience 2002;115:1119–26.

101. Korz V, Frey JU. Stress-related modulation of hippocampal long-term potentiation in rats: involvement of adrenal steroid receptors. J Neurosci 2003;23(19): 7281–7.

102. Avital A, Segal M, Richter-Levin G. Contrasting roles of corticosteroid receptors in hippocampal plasticity. J Neurosci 2006;26:9130–4.

103. Joels M, De Kloet ER. Control of neuronal excitability by corticosteroid hormones. Trends Neurosci 1992;15(1):25–30.

104. Maquet P. Functional neuroimaging of normal human sleep by positron emission tomography. J Sleep Res 2000;9(3):207–31.

105. Kavushansky A, Richter-Levin G. Effects of stress and corticosterone on activity and plasticity in the amygdala. J Neurosci Res 2006;84(7):1580–7.

106. Akirav I, Richter-Levin G. Mechanisms of amygdala modulation of hippocampal plasticity. J Neurosci 2002;22(22):9912–21.

107. Paz R, Pelletier JG, Bauer EP, et al. Emotional enhancement of memory via amygdala-driven facilitation of rhinal interactions. Nat Neurosci 2006;9:1321–9.

Insomnia Treatment Options for Women

Judith R. Davidson, PhD[a,b,c,]*

KEYWORDS

- Insomnia • Insomnia treatment • Sleep • Women
- Cognitive–behavioral therapy

Recognition of the special circumstances in which women develop insomnia is important for understanding, supporting, and treating women when they seek help for sleep difficulty. Insomnia, by definition, is difficulty falling asleep or staying asleep, waking up too early, or nonrestorative sleep, with associated fatigue, distress, or impairment in functioning.[1–3] Insomnia may be situational, intermittent, or persistent. It also can be a symptom of, or be concurrent with, another sleep disorder, a medical condition, a psychiatric disorder, emotional distress, or substance use. It is especially important to treat persistent insomnia, because it tends not to resolve on its own and it degrades quality of life.[4,5] Persistent insomnia increases the risk of subsequent psychiatric conditions, especially depression.[6–9] It also predicts a rise in health care use, including number of physician visits.[10–12] Fortunately, several effective pharmacologic and non-pharmacologic interventions are available for improving sleep in the short term and for reversing persistent insomnia.

Any given case of insomnia is likely to involve a diathesis for sleep difficulty combined with circumstances or events that trigger a bout of poor sleep, followed by phenomena that maintain the poor sleep. The factors associated with these phases in the development of insomnia have been termed, respectively, predisposing, precipitating, and perpetuating factors.[13]

PREDISPOSING FACTORS

Women are 1.4 to 2.0 times more likely to report insomnia than are men.[14–18] Depending on how insomnia is defined in a survey, the prevalence in women can range from 2% (stringently defined disorder of initiating or maintaining sleep)[19]

This is an updated version of the article "Insomnia: Therapeutic Options for Women," which appeared in *Sleep Medicine Clinics* (Volume 3, Issue 1, March 2008).

[a] Department of Psychology, Queen's University, 62 Arch Street, Kingston, ON, Canada K7L 3N6

[b] Department of Oncology, Queen's University, Kingston, ON, Canada K7L 3N6

[c] Kingston Family Health Team, 797 Princess Street, Suite 206, Kingston, ON, Canada K7L 1G1

* Department of Psychology, Queen's University, 62 Arch Street, Kingston, ON, Canada K7L 3N6.

E-mail address: davidsnj@queensu.ca

Obstet Gynecol Clin N Am 36 (2009) 831–846

doi:10.1016/j.ogc.2009.10.004

0889-8545/09/$ – see front matter © 2009 Elsevier Inc. All rights reserved.

obgyn.theclinics.com

to 61% (report of regular insomnia or trouble sleeping during the past 12 months).[14] In a telephone survey with detailed questions to establish an insomnia designation consistent with psychiatric (*Diagnostic and Statistical Manual of Mental Disorders, 4th Edition* [DSM-IV])[2] and World Health Organization (*International Classification of Diseases and Related Health Problems, 10th Revision* [ICD-10])[3] criteria—including sleep difficulty at least 3 nights per week for a minimum of 1 month with associated impairment or distress—the estimated prevalence of insomnia syndrome in Quebec women was 11%.[18] Many more women than this are dissatisfied with their sleep, but their symptoms do not meet clinical definitions of insomnia.[18,20] The higher rates in women as compared with men may be related to greater symptom awareness in women, socialization that encourages women more than men to acknowledge and report distress, biologic differences (eg, reproductive hormones, pregnancy, menstruation, menopause), possible greater involvement in nighttime child care and elder care, and the greater prevalence of anxiety and depression in women.[21,22]

A family history of insomnia appears to increase the likelihood of developing insomnia, especially if one's mother had insomnia.[23] The extent to which this represents genetic predisposition or the environment in which one grows up is unknown. The prevalence of insomnia increases with age, and, in women, there appears to be a steep rise at midlife.[20,24] Being prone to cognitive and emotional hyperarousal[25] and overactivation of the hypothalamic-pituitary-adrenal axis[26] are believed to increase vulnerability to insomnia.

PRECIPITATING FACTORS

Commonly reported precipitants of insomnia include stressful life events, such as death of a loved one or other personal loss; illness; work or school stress; family concerns; and interpersonal conflict.[24,27,28] It appears that arousal and distress, rather than the stressful events themselves, are associated with insomnia.[29,30] Japanese women reported that aging, living with a child under age 6, undergoing medical treatment, experiencing major life events, following irregular bedtimes, having sleep apnea-type symptoms, and living near heavy traffic were associated with insomnia.[31] Pregnancy, childbirth, and caring for an infant are times when a woman's sleep is bound to be disturbed. Women who develop chronic insomnia sometimes identify childbirth as the initial precipitant of their poor sleep. At insomnia clinics, mothers of infants frequently describe the reciprocal influence of infant and maternal sleep–wake patterns. Surprisingly, however, there is little research on the interaction of child and parent sleep. Meijer and van der Wittenboer[32] found that a mother's insomnia was worse than the father's before childbirth, and it remained worse over the first year. A mother is often nocturnally vigilant for her baby's crying and responsive to nighttime feeding needs. The sleep quality of young children influences the mother's sleep and daytime functioning. Meltzer and Mindell[33] found, for example, that the quality of children's sleep predicted the quality of maternal sleep, and that poor sleep in the child and mother was associated with maternal stress, mood disturbance, and fatigue. When children reach adolescence, parents may stay awake until their son or daughter returns home late at night. During perimenopause and menopause, women's sleep may be disrupted by nocturnal hot flashes.[34,35] During the menopausal transition, and at midlife in general, psychological distress is associated with sleep difficulty.[30,36] A high proportion of postmenopausal women have some level of sleep-disordered breathing.[37] Snoring bed partners are another potential precipitant of sleep difficulty. Caring for aging parents or an aging spouse, or caring for anyone with a disordered sleep schedule (eg, a person with Alzheimer's disease) will disrupt the caregiver's sleep. One's own illness or pain syndrome can precipitate a bout of poor sleep.

PERPETUATING FACTORS

Insomnia can be maintained by various physiologic, behavioral, emotional, and cognitive factors. Sometimes a precipitant of poor sleep, such as pain or ongoing worries about life circumstances, will persist, leading to chronic insomnia. In addition to ongoing precipitants, however, several perpetuating factors tend to develop over time, often independent of the initial precipitant. Typical perpetuating factors are: maladaptive sleep–wake habits, especially sleep scheduling; learned associations of the bed with sleeplessness; and dysfunctional cognitions that prevent sufficient presleep reduction in arousal.

Maladaptive sleep–wake habits include a tendency to go to bed early or to stay in bed later in the morning in an attempt to make up for poor sleep. This strategy tends to backfire, leading to increased sleep disruption and more nights of poor sleep. Similarly, sleep tends to remain poor for those who have inconsistent sleep times and wake times (for example, those who rise at different times each day or those who nap at various times during the day). In these cases, the homeostatic and circadian processes that regulate sleep[38] are being reset constantly. This ongoing desynchronization between sleep need (homeostatic) and the time of day (circadian) prevents sleep from improving.

Learned associations of the bed with sleeplessness develop when a person stays in bed when she is not sleeping. After several nights of not sleeping well in one's bed, there is an association of the bed and bedroom with being awake, and sometimes with frustration and dread. In classical conditioning terms, the bed and the bedroom are stimuli that elicit a conditioned arousal response that is incompatible with sleep. In such cases, the person sometimes discovers that she can fall asleep on the sofa, in another bed, or when away from home. Thus, the difficulty with sleeping in her own bed and bedroom persists. This phenomenon, although commonly accepted, has been the subject of very little research. A recent study found supportive but nonspecific evidence for insomnia-associated classical conditioning.[39]

Dysfunctional cognitions that perpetuate poor sleep tend to be troubling thoughts about the feared consequences of not sleeping. Some typical worries are

Here I go again! why can't I sleep? There must be something wrong with me.
I won't be able to function tomorrow.
I'll get sick. I am making myself prone to cancer.

Naturally, these troubling thoughts are associated with cognitive and emotional arousal, preventing the reduction in arousal that allows sleep to come.

THERAPEUTIC OPTIONS

Women make up most participants in insomnia trials[40,41] and are more likely than men to be using prescribed hypnotics.[42] Subsequently, much of the outcome data for insomnia treatments of all kinds are based on the experiences of women. Various pharmacologic and nonpharmacologic interventions have been shown to be efficacious for improving sleep.[43] The choice of intervention is influenced by many factors, including the nature of the insomnia, especially whether it is acute or chronic; age; the presence of medical or psychiatric comorbidity; condition of pregnancy or nursing;

concurrent medications and substances; availability of treatments; time; cost; and personal preference.

PHARMACOTHERAPY

Pharmacotherapy is a treatment option for acute, situational insomnia. The most commonly prescribed hypnotic medications are the broad class of benzodiazepine receptor agonists. These agents bind to the benzodiazepine site of the γ-aminobutyric acid A (GABA$_A$) receptor complex. In doing so, they enhance GABA-induced neuronal inhibition. The benzodiazepine receptor agonists include the traditional benzodiazepines (eg, flurazepam, estazolam, temazepam, and triazolam) and the newer nonbenzodiazepine agents (eg, zolpidem, zaleplon, zopiclone, and eszopiclone), hereafter referred to as the nonbenzodiazepines. Nonbenzodiazepines may bind selectively to the α1 subunit of the GABA$_A$ receptor complex[44] or have a totally separate binding site on the benzodiazepine receptor complex.[45] Whereas the traditional benzodiazepines have sedative and hypnotic properties, the nonbenzodiazepines have more specific hypnotic properties.

Benzodiazepines

The benzodiazepines are effective at increasing sleep duration and in reducing patient-reported time to sleep onset.[46] They also have some less desirable effects, however, including

Altered sleep stage composition (usually an increase in stages 1 and 2 and a reduction in slow wave sleep)
Tolerance after 1 to 3 weeks
Potential for dependence
Rebound insomnia after discontinuation
Next-day hangover
Effects on vigilance, concentration, and memory
Respiratory depression[47]

The benzodiazepines, especially alprazolam, should be avoided during pregnancy and nursing because of risks to the fetus, including congenital defects.[48] Temazepam is contraindicated in pregnancy according to the US Food and Drug Administration (FDA).[49] Benzodiazepines and the nonbenzodiazepines should be used with caution by women 60 years old or older. Although the benzodiazepine receptor agonists improve sleep in this age group, they are associated with dangerous cognitive and psychomotor adverse effects, including memory problems, confusion, disorientation, dizziness, loss of balance, and falls.[50]

Nonbenzodiazepines

Zolpidem and zaleplon show efficacy for reducing sleep latency. Zopiclone and eszopiclone (an isomer of racemic zopiclone) show efficacy for reducing sleep latency, number of awakenings, and wake time after sleep onset, and for increasing sleep duration and depth of sleep.[45,51,52] Dorsey and colleagues[53] found zolpidem to be useful for treating perimenopausal insomnia. Tolerance and rebound insomnia are unlikely with the nonbenzodiazepines.[45,52,54–56] Potential adverse effects of zolpidem include headache, dizziness, drowsiness, and nausea.[52] Zopiclone and eszopiclone have a bitter taste,[54,57] and patients taking eszopiclone are more likely than placebo-taking patients to experience somnolence and myalgia.[58] The literature is mixed about whether the nonbenzodiazepines are safer than benzodiazepines for older patients.[40,50]

Caution should be exercised in taking nonbenzodiazepines during pregnancy and nursing.[45,47] In the labeling of drugs for use in pregnancy, the FDA gives better ratings to zolpidem and zaleplon than to the benzodiazepines. Also, Diav-Citrin and colleagues[59] found that zopiclone taken during the first trimester was not associated with an increase in the rate of malformations. Because the safety information is very limited, however, current recommendations for the use of nonbenzodiazepines during pregnancy and nursing are that they be used only if the potential benefits to the mother justify the potential risks to the fetus.[45]

Melatonin

Although there are very few studies, the available research indicates that exogenous melatonin is not useful for insomnia. It appears to help sleep only for naps or sleep that is taken at times other than during the usual nocturnal sleep period, such as during the daytime or in the period just before normal bedtime called the "wake maintenance zone."[60,61] Melatonin can be useful for preventing eastbound jet lag and for night-shift work,[62,63] but only if taken at a very specific time with respect to the circadian rhythm of sleep–wakefulness. It should be used with caution unless the timing of administration with respect to circadian phase is planned carefully.

Ramelteon

Ramelteon is a melatonin receptor agonist that reduces sleep latency and sometimes increases sleep duration. It generally is tolerated well by patients, including those aged 65 and older.[64] Patients do not show signs of cognitive impairment, rebound insomnia, or withdrawal effects.[64,65] Potential adverse effects include headache, dizziness, somnolence, fatigue, and nausea. Patients with severe hepatic impairment should avoid ramelteon.[66] In pregnancy, it should be used only if the benefits clearly outweigh the risks to the fetus.[67]

Sedating Antidepressants

There have been few trials of sedating antidepressants in people with insomnia who are not depressed.[68] Walsh and colleagues[69] found trazodone to be somewhat useful, but less so than zolpidem, for treating primary insomnia, as measured by patient self-report. There has been a surge of prescription of trazodone as a hypnotic.[70] Although this antidepressant increases sleep duration in people with major depressive disorder, there appears to be no efficacy or tolerance data for trazodone as a hypnotic in nondepressed individuals.[71] Potential adverse effects include dizziness, arrhythmias, sedation, and psychomotor impairment.[68] Concern about safety, especially in elderly patients, is higher with trazodone than with the conventional hypnotics.[71] In sum, the scant literature supports the use of trazodone for insomnia only in patients with depressive tendencies.[72,73]

Antihistamines as Hypnotics

Most over-the-counter sleep remedies contain the antihistamine diphenhydramine. These remedies can cause daytime sleepiness, but there is little evidence that they are useful for people with chronic insomnia.[44] Placebo-controlled trials of diphenhydramine have shown some efficacy for self-reported or physician-reported measures of insomnia symptoms in the short term (1 to 2 weeks).[74–76] With polysomnographic measures, Morin and colleagues[76] found that diphenhydramine improved sleep efficiency over placebo in patients with mild insomnia during the first 2 weeks of treatment. Diphenhydramine can cause some psychomotor performance deficits and daytime sedation, both of which diminish after 3 to 4 days.[44,77] The hypnotic effects also recede, although the time course is unclear.[77,78] Diphenhydramine may offer help for those with mild insomnia, but its effects seem to be short-lived. Although not marketed for sleep, some patients take dimenhydrinate (Gravol) which contains diphenhydramine and 8-chlorotheophylline, a stimulant. The efficacy of this compound for insomnia is not well studied, and its chronic use for sleep has raised some safety concerns.[79,80]

Herbal Therapies

Fifteen percent of a Canadian community sample reported the use of herbal or dietary products for insomnia within the previous year.[18] Data from the US National Health Interview indicated that 82% of people with sleep trouble who had tried herbal therapies found them to be helpful.[14] Various herbal preparations are purported to help with sleep, including valerian root, lavender, hops, kava kava, and chamomile.[81,82] The efficacy of these therapies has been difficult to evaluate because of their unstandardized formulation and the paucity of sound clinical research.[81,82] A recent review of valerian as a sleep aid concluded that there is, as yet, no evidence of clinical efficacy.[83] Currently, there is insufficient or absent evidence of efficacy for most herbal products for insomnia.[82] Although some herbal therapies appear to be generally well tolerated (eg, valerian),[83] others are associated with adverse effects (eg, risk of hepatotoxicity with kava kava).[82]

NONPHARMACOLOGIC INTERVENTIONS

Insomnia-specific cognitive and behavioral treatments are the interventions of choice for insomnia that lasts for 1 month or longer. These treatments are not only efficacious, they are also safer than medication. They are associated with a higher degree of acceptance and satisfaction by patients as compared with hypnotic medication.[84,85]

The efficacy of these insomnia-specific therapies is believed to be due specifically to their ability to alter the main factors that perpetuate poor sleep. Perpetuating factors, as described previously, include maladaptive sleep–wake habits, especially sleep scheduling; learned associations of the bed with sleeplessness; and dysfunctional cognitions that prevent sufficient presleep reduction in arousal.

Interventions are designed to adjust sleep–wake scheduling to achieve rapid sleep onset and uninterrupted sleep, or to maximize the association of bedtime with reduced arousal and increased sleep tendency. Some of the interventions improve the conditions for the homeostatic and circadian processes that regulate sleep propensity. In doing so, they increase the likelihood of sleep and wakefulness occurring at desired hours. Insomnia-specific therapies generally fall into five categories: stimulus control therapy, sleep restriction, relaxation training, cognitive therapy, and sleep hygiene education.

Stimulus Control Therapy

As previously described, people with insomnia often come to associate their bed and bedroom with sleeplessness rather than with sleep. Stimulus control therapy[86] is a brief set of instructions for going to and getting up from bed, designed to maximize the association of the bed with sleepiness and sleep. It also emphasizes a consistent rise time, which helps support the circadian component of the rhythm of sleep tendency. The standard stimulus control instructions are

- Go to bed only when sleepy.
- Use the bed only for sleeping. Sexual activity is the only exception.

- Leave the bed and the bedroom if sleep does not come within 15 to 20 minutes. Return when sleepy. Repeat this step as often as necessary during the night.
- Maintain a regular rising time in the morning.
- Do not nap, or limit naps to the midafternoon.[a]

Sleep Restriction Therapy

Sleep restriction therapy[89] is the prescription of a specific amount of time in bed that is as close as possible to the actual sleep time. This procedure is designed to curtail the time in bed that is spent awake. Restriction of sleep builds up the homeostatic component of the sleep drive, and is therefore conducive to a rapid sleep onset and reduced time awake during the night. With this technique, time in bed is gradually increased as sleep becomes more consolidated. Sleep diaries are used to guide the prescription of time in bed. The steps for sleep restriction are

- Calculate mean daily subjective total sleep time from sleep diaries kept for at least 1 week.
- Prescribe time in bed as the mean total sleep time or 5 hours, whichever is greater.
- The patient chooses a rise time that is sustainable.
- Work backward (rise time minus time in bed) to establish the bedtime.
- For 1 week, the patient goes to bed no earlier than the prescribed bedtime and rises no later than the prescribed rise time. This interval is the sleep window.
- At the end of the week, adjust the sleep window based on that week's mean sleep efficiency (time asleep divided by time in bed times 100%) as follows: (1) If sleep efficiency is 90% or more, then increase time in bed by 15 minutes; (2) if sleep efficiency is between 85% and 90%, then keep time in bed constant; (3) if sleep efficiency is less than 85%, then decrease time in bed by 15 minutes. Adjustments to the window usually are made by altering the bedtime rather than the rise time.
- Make weekly adjustments until optimal sleep efficiency and duration are reached with minimal daytime sleepiness.

Relaxation-based Interventions

Relaxation techniques for insomnia include various approaches to release somatic and mental tension, thereby reducing physiologic, cognitive, and emotional arousal that interferes with sleep onset. Several relaxation techniques have been shown to be effective in treating insomnia. These include progressive muscle relaxation, imagery, meditation, and autogenic training.[90] Relaxing music has shown some potential for assisting sleep in older adults,[91,92] but more research is required.

Cognitive Therapy

The goal of cognitive therapy in the context of insomnia is to identify and alter maladaptive thinking patterns associated with arousal and the maintenance of sleep difficulty. For example, patients sometimes believe that they must get 8 hours of sleep per night, or that, if they do not sleep well, they will be unable to function the next day. Such thoughts lead to increased worry and arousal, thereby perpetuating the sleep disturbance. The Dysfunctional Beliefs and Attitudes Scale[93] is useful to help patients identify

---

[a] This is a variation of the original instruction to avoid napping altogether. An afternoon nap, no longer than 1 hour, starting before 3 PM, can be taken if sleepiness is overwhelming. A brief midafternoon nap is unlikely to interfere with nighttime sleep.[87,88]

their own particular sleep-related worries. The aim of insomnia-specific cognitive therapy is for the patient to replace the maladaptive sleep-related cognitions with ones that are realistic but less worrisome and arousing. This decatastrophization works well with empathy and education about the particular sleep-related fears. For example, it may be helpful to discuss interindividual variation in sleep need or changes in sleep with aging. Patients whose fears arise from an expectation of their inability to function after a sleepless night often benefit from knowing that fatigue, mood effects, and increased perceived exertion may occur, but that objective measures of performance generally show only subtle deficits with sleep loss.[94] Paradoxical intention can be useful for some people who try too hard to fall asleep, believing that they "must sleep." This technique involves instructing the patient to try to stay awake, rather than try to sleep, thereby reducing performance anxiety.

Sleep Hygiene Education

Sleep hygiene education involves provision of information about sleeping conditions and lifestyle habits that promote sleep or minimize sleep interference. A typical set of sleep hygiene recommendations follows:

- Avoid stimulants, including caffeine and nicotine, several hours before bed. Caffeine and nicotine can impede sleep onset and reduce sleep quality.
- Do not drink alcohol 4 to 6 hours before bedtime. Alcohol can lead to fragmented sleep and early morning awakenings.
- Avoid heavy meals within 2 hours of bedtime. These can interfere with sleep. A light snack, however, may be sleep-inducing.
- Regular exercise in the late afternoon or early evening may deepen sleep. However, exercise too close to bedtime may have a stimulating effect and may delay sleep onset.
- Keep the bedroom environment quiet, dark, and comfortable.

Treatment Format

Insomnia-specific cognitive and behavioral interventions can be offered as part of individual therapy or group programs. In individual therapy, interventions are tailored to the set of factors believed to perpetuate that person's insomnia based on the assessment. The various interventions are compatible and can be easily introduced sequentially. The patient continues to track progress with the use of sleep diaries. Typically, group programs involve a combination of sleep hygiene education, stimulus control therapy and/or sleep restriction, relaxation techniques, and cognitive therapy. There may be four to seven patients and one or two therapists per group. Group programs have the advantages of lower costs in therapist time and the mutual support provided by group members.

Evidence Base for Nonpharmacologic Interventions

The benefits of insomnia-specific cognitive and behavioral treatments for insomnia are well established from research with people who have primary insomnia, who are from the community at large, who are predominantly women (approximately 60%) with mean age in the early 40s, and who are healthy, nonusers of hypnotics, with mean insomnia duration of 11 years.[41,95] There is sound empiric support for the efficacy of stimulus control therapy, relaxation training, paradoxic intention, sleep restriction, biofeedback, and multicomponent cognitive–behavioral therapy for treating insomnia.[90,96] Sleep hygiene education, on its own, appears to have limited therapeutic value for people with insomnia.[96–98] The relation between sleep hygiene practices by midlife women and sleep variables is low,[99] suggesting that good sleep hygiene plays a fairly small role in predicting the quality of sleep.

On average, with insomnia-specific cognitive and behavioral interventions, patients with chronic insomnia see a reduction of about 30 minutes in sleep latency or 30 minutes in time awake after sleep onset.[41] Sleep duration is increased, on average, by approximately 30 minutes. Patients' ratings of sleep quality and satisfaction with sleep are enhanced significantly. Improvements in sleep are well maintained and sometimes further improved at follow-up 6 to 8 months after treatment. There is evidence of maintenance of gains even at 24 months[85] after treatment. The limited data on the effect of these interventions on daytime functioning suggest that depressive and anxiety symptoms are reduced,[100] but more research is required on other aspects of functioning, including fatigue, cognitive performance, and quality of life. Patients who participate in group programs achieve results broadly comparable to those of patients who participate in individual sleep therapy.[101] Self-help programs are associated with significant but modest improvements in sleep.[102,103]

There is abundant evidence that older adults benefit from insomnia-specific cognitive and behavioral techniques.[96,104] Patients who use hypnotic medications also see improvements to their sleep with the use of these techniques.[90,96] It is becoming clear that these interventions are helpful for patients whose insomnia is associated with medical or psychiatric illness.[96,105] In the past, insomnia in patients with comorbid conditions was often called "secondary" insomnia, and clinicians sometimes hesitated to treat it, focusing instead on the underlying problem. The temporal and causal relations between illness and insomnia are usually quite difficult to discern, however, and there is a move to favor the term "comorbid" insomnia for insomnia with another condition.[106] For medical conditions, the efficacy of insomnia-specific cognitive and behavioral treatments has been demonstrated for people with chronic pain[107] and for people with cancer.[108] For psychiatric conditions, the scant literature suggests that patients with depressive disorders can benefit from insomnia-specific cognitive and behavioral interventions for insomnia,[109,110] both in terms of sleep improvement and mood improvement. Patients with subclinical anxiety or depressive symptoms also appear to benefit.[100] Therefore, for several medical and mental health problems, there seems little reason to delay insomnia treatment if the patient wishes to improve sleep. Patients with bipolar disorder or seizures, however, should avoid sleep restriction because of the possibility of triggering mania or a seizure.[105]

CHOICE OF TREATMENT

Insomnia-specific pharmacologic and psychological interventions are both efficacious.[43] The timing of their benefits differs, however. Whereas medications (benzodiazepine receptor agonists) work immediately to improve sleep, and are useful in the short-to-medium term (generally 1 day to 4 weeks, although some newer agents have potential for use over longer periods), the cognitive and behavioral approaches are useful in the medium-to-long term (1 to 2 weeks to at least 2 years). Nonpharmacologic interventions are not without adverse effects. Patients using sleep restriction or stimulus control therapy may experience daytime sleepiness in the first few days or weeks of treatment. They should be warned about the dangers of driving or operating dangerous equipment while sleepy. The nonpharmacologic interventions are initially more time-consuming and expensive than hypnotic medication (because of clinician's time), but they have longer-term benefits. Unfortunately, few clinicians have training in the nonpharmacologic treatments, so the availability of these interventions is limited in many communities.

CLINICAL CONSIDERATIONS

For patients with severe depression, anxiety disorders, or substance abuse problems, the need to receive treatment for those disorders is a priority. Sleep disorders other than insomnia—such as sleep apnea, hypopneas, restless legs syndrome and periodic limb movement disorder—should be screened for and treated if present. Circadian rhythm disorders need to be kept in mind. For example, occasionally a complaint of chronic sleep initiation problems arises from delayed sleep phase syndrome. When sleep is disturbed by nocturnal hot flashes, treatment directed at the hot flashes themselves can be considered.[111,112] If the disturbance persists, cognitive and behavioral techniques aimed at reducing the duration of awakenings may be helpful. Insomnia often occurs with medical conditions,[113] and, if the direct cause of the problem is treatable (eg, hyperthyroidism, acute pain due to injury), then medical treatment is the first course of action. Of course, sleep difficulty associated with stimulants (eg, amphetamines and caffeine) or medications (eg, certain antihypertensives, levothyroxine) needs to be ruled out.

When the patient works on rotating shifts, designing an insomnia treatment protocol can be especially challenging because of the instability of the circadian rhythm of sleep and wakefulness. Also, for individuals who are using such techniques as stimulus control therapy and sleep restriction, vacations and travel to other time zones can complicate and prolong the treatment process. For users of hypnotics, decisions need to be made about whether, when, and how to withdraw from the medication. If the decision is to withdraw, it is preferable to do so in parallel with insomnia-specific cognitive and behavioral treatment. The withdrawal program should be systematic and medically supervised. A withdrawal protocol is outlined by Morin and Espie.[93]

Useful areas of future clinical research are the prevention of insomnia; the cotreatment of mothers and young children; the treatment of insomnia with comorbid mental health issues; raising awareness of nonpharmacologic treatments; and making nonpharmacologic treatments available through the health care system.[114,115]

SUMMARY

Women are at greater risk of developing insomnia than are men, and the circumstances of pregnancy, childbirth, midlife, and menopause are key times of sleep disturbance. These are opportunities to prevent sleep disruption from transforming into chronic insomnia. For immediate relief of acute insomnia, short-term use of nonbenzodiazepine hypnotics can be helpful. To restore and maintain healthy sleep patterns, several insomnia-specific cognitive and behavioral interventions are recommended. The choice of a specific treatment depends on the nature and duration of insomnia, the presence of medical or mental health problems, the stage of a woman's life, the availability of the treatments, and personal preference.

ACKNOWLEDGMENTS

The author thanks Richard J. Beninger and Brenda Bass for their helpful comments on earlier versions of this manuscript. Thanks also to Petrus de Villiers for reviewing the pharmacologic sections.

REFERENCES

1. American Sleep Disorders Association. The International classification of sleep disorders, revised: diagnostic and coding manual. Rochester (MN): American Sleep Disorders Association; 1997.

2. American Psychiatric Association. Diagnostic and statistical manual of mental disorders. 4th edition. Washington, DC: American Psychiatric Association; 1994.
3. World Health Organization. International statistical classification of diseases and related health problems, 10th revision. Geneva (Switzerland): World Health Organization; 2007.
4. Zammit GK, Weiner J, Damato N, et al. Quality of life in people with insomnia. Sleep 1999;22:S379–85.
5. Roth T, Ancoli-Israel S. Daytime consequences and correlates of insomnia in the United States: results of the 1991 National Sleep Foundation Survey II. Sleep 1999;22:S354–8.
6. Ford DE, Kamerow DB. Epidemiologic study of sleep disturbances and psychiatric disorders. JAMA 1989;262:1479–84.
7. Breslau N, Roth T, Rosenthal L, et al. Sleep disturbance and psychiatric disorders: a longitudinal epidemiological study of young adults. Biol Psychiatry 1996;39:411–8.
8. Roberts RE, Shema SJ, Kaplan G, et al. Sleep complaints and depression in an aging cohort: a prospective perspective. Am J Psychiatry 2000;157:81–8.
9. Perlis ML, Giles DE, Buysse DJ, et al. Self-reported sleep disturbance as a prodromal symptom in recurrent depression. J Affect Disord 1997;42: 209–12.
10. Simon GE, VonKorff M. Prevalence, burden, and treatment of insomnia in primary care. Am J Psychiatry 1997;154:1417–23.
11. Weissman MM, Greenwald S, Nino-Murcia G, et al. The morbidity of insomnia uncomplicated by psychiatric disorders. Gen Hosp Psychiatry 1997;19:245–50.
12. Weyerer S, Dilling H. Prevalence and treatment of insomnia in the community: results from the Upper Bavarian field study. Sleep 1991;14:392–8.
13. Spielman AJ, Glovinsky PB. Introduction: the varied nature of insomnia. In: Hauri PJ, editor. Case studies in insomnia. New York: Plenum; 1991. p. 1–15.
14. Pearson NJ, Johnson LL, Nahin RL. Insomnia, trouble sleeping, and complementary and alternative medicine. Arch Intern Med 2006;166:1775–82.
15. Leger D, Guilleminault C, Dreyfus JP, et al. Prevalence of insomnia in a survey of 12,778 adults in France. J Sleep Res 2000;9:35–42.
16. Stewart R, Besset A, Bebbington P, et al. Insomnia comorbidity and impact and hypnotic use by age group in a national survey population aged 16 to 74 years. Sleep 2006;29:1391–7.
17. Ohayon MM, Caulet M, Guilleminault C. How a general population perceives its sleep and how this relates to the complaint of insomnia. Sleep 1997;20:715–23.
18. Morin CM, Leblanc M, Daley M, et al. Epidemiology of insomnia: prevalence, self-help treatments, consultations, and determinants of help-seeking behaviors. Sleep Med 2006;7:123–30.
19. Liljenberg B, Almqvist M, Hetta J, et al. The prevalence of insomnia: the importance of operationally defined criteria. Ann Clin Res 1988;20:393–8.
20. Ohayon MM. Epidemiology of insomnia: what we know and what we still need to learn. Sleep Med Rev 2002;6:97–111.
21. Barsky AJ, Peekna HM, Borus JF. Somatic symptom reporting in women and men. J Gen Intern Med 2001;16:266–75.
22. Soares CN. Insomnia in women: an overlooked epidemic? Arch Womens Ment Health 2005;8:205–13.
23. Bastien C, Morin CM. Familial incidence of insomnia. J Sleep Res 2000;9:49–54.
24. Tjepkema M. Insomnia. catalogue 82-003. Health Reports, Statistics Canada 2005;17:9–25.

25. Espie CA. Insomnia: conceptual issues in the development, maintenance and treatment of sleep disorder in adults. Annu Rev Psychol 2002;53:1–44.

26. Vgontzas AN, Chrousos GP. Sleep, the hypothalamic-pituitary-adrenal axis, and cytokines: multiple interactions and disturbances in sleep disorders. Endocrinol Metab Clin North Am 2002;31:15–36.

27. Bastien CH, Vallieres A, Morin CM. Precipitating factors of insomnia. Behav Sleep Med 2004;2:50–62.

28. Healey ES, Kales A, Monroe LJ, et al. Onset of insomnia: role of life-stress events. Psychosom Med 1981;43(5):439–51.

29. Morin CM, Rodrigue S, Ivers H. Role of stress, arousal, and coping skills in primary insomnia. Psychosom Med 2003;65:259–67.

30. Shaver JLF, Johnston SK, Lentz MJ, et al. Stress exposure, psychological distress, and physiological stress activation in midlife women with insomnia. Psychosom Med 2002;64:793–802.

31. Kageyama T, Kabuto M, Nitta H, et al. A population study on risk factors for insomnia among adult Japanese women: a possible effect of road traffic volume. Sleep 1997;20:963–71.

32. Meijer AM, van den Wittenboer GLH. Contribution of infants- sleep and crying to marital relationship of first-time parent couples in the 1st year after childbirth. J Fam Psychol 2007;21:49–57.

33. Meltzer LJ, Mindell JA. Relationship between child sleep disturbances and maternal sleep, mood, and parenting stress: a pilot study. J Fam Psychol 2007;21:67–73.

34. Shaver JLF, Zenk SN. Sleep disturbance and menopause. J Womens Health Gend Based Med 2000;9:109–18.

35. Savard J, Davidson JR, Ivers H, et al. The association between nocturnal hot flashes and sleep in breast cancer survivors. J Pain Symptom Manage 2004; 27:513–22.

36. Kloss JD, Tweedy K, Gilrain K. Psychological factors associated with sleep disturbance among perimenopausal women. Behav Sleep Med 2004;2: 177–90.

37. Guilleminault C, Palombini L, Poyares D, et al. Chronic insomnia, postmenopausal women, and sleep-disordered breathing: part 1. Frequency of sleep-disordered breathing in a cohort. J Psychosom Res 2002;53:611–5.

38. Borbely AA. Sleep mechanisms. Sleep Biol Rhythms 2004;2:S67–8.

39. Robertson JA, Broomfield NM, Espie CA. Prospective comparison of subjective arousal during the presleep period in primary sleep-onset insomnia and normal sleepers. J Sleep Res 2007;16:230–8.

40. Dolder C, Nelson M, McKinsey J. Use of nonbenzodiazepine hypnotics in the elderly. Are all agents the same? CNS Drugs 2007;21:389–405.

41. Morin CM, Culbert JP, Schwartz SM. Nonpharmacological interventions for insomnia: a meta-analysis of treatment efficacy. Am J Psychiatry 1994;151: 1172–80.

42. Kassam A, Patten SB. Hypnotic use in a population-based sample of over thirty-five thousand interviewed Canadians. Popul Health Metr 2006;4:15–5. DOI: 10.1186/1478-7954-4-15.

43. Smith MT, Perlis ML, Park A, et al. Comparative meta-analysis of pharmacotherapy and behaviour therapy for persistent insomnia. Am J Psychiatry 2002; 159:5–11.

44. Mendelson WB, Roth T, Cassella J, et al. The treatment of chronic insomnia: drug indications, chronic use, and abuse liability. Sleep Med Rev 2004;8:7–17.

45. Najib J. Eszopiclone, a nonbenzodiazepine sedative-hypnotic agent for the treatment of transient and chronic insomnia. Clin Ther 2006;28:491–516.
46. Holbrook AM, Crowther R, Lotter A, et al. Meta-analysis of benzodiazepine use in the treatment of insomnia. Can Med Assoc J 2000;162:225–33.
47. Montplaisir J, Hawa R, Moller H, et al. Zopiclone and zaleplon vs benzodiazepines in the treatment of insomnia: Canadian consensus statement. Hum Psychopharmacol 2003;18:29–38.
48. Iqbal MM, Sobhan T, Ryals T. Effects of commonly used benzodiazepines on the fetus, the neonate, and the nursing infant. Psychiatr Serv 2002;53:39–49.
49. Santiago JR, Nolledo MS, Kinzler W, et al. Sleep and sleep disorders in pregnancy. Ann Intern Med 2001;134:396–408.
50. Glass J, Lanctot KL, Herrmann N, et al. Sedative hypnotics in older people with insomnia: meta-analysis of risks and benefits. Br Med J 2005;331:1169.
51. Benca R. Diagnosis and treatment of chronic insomnia: a review. Psychiatr Serv 2005;56:332–43.
52. Swainston Harrison T, Keating GM. Zolpidem: a review of its use in the management of insomnia. CNS Drugs 2005;19:65–89.
53. Dorsey CM, Lee KA, Scharf MB. Effect of zolpidem on sleep in women with perimenopausal and postmenopausal insomnia: a 4-week, randomized, multicenter, double-blind, placebo-controlled study. Clin Ther 2004;26:1578–86.
54. Melton ST, Wood JM, Kirkwood CK. Eszopiclone for insomnia. Ann Pharmacother 2005;39:1659–65.
55. Krystal AD, Walsh JK, Laska E, et al. Sustained efficacy of eszopiclone over 6 months of nightly treatment: results of a randomized, double-blind, placebo-controlled study in adults with chronic insomnia. Sleep 2003;26:793–9.
56. Roth T, Walsh JK, Krystal AD, et al. An evaluation of the efficacy and safety of eszopiclone over 12 months in patients with chronic primary insomnia. Sleep Med 2005;6:487–95.
57. Hajak G. A comparative assessment of the risks and benefits of zopiclone. A review of 15 years' clinical experience. Drug Saf 1999;21:457–69.
58. Walsh JK, Krystal AD, Amato DA, et al. Nightly treatment of primary insomnia with eszopiclone for six months: effect on sleep, quality of life, and work limitations. Sleep 2007;30:959–68.
59. Diav-Citrin O, Okotore B, Lucarelli K, et al. Pregnancy outcome following first-trimester exposure to zopiclone: a prospective controlled cohort study. Am J Perinatol 1999;16:157–60.
60. Wyatt JK, Dijk D-J, Ritz-de Cecco A, et al. Sleep-facilitating effect of exogenous melatonin in healthy young men and women is circadian-phase dependent. Sleep 2006;29:609–18.
61. Scheer FAJL, Czeisler CA. Melatonin, sleep, and circadian rhythms. Sleep Med Rev 2005;9:5–9.
62. Burgess HJ, Sharkey KM, Eastman CI. Bright light, dark and melatonin can promote circadian adaptation in night shift workers. Sleep Med Rev 2002;6:407–20.
63. Revell VL, Eastman CI. How to trick mother nature into letting you fly around or stay up all night. J Biol Rhythms 2005;20:353–65.
64. Roth T, Seiden D, Sainati S, et al. Effects of ramelteon on patient-reported sleep latency in older adults with chronic insomnia. Sleep Med 2006;7:312–8.
65. Erman M, Seiden D, Zammit G, et al. An efficacy, safety, and dose-response study of ramelteon in patients with chronic primary insomnia. Sleep Med 2006;7:17–24.

66. Borja NL, Daniel KL. Ramelteon for the treatment of insomnia. Clin Ther 2006;28: 1540–55.
67. Rozerem (ramelteon) prescribing information. Available at: http://hcp.rozerem. com. Accessed October 17, 2009.
68. Mendelson WB. A review of the evidence for the efficacy and safety of trazodone in insomnia. J Clin Psychiatry 2005;66:469–76.
69. Walsh JK, Erman M, Erwin CW, et al. Subjective hypnotic efficacy of trazodone and zolpidem. Hum Psychopharmacol 1998;13:191–8.
70. Walsh JK, Schweitzer PK. Ten-year trends in the pharmacological treatment of insomnia. Sleep 1999;22:371–5.
71. James SP, Mendelson WB. The use of trazodone as a hypnotic: a critical review. J Clin Psychiatry 2004;65:752–5.
72. Weigand MH. Antidepressants for the treatment of insomnia. A suitable approach? Drugs 2008;68(17):2411–7.
73. DeMartinis NA, Winokur A. Effects of psychiatric medications on sleep and sleep disorders. CNS Neurol Disord Drug Targets 2007;6:17–29.
74. Kudo Y, Kurihara M. Clinical evaluation of diphenhydramine hydrochloride for the treatment of insomnia in psychiatric patients: a double-blind study. J Clin Pharmacol 1990;30:1041–8.
75. Rickels K, Morris RJ, Newman H, et al. Diphenhydramine in insomniac family practice patients: a double-blind study. J Clin Psychiatry 1983;23:235–42.
76. Morin CM, Koetter U, Bastien C, et al. Valerian-hops combination and diphenhydramine for treating insomnia: a randomized placebo-controlled clinical trial. Sleep 2005;28:1465–71.
77. Barbier AJ, Bradbury MJ. Histaminergic control of sleep-wake cycles: Recent therapeutic advances for sleep and wake disorders. CNS Neurol Disord Drug Targets 2007;6:31–43.
78. Richardson GS, Roehrs TA, Rosenthal L, et al. Tolerance to daytime sedative effects of H1 antihistamines. J Clin Pharmacol 2002;22:511–5.
79. Sproule BA, Busto UA, Buckle C, et al. The use of nonprescription sleep products in the elderly. Int J Geriatr Psychiatry 1999;14:851–7.
80. Craig DF, Mellor CS. Dimenhydrinate dependence and withdrawal. CMAJ 1990; 142:970–3.
81. Wheatley D. Medicinal plants for insomnia: a review of their pharmacology, efficacy, and tolerability. J Psychopharmacol 2005;19:414–21.
82. Meoli AL, Rosen C, Kristo D, et al. Oral nonprescription treatment for insomnia: an evaluation of products with limited evidence. J Clin Sleep Med 2005;1:173–87.
83. Taibi DM, Landis CA, Petry H, et al. A systematic review of valerian as a sleep aid: safe but not effective. Sleep Med Rev 2007;11:209–30.
84. Morin CM, Gaulier B, Barry T, et al. Patients' acceptance of psychological and pharmacological therapies for insomnia. Sleep 1992;15:302–5.
85. Morin CM, Colecchi C, Stone J, et al. Behavioral and pharmacological therapies for late-life insomnia. A randomized controlled trial. JAMA 1999;281:991–9.
86. Bootzin RR, Epstein D, Wood JM. Stimulus control instructions. In: Hauri P, editor. Case Studies in Insomnia. New York: Plenum Press; 1991. p. 19–28.
87. Aber R, Webb WB. Effects of a limited nap on night sleep in older subjects. Psychol Aging 1986;1:300–2.
88. Aschoff J. Naps as integral parts of the wake time within the human sleep-wake cycle. J Biol Rhythms 1994;9:145–55.
89. Spielman AJ, Saskin P, Thorpy MJ. Treatment of chronic insomnia by restriction of time in bed. Sleep 1987;10(1):45–56.

90. Morin CM, Bootzin RR, Buysse DJ, et al. Psychological and behavioral treatment of insomnia: update of the recent evidence (1998–2004). Sleep 2006;29: 1398–414.
91. Lai H-L, Good M. Music improves sleep quality in older adults. J Adv Nurs 2005; 49:234–44.
92. Johnson JE. The use of music to promote sleep in older women. J Community Health Nurs 2003;20:27–35.
93. Morin CM, Espie CA. Insomnia: a clinical guide to assessment and treatment. New York: Kluwer Academic/Plenum Publishers; 2003.
94. Riedel BW, Lichstein KL. Insomnia and daytime functioning. Sleep Med Rev 2000;4:277–98.
95. Murtagh DR, Greenwood KM. Identifying effective psychological treatments for insomnia: a meta-analysis. J Consult Clin Psychol 1995;63:79–89.
96. Morgenthaler T, Kramer M, Alessi C, et al. Practice parameters for the psychological and behavioural treatment of insomnia: an update. An American Academy of Sleep Medicine report. Sleep 2006;29:1415–9.
97. Schoicket SL, Bertelson AD, Lacks P. Is sleep hygiene a sufficient treatment for sleep-maintenance insomnia? Behav Ther 1988;19:183–90.
98. Engle-Friedman M, Bootzin RR, Hazlewood L, et al. An evaluation of behavioral treatments for insomnia in the older adult. J Clin Psychol 1992;48:77–90.
99. Cheek RE, Shaver JL, Lentz MJ. Lifestyle practices and nocturnal sleep in midlife women with and without insomnia. Biol Res Nurs 2004;6:46–58.
100. Vallieres A, Bastien CH, Ouellet M, et al. Cognitive–behaviour therapy for insomnia associated with anxiety or depression [abstract]. Sleep 2000;23(Suppl 2):A311.
101. Bastien C, Morin C, Ouellet M-C, et al. Cognitive-behavioral therapy for insomnia: comparison of individual therapy, group therapy, and telephone consultations. J Consult Clin Psychol 2004;72:653–9.
102. Strom L, Pettersson R, Andersson G. Internet-based treatment for insomnia: a controlled evaluation. J Consult Clin Psychol 2004;72:113–20.
103. Morin CM, Beaulieu-Bonneau S, Leblanc M, et al. Self-help treatment for insomnia: a randomized controlled trial. Sleep 2005;28:1319–27.
104. Irwin MR, Cole JC, Nicassio PM. Comparative meta-analysis of behavioral interventions for insomnia and their efficacy in middle-aged adults and in older adults 55+ years of age. Health Psychol 2006;25:3–14.
105. Smith MT, Huang MI, Manber R. Cognitive behavior therapy for chronic insomnia occurring within the context of medical and psychiatric disorders. Clin Psychol Rev 2005;25:559–92.
106. Leshner AI, Baghdoyan HA, Bennett SJ, et al. National Institutes of Health State of the Science Conference statement; manifestations and management of chronic insomnia in adults. Sleep 2005;28:1049–57.
107. Currie SR, Wilson KG, Pontefract AJ, et al. Cognitive–behavioral treatment of insomnia secondary to chronic pain. J Consult Clin Psychol 2000;68:407–16.
108. Savard J, Simard S, Ivers H, et al. Randomized study of the efficacy of cognitive-behavioural therapy for insomnia secondary to breast cancer. Part I: sleep and psychological effects. Am J Clin Oncol 2005;23:6083–96.
109. Morawetz D. Insomnia and depression: which comes first? Sleep Res Online 2003;5:77–81.
110. Dashevsky B, Kramer M. Behavioral treatment of chronic insomnia in psychiatrically ill patients. J Clin Psychiatry 1998;59:693–9.
111. Hickey M, Davis SR, Sturdee DW. Treatment of menopausal symptoms: What shall we do now? Lancet 2005;366:409–21.

112. Polo-Kantola P. Dealing with menopausal sleep disturbances. Sleep Med Clin 2008;3:121–31.
113. Taylor DJ, Mallory LJ, Lichstein KL, et al. Comorbidity of chronic insomnia with medical problems. Sleep 2007;30:213–8.
114. Espie CA, Inglis SJ, Tessier S, et al. The clinical effectiveness of cognitive behaviour therapy for chronic insomnia: implementation and evaluation of a sleep clinic in general medical practice. Behav Res Ther 2001;39:45–60.
115. Davidson JR, Feldman-Stewart D, Brennenstuhl S, et al. How to provide insomnia interventions to people with cancer: insights from patients. Psychoon-cology 2007;16(11):1028–38.

Intimate Partner Violence

Adam J. Zolotor, MD, MPH[a,b,*], Amy C. Denham, MD, MPH[a], Amy Weil, MD[c,d]

KEYWORDS
- Intimate partner violence • Domestic violence
- Child abuse and neglect

Intimate partner violence (IPV) is a common, serious, and preventable public health problem. IPV includes psychologic, physical, or sexual harm by a current or former partner or spouse. It occurs between married and unmarried couples and between heterosexual and same-sex couples. In defining IPV, the Centers for Disease Control and Prevention (CDC) includes the following forms of violence in its definition of IPV:

Psychologic/emotional violence: This involves trauma to a victim caused by acts, threats of acts, or coercive tactics.

Psychologic/emotional abuse: This can include, but is not limited to, humiliating a victim, controlling what a victim can and cannot do, withholding information from a victim, deliberately doing something to make a victim feel diminished or embarrassed, isolating a victim from friends and family, and denying a victim access to money or other basic resources.

Physical violence: This is the intentional use of physical force with the potential for causing disability, injury, harm, or death. Physical violence includes, but is not

---

This work was support by the Sunshine Lady Foundation Child Maltreatment Doctoral Fellowship.

This is an updated version of the article "Intimate Partner Violence," which appeared in *Primary Care: Clinics in Office Practice* (Volume 36, Issue 1, March 2009).

[a] Department of Family Medicine, University of North Carolina School of Medicine, CB# 7595, Chapel Hill, NC 27599-7595, USA

[b] Injury Prevention Research Center, CB# 7505, University of North Carolina, Chapel Hill, NC, USA

[c] Department of Medicine, Division of General Medicine and Epidemiology, University of North Carolina School of Medicine, 5039 Old Clinic Building, CB# 7110, Chapel Hill, NC 27599-7110, USA

[d] Beacon Child and Family Program, CB# 7600, University of North Carolina School of Medicine, Chapel Hill, NC 7595-7600, USA

* Corresponding author. Department of Family Medicine, University of North Carolina School of Medicine, CB#7595, Chapel Hill, NC 27599-7595.

E-mail address: ajzolo@med.unc.edu (A.J. Zolotor).

limited to, scratching, pushing, shoving, throwing, grabbing, biting, strangulating, shaking, slapping, punching, burning, using a weapon, and using restraints or one's body, size, or strength against another person.

Sexual violence: This is divided into three categories: (1) use of physical force to compel a person to engage in a sexual act against his or her will whether or not the act is completed; (2) attempted or completed sex act involving a person unable to understand the nature or condition of the act, to decline participation, or to communicate unwillingness to engage in the sexual act (eg, because of illness, disability, or the influence of alcohol or other drugs, or because of intimidation or pressure); and (3) abusive sexual contact.[1]

EPIDEMIOLOGY

IPV is pervasive. Population-based estimates demonstrate that 32 million Americans have been affected by IPV.[2] The prevalence and incidence of IPV can be measured on a continuum from rare events, such as death, to more common events, such as self-reported pushing, slapping, and intimidation. It also is useful to consider how this pervasive phenomenon affects clinical practice.

The ecologic model of IPV considers IPV a result of a complex set of circumstances from risk factors that occur at the level of the victim, the perpetrator, their relationship, the family, the community, and society. Risk factors at the level of individual victims include female gender, young age, history of IPV, history of sexual assault, history of child abuse victimization, heavy alcohol or drug use, unemployment, depression, and racial or ethnic minority status.[2–4] Relationship level risk factors include income or educational disparity and male control of relationship (eg, psychologic or economic).[5] Community level risk factors include poverty, poor social cohesion, and weak sanctions, including minimal legal penalties or rare successful prosecutions.[6] Societal level risk factors include traditional gender norms and general acceptance of violence for conflict resolution.

Anonymous telephone surveys afford the best estimate of incident and prevalent IPV. The most comprehensive national assessment of IPV from a national telephone survey is from the Behavioral Risk Factor Surveillance System 2005 IPV module. This survey of more than 70,000 United States adults demonstrated that one in four women and one in seven men report a lifetime threatened or completed physical or sexual IPV. In the same survey, 1.4% of women and 0.7% of men reported such victimization within the past year. When IPV is defined more broadly to include a variety of physical and psychologic acts of violence, estimates for any IPV are as high as one in five men and women.[7] Telephone surveys, however, may underestimate the true extent of IPV because of recall bias and social desirability bias, and the estimates for IPV may vary because of survey instruments, operational definitions, and arbitrary cut points.

The National Crime Victimization Survey estimates that 467,000 people are victims of criminal IPV each year. The survey includes only IPV reported to law enforcement authorities and, therefore, most likely grossly underestimates IPV. More than 80% of IPV incidents reported to law enforcement involve female victims.[8] Death by IPV is a rare but tragic event. Using data from the National Violent Death Reporting System in 16 states, the CDC estimated that 1200 IPV homicides occurred in 2005. The rate of IPV homicide is 0.8 per 100,000 persons. The rate is higher among African Americans (1.5 per 100,000 persons) and American Indians (2 per 100,000 persons) than among Caucasians (0.6 per 100,000 persons). The majority of IPV victims are women, estimated at 65%.[9] Victims are at a higher risk for mortality if a perpetrator has access to a gun, has previously threatened the victim with a weapon, or uses illicit drugs. If perpetrator and victim have recently separated or if a victim has asked the perpetrator to leave the mutual dwelling, then the victim also is at higher risk for mortality.[10] Clinicians should be alert to these high-risk situations in counseling individuals affected by IPV.

Clinicians may see high number of patients who have a history of current or former IPV in medical offices. A recent large study of women enrolled in health maintenance organizations found that 44% had a history of IPV.[11] One study of women in pediatric clinics found that 14% of mothers screened positive for at least one of three questions related to severe IPV. Using a longer standard instrument, however, 76% of mothers reported a history of being a victim of psychologic aggression, 32% reported physical assault, 9% reported resultant injury, and 29% reported sexual coercion within the past year.[12] These data suggest that obstetrics and gynecology physicians should consider patients presenting in an ambulatory care practice setting as having very high risk for current or past IPV.

HEALTH EFFECTS OF INTIMATE PARTNER VIOLENCE

IPV has a significant effect on victims' health, influencing many aspects of physical and mental health. Individuals affected by IPV consistently are more likely than individuals not affected by IPV to report poor health,[13–15] a measure that correlates with long-term morbidity and mortality. Physical and mental health effects of IPV persist for many years beyond the period of abuse,[5,14] and a longer duration of abuse is associated with worse health outcomes.[16] Physical, sexual, and psychologic/emotional IPV all have adverse health effects.[14–16] The physical and mental health consequences of IPV occur in male and female victims, but women are more likely to report negative physical and mental health effects.[15]

Physical Health

Injuries
Injury is a direct health effect of IPV. Approximately 2 million injuries in women are attributable to IPV each year.[17] Approximately 42% of women who experience IPV report that they suffered an injury during their most recent victimization, although less than one third of these injuries are brought to the attention of health care providers. Women are more likely than men to be injured when victimized by an intimate partner, and they tend to have a greater severity of injury. Minor injuries, such as scratches and bruises, are most common, but more serious injuries, such as lacerations, broken bones, sprains, strains, and head injuries, also occur in a significant proportion of victims of IPV.[2]

There is no pathognomonic pattern of injury that suggests IPV; however, certain patterns of injury are suggestive and should raise clinicians' suspicion of intentional injury. Central injuries, such as injuries to the head, neck, breast, or abdomen, are more likely the result of IPV.[18] Trauma to the face, orbital fractures, and dental injuries are especially common.[18,19] Musculoskeletal injuries to the extremities, including fractures, sprains, or dislocations, account for more than one quarter of injuries attributable to IPV.[19] Clinicians should maintain an index of suspicion for IPV when patients present with these types of injuries.

In addition to the acute effects of injury, survivors of IPV also suffer long-term sequelae of inflicted injury. For example, women who have had repeated head trauma may have long-term symptoms of traumatic brain injury. Victims who have sustained injuries from strangulation may have problems with swallowing or speech.[20]

Other physical health effects

Individuals exposed to IPV experience increased risk for several acute and chronic health conditions not directly attributable to trauma, such as sexually transmitted infections,[20,21] cervical dysplasia,[20] unplanned pregnancy,[21] arthritis,[17] migraine,[22] asthma,[17,22] stroke, high cholesterol, heart disease,[17] irritable bowel syndrome and functional gastrointestinal disorders,[13,23] fibromyalgia, chronic fatigue syndrome, and temporomandibular joint syndrome.[17] Victims of IPV also are more likely to have chronic pain syndromes[20,24] and are more likely to have multiple somatic complaints, including stomach pain, back pain, menstrual problems, headaches, chest pain, dizziness, fainting spells, palpitations, shortness of breath, constipation, generalized fatigue, and insomnia.[22]

For many of these health conditions, the mechanism through which IPV increases risk is unknown but probably is multifactorial. Contributing factors may include the direct effect of physical trauma, the long-term accumulated stress of physical and psychologic trauma, and increased prevalence of behavioral risk. Regardless of etiology, it is useful for clinicians to know the constellation of conditions and symptoms that frequently present in victims of IPV. When a patient presents with frequent somatic complaints or other conditions consistent with IPV, a clinician should consider inquiring about IPV not only because intervention may be beneficial to a patient but also because knowledge of IPV could influence the treatment plan and help the clinician understand barriers to treatment adherence.

Intimate Partner Violence and Pregnancy

Maternal morbidity and mortality

It is not uncommon for IPV to continue during pregnancy, putting women at risk for several pregnancy-related complications. Women who experience IPV during pregnancy are at increased risk for spontaneous abortion,[20] preterm labor, hypertensive disorders of pregnancy, vaginal bleeding, placental abruption, severe nausea and vomiting, dehydration, diabetes, urinary tract infection, and premature rupture of membranes.[25] Pregnancies of couples affected by IPV also are more likely to have been unplanned.[20] IPV is associated with a short interpregnancy interval in adolescents.[20] Late entry into prenatal care is common among women who are victims of IPV, and the possibility of IPV should be considered in women who receive late or no prenatal care.[20] IPV-related homicide is the leading cause of maternal mortality, accounting for 13% to 24% of all deaths in pregnancy.[20]

Infant morbidity and mortality

Infants affected by IPV during pregnancy also are at risk. Although studies have shown conflicting results, it seems that there is an association between IPV and low birth weight.[25–30] Abuse during pregnancy also seems to increase the risk for prematurity and perinatal death.[29–32]

Mental Health

In addition to the physical health effects (described previously), victims of IPV frequently suffer chronic mental illness.[15] Although mental health consequences are seen whether abuse is physical, sexual, or psychologic, some data suggest that mental health outcomes are the worst for individuals who experience sexual IPV.[14]

Individuals who experience IPV are at increased risk for depression,[24] an effect seen with physical, sexual, and emotional IPV.[14–16] They also are at increased risk for suicidal thoughts and attempts.[13] Alcohol abuse and illicit drug use also are more common among individuals who experience IPV.[15–17,20]

Posttraumatic stress disorder (PTSD) is prevalent, occurring in 31% to 84% of women exposed to IPV.[31] Symptoms of PTSD, including emotional detachment, sleep disturbances, flashbacks, and mentally replaying episodes of assault, may persist long after the violence is no longer present in a woman's life. Higher rates of PTSD are seen with sexual and physical IPV than with physical IPV alone,[21] and a greater severity and frequency of violence correlates with greater risk for PTSD.[24] The high prevalence of PTSD among survivors of IPV may be a key factor in explaining the relationship between violence and physical health symptoms.[32]

Disability

A marker of the long-term toll of IPV is the high rate of disability among IPV survivors, approximately twice that of individuals not exposed to IPV.[33] Women who have a history of exposure to IPV report higher rates of disability because of chronic pain, nervous system injuries or disorders, mental illness or depression, chronic disease, and blindness.[33] Victims of IPV report higher use of disability equipment, such as canes or wheelchairs, and are more likely to report activity limitations due to health problems.[17]

Health Risk Behaviors

IPV is associated with several behaviors that confer health risk, which may contribute to the increased physical, mental, and pregnancy-related health risk seen in victims of IPV. More severe violence correlates more strongly with negative health behaviors by victims. IPV victims are more likely to abuse substances, including tobacco, alcohol, and other drugs.[15–17,20] They are more likely to engage in risky sexual behaviors, including unprotected sex, early sexual initiation, multiple sex partners, and trading sex for food, money, or other items.[17,20] Women who are abused are more likely to engage in disordered eating patterns, including overeating and vomiting or use of laxatives for weight control.[20]

Women who have a history of IPV may be perceived to overuse the health care system, with high rates of primary care and emergency department use; however, they commonly report unmet health care needs and troubled patient-physician communication.[20] What providers perceive as a lack of motivation to adhere to health recommendations could be related to the dynamics of violence. Many survivors report that partners interfere with their receipt of health care services,[34] one component in an overall pattern of control of victims' lives by their partners. Recognizing IPV should help providers understand the barriers and challenges that patients face, allowing them to form a more constructive therapeutic relationship.

SCREENING FOR INTIMATE PARTNER VIOLENCE

As providers become more aware of IPV as a common problem with myriad health consequences, many have begun to screen routinely for IPV. Screening practices among providers vary as there is no gold standard test for IPV. A recent review of more than 35 screening tools underscores the range and confusion in screening for IPV in clinical settings. Many of the tools are too long for practical use in a busy clinic and are more appropriate for research. Shorter tools often lack adequate sensitivity or require follow-up discussion to improve diagnostic usefulness.[35] One study demonstrated that the use of a computer to complete survey-based screening tools is a practical option in emergency department settings.[36]

In parallel, many physicians are reluctant to integrate screening into practice. They are uncomfortable asking about "private" matters, do not feel well equipped to discuss or assist with IPV, or are worried about time, privacy, legal issues, and personal safety. Although many national groups have recommended screening for IPV, rates of screening in primary care settings are estimated at 9% to 11%, depending on the type of clinic visit.[37] A recent study noted more discomfort among male physicians and among those in private practice and less discomfort among obstetrician/gynecologists, among clinicians practicing for 5 to 10 years, and among those working in a hospital setting.[38]

Controversy

In 2004, the US Preventive Services Task Force (USPSTF) assigned screening for IPV a recommendation of level I (insufficient evidence), citing methodologic problems with many studies and lack of proved efficacy of interventions to assist patients. The USPSTF defined successful intervention for IPV in adults as shelter use or leaving the abusive relationship. They found[39]

- No direct evidence that screening leads to decreased disability or premature death
- No existing studies that determine the accuracy of screening tools for identifying family and IPV among children, women, or older adults in general populations
- Fair to good evidence that interventions reduce harm to children when child abuse or neglect has been assessed
- No studies that have directly assessed the harm of screening and interventions for the family, so cost-benefit analysis cannot be conducted

This rigid evaluation of evidence is difficult to apply to IPV screening for several reasons. Screening for IPV should not be compared with radiographic tests for breast cancer or sigmoidoscopy for colon cancer screening but rather to the type of analysis used for more similar and morbid conditions, such as counseling for depression.[40] Many clinicians agree that good evidence for screening for IPV might be hard to obtain. Some clinicians worry that the "insufficient" recommendation would cause even lower detection rates of IPV than before,[41] whereas advocates urge more research to be done. Although evidence does not exist to definitively prove that knowing about IPV reduces harm, common sense and prior experience suggest that knowing about such a difficult, potentially dangerous situation would be helpful toward understanding and assisting patients with health problems and would even prevent needless deaths. Smoking cessation counseling may be a good analogy, as described by Janssen and colleagues[42]:

> When primary care physicians routinely ask about smoking as part of patient history taking, they do not do so in the belief that asking the question will stop their patients from smoking. Instead, knowledge of smoking status may guide the physician to undertake more frequent monitoring of cardiovascular and pulmonary health status, including measurement of blood pressure, evaluation of exercise tolerance, etc. Similarly, asking about intimate partner violence and obtaining a positive response identifies an opportunity for prevention of health-related sequelae.

One can particularly see how inquiry would be important before embarking on sensitive examinations, such as the breast and pelvic examinations, where retraumatization can easily occur.

Many clinicians were skeptical about the shelter use and departure end points identified by the USPSTF. Substantial numbers of patients remain in adverse relationships over time, yet may have improved health, especially after disclosure and care of

IPV-related medical problems. The American College of Obstetricians and Gynecologists, the American Medical Association, and the American Academy of Family Physicians recommend IPV screening, while the Joint Commission mandates patient safety screening for hospital accreditation.

WHAT PATIENTS WANT REGARDING SCREENING

A recent meta-analysis evaluated qualitative studies regarding women's preferences for IPV screening.[43] Women wanted caregivers to be nonjudgmental, compassionate, and confidential. They wanted the professional to understand the complex, long-term nature of IPV and to understand its social and psychologic ramifications. Women wanted providers to avoid medicalizing the issue and to raise it in a confident, unrushed manner. They wanted confirmation that violence was unacceptable and undeserved and that abuse was not their fault. They hoped the health care professional would bolster their confidence and allow them to progress at their own pace. They did not want to be pressured to disclose, leave the relationship, or press charges. Women wanted to share decision-making with providers.[43] They did not want to be told to leave the situation or make use of a shelter, the specific end points the USPSTF emphasized. Women prefer to be queried in a patient-centered interview format where a clinician follows up on a patient's own cues rather than following a checklist.[44] Ninety percent of the teens would not mind being screened by a health care provider; however, those who were most likely to object to screening were victims of physical violence or victims or perpetrators of sexual violence.[45]

RESOLUTION OF THE CONFLICT

IPV may contribute directly to the health problem (a current injury), exacerbate or cause somatic and psychologic states (PTSD, depression, and anxiety), or explain patient nonadherence (control by perpetrator). Thus, knowing about a woman's experience can be critical to diagnosing and treating her complaints. Asking about violence also educates patients about IPV, may increase recognition of their situation in the future,[46] and informs patients that providers can offer help for these problems. Even though the majority of patients are not currently in an abusive relationship, many have or will experience abuse at some point.

Because it is important to know about violence when providing care, it is recommended that providers assess for violence in all new patients and when it could play a role in determining the differential diagnosis of a medical condition (**Boxes 1** and **2**). Asking about violence before performing a genital examination or during a yearly examination is reasonable. Some institutions have nurses inquire at

---

Box 1
Characteristics of good intimate partner violence screening techniques

Always ask about violence in privacy and assure confidentiality

Provide a preface that contextualizes and normalizes your query for the patient

Ask about the past and the present situation

Ask about psychologic and control factors and physical and sexual violence

Ask like you want to know the answer

Ask again if you have clinical suspicion, as patients often will not answer positively to your inquiry the first time or may downplay physical or sexual violence

> **Box 2**
> **Samples of intimate partner violence screening questions**
>
> Because violence is such a common and difficult problem, I ask all my patients if they have ever been harmed emotionally, physically, or sexually in the past or present.
>
> Many times people complaining of _____ have worse symptoms/more trouble recovering from _____ if they have been exposed to traumatic events. Have you ever been hurt emotionally, physically, or sexually in the past or recently?
>
> Do you feel threatened or controlled by a partner, ex-partner, or anyone else in your life?
>
> Has your partner or anyone else ever hurt you physically, for example by pushing, shoving, hitting, slapping, or kicking you, or by forcing you to have sex?

each appointment in triage when patients are alone. IPV can manifest as many different complaints or problems. Multiple physical complaints, chronic pain, depression, anxiety, substance abuse, or PTSD should prompt consideration of IPV, especially if the examination is inconsistent or treatment is not working.[47–53]

If They Say "Yes," Then What?

A positive answer to an IPV screen can feel like a crisis moment because of anxiety generated in a clinician. Most often, abuse is psychologic and ongoing and may not necessitate crisis-type intervention and, like other chronic problems, it can be worked on over time. Cementing the therapeutic doctor–patient relationship is crucial and facilitates assessing whether or not a patient is in imminent danger. Patients who may be in severe, acute danger may benefit from seeking additional help if available. Help may come in the form of a hospital-based program, law enforcement (to press formal charges or to begin the process of obtaining a restraining order), community-based IPV organizations that can provide ongoing advocates, or a shelter if patients are worried for their immediate safety. The Violence Against Women Act offers many protections to victims of abuse, independent of their immigration status. Knowing about this law often can assuage patient fears regarding legal action.[54] Frequent office visits can be helpful to continue to care for medical problems, offer support, and assess for safety (**Box 3**).

Safety Assessment

Do patients believe they are in imminent danger? If they answer "yes," consider contacting the IPV program, law enforcement, or a shelter if available in the community. If possible, empower patients to make these calls. Unfortunately, although patients often know when they are in danger, they are not always correct when they say they are not in danger.[55] One large case-controlled study found that more than one half of the victims of attempted or completed IPV homicides did not suspect they

> **Box 3**
> **Responding to a positive screen for intimate partner violence**
>
> Respond with empathy
>
> Establish/continue a collaborative, noncontrolling therapeutic relationship that does not replicate the pattern of abuse
>
> Assist with health
>
> Assess for safety

were at risk for harm.[56] To clarify patient safety, clinicians should assess for increasing frequency or severity of violence, prior use or threat of use of a weapon (eg, a knife or gun), assailant use of alcohol or illegal drugs, threat of homicide or suicide, or recent separation. Such patients may be in mortal danger and may benefit from seeking additional help if available.

EFFECTS ON CHILDREN

IPV and child maltreatment have many overlapping features, risk factors, and consequences. In many cases, they are final common outcomes from family dysfunction, stress, and societal tolerance of violence. In some cases, the best interest of children and parent victims may not be served in the same way.

Co-occurrence of Intimate Partner Violence and Child Maltreatment

IPV that occurs between partners, one of whom is a parent, often occurs in households with child maltreatment. Child maltreatment broadly encompasses child physical abuse, psychologic abuse, neglect, and sexual abuse. Studies that screened for IPV in a population of families affected by child maltreatment or for child maltreatment in families affected by IPV have clearly demonstrated that IPV and child maltreatment often occur in the same homes. Approximately 26% to 73% of families reported to child protective services for child maltreatment also are affected by IPV.[57–59] Conversely, families in which a woman is victimized by IPV have rates of child maltreatment between 30% and 60%,[57] with some studies reporting rates as high as 100%.[60] Past research estimating rates of co-occurrence of IPV and child maltreatment, however, may suffer significantly from selection bias and the lack of an appropriate comparison group. Recently, by using more appropriate comparison populations, several studies have demonstrated relationships between IPV and physical abuse, sexual abuse, and neglect.[61–65]

Harmful Effects of Intimate Partner Violence to Children

IPV can harm children physically and mentally. Children can be considered "collateral damage" in an assault between intimate partners. Nearly one half of homes with child maltreatment fatalities have reported IPV.[57,60,62] A single study of child injuries presenting to a pediatric emergency department in a large city demonstrates the range of these collateral injuries. One half of the child victims were under age 2, and 59% were being held by a caregiver when injured. Most of the injuries to the child were to the head (25%), face (19%), and eyes (12%). The child's father was most often responsible for the injury (50%), with the child's mother (13%) or mother's boyfriend (10%) found responsible in a smaller percentage of cases.[66] Two studies have demonstrated high emergency department use rates in children whose mothers have a history of IPV.[67,68]

Several longitudinal studies have demonstrated important associations between child and subsequent adult mental health. Child reports of witnessed IPV are associated with increased odds of suicidal ideation[69] and 2.6 times increased odds of suicide attempt.[70] Two reports from a high-risk cohort study have shown that witnessing IPV during childhood leads to more mental health symptoms and more clinical depression, anxiety, and anger.[71,72]

Legal Ramifications

IPV is increasingly important to child welfare agencies because of the direct effects of harm to children (physical and mental) and the risk it poses for child maltreatment. At least 40 states, 3 territories, and the District of Columbia include children as a class of protected persons in definitions of IPV. In many states, an act of IPV in the presence of a child confers a harsher penalty. Some states require the reporting of IPV to child welfare agencies under some circumstances.[73]

Practicing women's health care professionals should understand that IPV is common, it can be harmful to a child's mental and physical health, and it has pervasive psychologic consequences that may be lifelong. It also is related closely to the risk for all forms of child maltreatment. Clinicians should understand the IPV reporting laws in their state as issued by child welfare agencies. They also should consider IPV in the differential diagnosis for children's behavioral problems as a cause or contributing factor and understand methods for eliciting a history of IPV from caregivers.

SUMMARY

IPV is a common problem affecting many women who present to obstetricians, gynecologists, and other women's health care professionals. It takes on many forms, including psychologic/emotional, physical, and sexual abuse, and its effects on the health of victims and their children vary. Although many physicians may be uncomfortable inquiring about IPV, a knowledge of patients' IPV victimization may help physicians develop a better understanding of patients' presenting symptoms and health risks, form more effective therapeutic relationships, and work toward reducing the myriad health risks associated with IPV.

REFERENCES

1. Centers for Disease Control and Prevention. National Center for Injury Prevention and Control. Intimate partner violence prevention scientific information: definitions. Available at: http://www.cdc.gov/ncipc/dvp/IPV/ipv-definitions.htm. Accessed July 3, 2008.
2. Tjaden P, Thoennes N. Full report of the prevalence, incidence, and consequences of violence against women: findings from the National Violence Against Women Survey. Washington, DC: US Department of Justice; 2000.
3. McCloskey LA, Lichter E, Ganz ML, et al. Intimate partner violence and patient screening across medical specialties. Acad Emerg Med 2005;12(8):712–22.
4. Lehrer JA, Buka S, Gortmaker S, et al. Depressive symptomatology as a predictor of exposure to intimate partner violence among US female adolescents and young adults. Arch Pediatr Adolesc Med 2006;160(3):270–6.
5. Bowen E, Heron J, Waylen A, et al. Domestic violence risk during and after pregnancy: findings from a British longitudinal study. BJOG 2005;112(8):1083–9.
6. Zolotor AJ, Runyan DK. Social capital, family violence, and neglect. Pediatrics 2006;117(6):e1124–31.
7. Straus MA, Gelles RJ. Physical violence in American families: risk factors and adaptations to violence in 8,145 families. New Brunswick (NJ): Transaction; 1990.
8. US Department of Justice. Crime victimization in the United States, 2005 statistical tables. Washington, DC: US Department of Justice; 2007.
9. Karch DL, Lubell KM, Friday J, et al. Surveillance for violent deaths—national violent death reporting system, 16 states, 2005. MMWR Surveill Summ 2008; 57(3):1–45.
10. Campbell JC, Webster D, Koziol-McLain J, et al. Risk factors for femicide in abusive relationships: results from a multisite case control study. Am J Public Health 2003;93(7):1089–97.

11. Thompson RS, Bonomi AE, Anderson M, et al. Intimate partner violence: prevalence, types, and chronicity in adult women. Am J Prev Med 2006;30(6):447–57.
12. Dubowitz H, Prescott L, Feigelman S, et al. Screening for intimate partner violence in a pediatric primary care clinic. Pediatrics 2008;121(1):e85–91.
13. Ellsberg M, Jansen HA, Heise L, et al. Intimate partner violence and women's physical and mental health in the WHO multi-country study on women's health and domestic violence: an observational study. Lancet 2008;371(9619):1165–72.
14. Bonomi AE, Anderson ML, Rivara FP, et al. Health outcomes in women with physical and sexual intimate partner violence exposure. J Womens Health (Larchmt) 2007;16(7):987–97.
15. Coker AL, Davis KE, Arias I, et al. Physical and mental health effects of intimate partner violence for men and women. Am J Prev Med 2002;23(4):260–8.
16. Bonomi AE, Thompson RS, Anderson M, et al. Intimate partner violence and women's physical, mental, and social functioning. Am J Prev Med 2006;30(6):458–66.
17. Centers for Disease Control and Prevention. Adverse health conditions and health risk behaviors associated with intimate partner violence—United States, 2005. MMWR Morb Mortal Wkly Rep 2008;57(5):113–7.
18. Allen T, Novak SA, Bench LL. Patterns of injuries: accident or abuse. Violence Against Women 2007;13(8):802–16.
19. Bhandari M, Dosanjh S, Tornetta P, et al. Musculoskeletal manifestations of physical abuse after intimate partner violence. J Trauma 2006;61(6):1473–9.
20. Plichta SB. Intimate partner violence and physical health consequences: policy and practice implications. J Interpers Violence 2004;19(11):1296–323.
21. McFarlane J, Malecha A, Watson K, et al. Intimate partner sexual assault against women: frequency, health consequences, and treatment outcomes. Obstet Gynecol 2005;105(1):99–108.
22. Eberhard-Gran M, Schei B, Eskild A. Somatic symptoms and diseases are more common in women exposed to violence. J Gen Intern Med 2007;22(12):1668–73.
23. Leserman J, Drossman DA. Relationship of abuse history to functional gastrointestinal disorders and symptoms: some possible mediating mechanisms. Trauma Violence Abuse 2007;8(3):331–43.
24. Dutton MA, Green BL, Kaltman SI, et al. Intimate partner violence, PTSD, and adverse health outcomes. J Interpers Violence 2006;21(7):955–68.
25. Silverman JG, Decker MR, Reed E, et al. Intimate partner violence victimization prior to and during pregnancy among women residing in 26 U.S. states: associations with maternal and neonatal health. Am J Obstet Gynecol 2006;195(1):140–8.
26. Murphy CC, Schei B, Myhr TL, et al. Abuse: a risk factor for low birth weight? A systematic review and meta-analysis. CMAJ 2001;164(11):1567–72.
27. Rosen D, Seng JS, Tolman RM, et al. Intimate partner violence, depression, and posttraumatic stress disorder as additional predictors of low birth weight infants among low-income mothers. J Interpers Violence 2007;22(10):1305–14.
28. McFarlane J. Intimate partner violence and physical health consequences: commentary on Plichta. J Interpers Violence 2004;19(11):1335–41.
29. Sharps PW, Laughon K, Giangrande SK. Intimate partner violence and the childbearing year: maternal and infant health consequences. Trauma Violence Abuse 2007;8(2):105–16.
30. Coker AL, Sanderson M, Dong B. Partner violence during pregnancy and risk of adverse pregnancy outcomes. Paediatr Perinat Epidemiol 2004;18(4):260–9.
31. Woods SJ. Intimate partner violence and post-traumatic stress disorder symptoms in women: what we know and need to know. J Interpers Violence 2005; 20(4):394–402.

32. Taft CT, Vogt DS, Mechanic MB, et al. Posttraumatic stress disorder and physical health symptoms among women seeking help for relationship aggression. J Fam Psychol 2007;21(3):354–62.

33. Coker AL, Smith PH, Fadden MK. Intimate partner violence and disabilities among women attending family practice clinics. J Womens Health (Larchmt) 2005;14(9):829–38.

34. McCloskey LA, Williams CM, Lichter E, et al. Abused women disclose partner interference with health care: an unrecognized form of battering. J Gen Intern Med 2007;22(8):1067–72.

35. Basile KC, Hertz MF, Back SE. Intimate partner violence and sexual violence victimization assessment instruments for use in health care settings: version1. Atlanta (GA): Centers for Disease Control and Prevention, National Center for Injury Control and Prevention; 2007.

36. Rhodes KV, Lauderdale DS, He T, et al. Between me and the computer: increased detection of intimate partner violence using a computer questionnaire. Ann Emerg Med 2002;40(5):476–84.

37. Rodriguez MA, Bauer HM, McLoughlin E, et al. Screening and intervention for intimate partner abuse: practices and attitudes of primary care physicians. JAMA 1999;282(5):468–74.

38. Jaffee KD, Epling JW, Grant W, et al. Physician-identified barriers to intimate partner violence screening. J Womens Health (Larchmt) 2005;14(8):713–20.

39. US Preventive Services Task Force. Screening for family and intimate partner violence: recommendation statement. Ann Intern Med 2004;140(5):382–6.

40. Lachs MS. Screening for family violence: what's an evidence-based doctor to do? Ann Intern Med 2004;140(5):399–400.

41. Marks JS, Cassidy EF. Does a failure to count mean that it fails to count? Addressing intimate partner violence. Am J Prev Med 2006;30(6):530–1.

42. Janssen P, Dascal-Weichhendler H, McGregor M. Assessment for intimate partner violence: where do we stand? J Am Board Fam Med 2006;19(4): 413–5.

43. Feder GS, Hutson M, Ramsay J, et al. Women exposed to intimate partner violence: expectations and experiences when they encounter health care professionals: a meta-analysis of qualitative studies. Arch Intern Med 2006;166(1): 22–37.

44. McCord-Duncan EC, Floyd M, Kemp EC, et al. Detecting potential intimate partner violence: which approach do women want? Fam Med 2006;38(6):416–22.

45. Zeitler MS, Paine AD, Breitbart V, et al. Attitudes about intimate partner violence screening among an ethnically diverse sample of young women. J Adolesc Health 2006;39(1):119, e111–18.

46. Nicolaidis C. Partner interference with health care: do we want one more piece of a complex puzzle? J Gen Intern Med 2007;22(8):1216–7.

47. Golding JM. Intimate partner violence as a risk factor for mental disorders: a meta-analysis. J Fam Violence 1999;14(2):99–132.

48. Coker AL, Smith PH, McKeown RE, et al. Frequency and correlates of intimate partner violence by type: physical, sexual, and psychological battering. Am J Public Health 2000;90(4):553–9.

49. McCauley J, Kern DE, Kolodner K, et al. The "battering syndrome": prevalence and clinical characteristics of domestic violence in primary care internal medicine practices. Ann Intern Med 1995;123(10):737–46.

50. Roberts GL, Lawrence JM, Williams GM, et al. The impact of domestic violence on women's mental health. Aust N Z J Public Health 1998;22(7):796–801.

51. Petersen R, Gazmararian J, Andersen Clark K. Partner violence: implications for health and community settings. Womens Health Issues 2001;11(2):116–25.
52. Thompson MP, Kaslow NJ, Kingree JB, et al. Partner abuse and posttraumatic stress disorder as risk factors for suicide attempts in a sample of low-income, inner-city women. J Trauma Stress 1999;12(1):59–72.
53. Brokaw J, Fullerton-Gleason L, Olson L, et al. Health status and intimate partner violence: a cross-sectional study. Ann Emerg Med 2002;39(1):31–8.
54. US House of Representatives. Violence Against Women Act. Available at: www.now.org/issues/violence/vawa/vawa1998.html. Accessed July 3, 2008.
55. Weisz A. Assessing the risk of severe domestic violence: the importance of survivor's predictions. J Interpers Violence 2000;15:75–90.
56. Campbell JC, Koziol-McLain J, Webster D, et al. Research results from a national study of intimate partner femicide: the danger assessment instrument. Washington, DC: National Institute of Justice; 2002.
57. Edleson JL. The overlap between child maltreatment and woman battering. Violence Against Women 1999;5:134–54.
58. English DJ, Edleson JL, Herrick ME. Domestic violence in one state's child protective caseload: a study of differential case dispositions and outcomes. Child Youth Serv Rev 2005;27:1183–201.
59. Hazen AL, Connelly CD, Kelleher K, et al. Intimate partner violence among female caregivers of children reported for child maltreatment. Child Abuse Negl 2004;28(3):301–19.
60. Appel AE, Holden GW. The co-occurrence of spouse and physical child abuse: a review and appraisal. J Fam Psychol 1998;12:578–99.
61. Lee LC, Kotch JB, Cox CE. Child maltreatment in families experiencing domestic violence. Violence Vict 2004;19(5):573–91.
62. Zolotor AJ, Theodore AD, Coyne-Beasley T, et al. Intimate partner violence and child maltreatment: overlapping risk. Brief Treat Crisis Interv 2007;7(4):305–21.
63. Tajima EA. The relative importance of wife abuse as a risk factor for violence against children. Child Abuse Negl 2000;24(11):1383–98.
64. Rumm PD, Cummings P, Krauss MR, et al. Identified spouse abuse as a risk factor for child abuse. Child Abuse Negl 2000;24(11):1375–81.
65. McGuigan WM, Pratt CC. The predictive impact of domestic violence on three types of child maltreatment. Child Abuse Negl 2001;25(7):869–83.
66. Christian CW, Scribano P, Seidl T, et al. Pediatric injury resulting from family violence. Pediatrics 1997;99(2):E8.
67. Duffy SJ, McGrath ME, Becker BM, et al. Mothers with histories of domestic violence in a pediatric emergency department. Pediatrics 1999;103(5 Pt 1):1007–13.
68. Casanueva C, Foushee V, Barth R. Intimate partner violence as a risk for children's use of the emergency room and injuries. Child Youth Serv Rev 2005;27(11):1223–42.
69. Thompson R, Briggs E, English DJ, et al. Suicidal ideation among 8-year-olds who are maltreated and at risk: findings from the LONGSCAN studies. Child Maltreat 2005;10(1):26–36.
70. Dube SR, Anda RF, Felitti VJ, et al. Childhood abuse, household dysfunction, and the risk of attempted suicide throughout the life span: findings from the Adverse Childhood Experiences Study. JAMA 2001;286(24):3089–96.
71. Dubowitz H, Black MM, Kerr MA, et al. Type and timing of mothers' victimization: effects on mothers and children. Pediatrics 2001;107(4):728–35.

72. Johnson RM, Kotch JB, Catellier DJ, et al. Adverse behavioral and emotional outcomes from child abuse and witnessed violence. Child Maltreat 2002;7(3): 179–86.
73. National Clearinghouse on Child Abuse and Neglect Information. Children and domestic violence. Washington, DC: US Department of Health and Human Services; 2004.

Female Sexual Dysfunction

Anita H. Clayton, MD[a],*, David V. Hamilton, MD, MA[b]

KEYWORDS

- Female sexual dysfunction • Sexual disorders
- Hypoactive sexual desire disorder
- Female sexual arousal disorder

The past 20 years has seen an explosion of research into female sexuality. Although rigorous epidemiologic study of female sexuality essentially began with publication of *Sexual Behavior of the Human Female*[1] in 1953, the specific study of postmenopausal sexuality did not begin in earnest until the 1990s. With the research, practitioners have come to understand that healthy, even satisfying, sexual function may extend throughout the life cycle.

SEXUAL RESPONSE CYCLE

Three models of the female sexual response cycle have been postulated: Masters and Johnson described stimulation leading to excitement, plateau, orgasm, and resolution, Kaplan articulated sexual desire, arousal, and orgasm as a pattern, and Basson suggested some women may participate in sexual activity for reasons other than desire, for example, motivated by a wish for emotional intimacy. In a study by Sand and Fisher, equal numbers of women endorsed each model, suggesting that the female sexual response is heterogenous,[2] with sexual dysfunction as measured by the Female Sexual Function Index (FSFI) more likely to occur in those identifying with the Basson model.

FEMALE SEXUAL PHYSIOLOGY

Regulation of the hormonal cycle involves complex interplay along the HPG axis: the hypothalamus, the anterior pituitary gland, and the ovaries. The hypothalamus releases gonadotropin-releasing hormone (GnRH), which induces the release of luteinizing

This is an advance version of an article that will appear in an issue of *Psychiatric Clinics of North America* devoted to Women's Mental Health (Volume 33, Issue 2, June 2010).

[a] Department of Psychiatry & Neurobehavioral Sciences, University of Virginia, 2955 Ivy Road, Northridge Suite 210, Charlottesville, VA 22903, USA

[b] Department of Psychiatry and Neurobehavioral Sciences, Institute for Law, Psychiatry, and Public Policy, University of Virginia, Charlottesville, VA, USA

* Corresponding author.

E-mail address: ahc8v@virginia.edu (A.H. Clayton).

hormone (LH) and follicle-stimulating hormone (FSH) from the anterior pituitary gland. LH stimulates ovarian theca cells to produce testosterone, some of which is converted to estrogen by the granulosa cells before release into circulation. FSH acts on granulosa cells in the ovary, producing estrogens and inhibin. As a regulating feedback mechanism, estrogen inhibits release of LH in the anterior pituitary, while inhibin decreases release of FSH (also at the anterior pituitary), keeping the system in balance.

Several factors complicate the detection of sexual dysfunction due to androgen insufficiency. Only bioavailable testosterone traverses the blood-brain barrier to exert an influence on the brain structures involved in sexual function (eg, hypothalamus, pituitary, amygdala). The majority of circulating testosterone is bound to the protein, sex hormone-binding globulin (SHBG). This chemical complex, too large to cross the blood-brain barrier, does not influence the central nervous system directly. Little is known about androgen effects in women relative to men. Assays used in determining the amount of both free and bound testosterone have relative ranges defined by androgen levels measured in men.[3]

Several neurotransmitters influence sexual function, evidenced by the number of centrally active medications that produce sexual side effects. Dopamine seems to mediate sexual desire and the subjective sense of arousal, as well as the drive to continue sexual activity once it begins.[4] In both the brain and the genitalia,[5] norepinephrine is the principal neurotransmitter regulating sexual arousal, which depends on central nervous system arousal via norepinephrine increases in excitation in the ventromedial hypothalamus.[6] Increased serotonergic transmission modulates dopamine and norepinephrine, diminishing the excitatory effects of both.[7] Serotonin seems to affect sexual arousal in peripheral tissues, by way of effects on vascular tone and blood flow. Serotonin may mediate uterine contractions during orgasm, may also interfere with arousal via negative effects on sensation and inhibition of the synthesis of nitric oxide (NO).[8] Finally, serotonin inhibits orgasm in some people by stimulation of 5-HT2 receptors, evidenced by selective serotonin reuptake inhibitor (SSRI)-induced anorgasmia and other problems with orgasm.[9]

Once sexual stimulation begins, the vasocongestion of clitoral tissue during arousal is positively mediated by NO[10] and vasoactive intestinal peptide (VIP).[11] Sufficient levels of free testosterone[12] are also required for NO to initiate vasocongestion with sexual stimulation. Acetylcholinergic nerve fibers innervate vascular smooth muscle in the vagina, allowing for vaginal engorgement during arousal, and subsequent lubrication.[13]

Multiple neurotransmitters must act in concert for adequate sexual functioning to occur. Drugs affecting sex steroids, such as estrogen and prolactin, or neurotransmitter function (eg, norepinephrine, serotonin, NO) also run the risk of impairing the ability to orgasm.[14,15] The most common medical conditions affecting these neurotransmitters include neurologic disorders, endocrine dysfunction, cardiovascular disease, and pelvic conditions. Depression, anxiety disorders, and eating disorders are also associated with sexual dysfunction. Medications that contribute to sexual dysfunction include histamine receptor (H2) blockers, narcotics, NSAIDs, oral contraceptives, thiazide diuretics, non-selective beta antagonists, and psychotropics such as antidepressants, antipsychotics, and benzodiazepines.[16] Studies have found that the SSRI antidepressants (ie, citalopram, escitalopram, fluvoxamine, fluoxetine, paroxetine, and sertraline), along with the serotonin-norepinephrine reuptake inhibiting (SNRI) antidepressant venlafaxine, confer the greatest risk of sexual dysfunction. Antidepressants that do not exploit serotonin reuptake as their primary therapeutic action, including bupropion, mirtazapine, and transdermal selegiline, do not significantly inhibit sexual function.[17,18] A special case appears to be the SNRI duloxetine, which

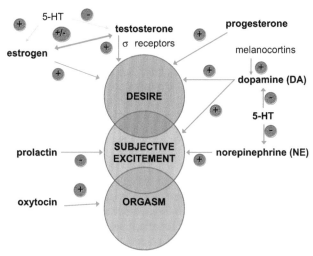

Fig. 1. Central effects on sexual function. + indicates a positive effect; − indicates a negative effect. (*Modified from* Clayton AH. Sexual function and dysfunction in women. Psychiatr Clin North Am 2003;26:673–82; with *Data from* Cohen AJ. Antidepressant-induced sexual dysfunction associated with low serum free testosterone. Mental Health Today 2000. http://www.mental-health-today.com/rx/testos.htm; with permission.)

has been demonstrated to have effects on sexual function intermediate to SSRIs and placebo (**Figs. 1** and **2**).[19]

DYSFUNCTIONS AND DISORDER

To properly detect and diagnose the presence of sexual disorders, it is critical to discern the distinction between *dysfunction* and *disorder*. Dysfunction describes the

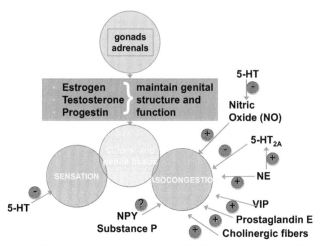

Fig. 2. Peripheral effects on sexual function. + indicates a positive effect; − indicates a negative effect. (*Modified from* Clayton AH. Sexual function and dysfunction in women. Psychiatr Clin North Am 2003;26:673–82; with permission.)

presence of medically relevant symptoms or signs of sexual function that is in some way not consistent with the medical understanding of healthy sexual functioning. However, the diagnosis of female sexual dysfunction (FSD) requires not only the presence of clinically significant sexual dysfunction but also that this dysfunction causes *distress* in the woman experiencing it. In brief, a diagnosis of FSD is not indicated if a putative symptom or sign of sexual dysfunction is not associated with distress. This necessity for distress in making the diagnosis of a sexual disorder is part of the *Diagnostic and Statistical Manual of Mental Disorders* (Fourth Edition, Text Revised) (DSM-IV-TR) diagnostic criteria for each FSD, typically delineated as criterion B.[20]

EPIDEMIOLOGY

Unfortunately, discussions regarding sexual functioning have not been a routine part of health care. Nusbaum and colleagues[21] found that only 14% to 17% of women reported that their doctor had brought up the subject of sexual function, and that most women had never spoken with their doctor about sex. If the topic had been raised, the patient was nearly twice as likely as the physician to have initiated the discussion, regardless of age group. The majority of women in each age category believed that their physician would not be receptive to discussing their sexual concerns, either because they felt their doctor simply lacked interest or they would be too embarrassed.

Few studies in the United States have specifically addressed the incidence and prevalence of sexual dysfunction among women. In one of the few studies to address the issue, Bancroft and colleagues[22] found that among Caucasian and African American women between 20 and 65 years old who were asked about their degree of distress associated with sexual problems, 24% of women reported distress about their sexual relationship, their own sexuality, or both. Although this study provided valuable preliminary results, it did not address whether menopausal status was associated with changes in sexual function.

A recent meta-analysis of international epidemiologic studies of the prevalence of FSD suggested that sexual dysfunctions are highly prevalent across cultures, with the incidence of sexual dysfunctions increasing directly with age for both men and women.[23] Whereas the frequency of symptoms increases with age, personal distress about those symptoms seems to diminish as women age.[24] Finally, the role of culture was not as important as the medical problems suffered by respondents in determining likelihood of participation in sexual activity.[23]

A large, recent epidemiologic survey, the Prevalence and Correlates of Female Sexual Disorders and Determinants of Treatment Seeking (PRESIDE), queried a representative sample of 50,002 United States women (n = 31,581 with 63% response rate) using the Changes in Sexual Functioning Questionnaire (CSFQ) to determine sexual dysfunctions, and the Female Sexual Distress Scale (FSDS) to evaluate level of distress.[25] Complaints of desire, arousal, and orgasm were reported in 38.7%, 26.1%, and 20.5%, respectively, with 44.2% of women describing any sexual problem. When marked distress was assessed as a cofactor, consistent with DSM-IV-TR criterion B, the prevalence rates decreased to 10%, 5.4%, and 4.7%, respectively, with 12% reporting any distressing sexual problem.

NEUROIMAGING

Recent advances in neuroimaging have demonstrated regions of the brain involved in sexual activity. Functional magnetic resonance imaging (fMRI) of 20 women with no history of sexual dysfunction (NHSD) was compared with 16 women with hypoactive sexual desire disorder (HSDD). Subjective arousal to erotic stimuli was significantly greater in the NHSD women, with different areas of the brain activated in women with NHSD versus HSDD. Cognitive/central sexual response or brain activation patterns were not significantly associated with peripheral sexual response in either group.[26]

In another study, positron emission tomography (PET) suggested that activation of the left lateral orbital frontal cortex is related to the level of behavioral inhibition during sex, with deactivation of the temporal lobe directly reflecting the level of arousal. The prefrontal cortex and the left temporal lobe showed decreased regional blood flow during orgasm in women. Glucose metabolism in the deep cerebellar nuclei was associated with orgasm-specific muscle contractions, with ventral midbrain and right caudate dopamine-containing areas also involved.[27] Other PET scans, coupled with magnetic resonance imaging (MRI), have shown increased activation at orgasm, compared with pre-orgasm sexual arousal in the paraventricular nucleus of the hypothalamus, the periaqueductal gray area of the midbrain, the hippocampus, and the cerebellum.[28] Subsequent hormonal spikes in prolactin and oxytocin have been associated with an overall sense of well-being, and perhaps facilitate bonding with a sexual partner.

GENETICS

Recent data support both a genetic and an environmental contribution to sexual function. Twin studies of 4037 women from the United Kingdom and 3080 Australian women supported a significant genetic influence on orgasmic capacity.[29,30] One-third of the women reported never or infrequently achieving orgasm during intercourse and 21% during masturbation. Genetic influences accounted for 34% and 32% among UK and Australian women, respectively of the variance in achieving orgasm with intercourse, with an estimated heritability of 45% and 51%, respectively for orgasm during masturbation. These results suggest that the wide variation in orgasmic function in women has a strong genetic basis, and cannot be attributed solely to sociocultural influences. However, high variability in traits suggests limited selection for functionality. For example, clitoral length is highly variable, whereas vaginal length is not. Given the association between the size of clitoral structures and ability to achieve orgasm, the marked variability in clitoral size is not suggestive of evolutionary selection bias for clitoral structure, and by inference, on female orgasm.[31]

Vulnerability to sexual dysfunction with antidepressant medications is also subject to genetic influences, related to 5-HT2A receptor polymorphisms.[32] Women with the II genotype for the SLC6A4 promoter region (5HTTLPR) were nearly 8 times more likely to have SSRI-associated sexual dysfunction if they were taking oral contraceptives.[33] In addition, dopamine (D4) receptor polymorphisms influence all phases of the sexual response cycle.[34]

HYPOACTIVE SEXUAL DESIRE DISORDER

The 2 key criteria for the diagnosis of HSDD are (1) the experiencing of difficulty in the desire phase of the sexual response cycle and (2) that this difficulty causes marked distress. Data from the PRESIDE study suggest rates of distressing low sexual desire (ie, HSDD) in the general population of 10%.[25] The most common co-occurring conditions were psychiatric (depression and anxiety), followed by thyroid problems and urinary incontinence. Comorbid arousal problems increased dramatically in postmenopausal women, with surgically induced menopause rates 54% higher and 34% higher in natural menopause women than in premenopausal women. In the Women's

International Study of Health and Sexuality (WISHeS), Leiblum and colleagues[35] reported on HSDD from data collected from 952 partnered United States women (46% response rate), employing 2 valid and reliable psychometric instruments to determine women with or without HSDD: the Profile of Female Sexual Function (PFSF) to assess sexual desire in women, and the Personal Distress Scale (PDS) to assess distress experienced by women due to low sexual desire. The WISHeS data demonstrated that HSDD ranged in prevalence from 14% in premenopausal women to 26% in surgically postmenopausal women aged 20 to 49 years. No significant differences were found in the prevalence of HSDD between surgically postmenopausal women, aged 50 to 70 years, and naturally postmenopausal women in the same age cohort. In addition, HSDD was associated with significantly lower sexual and partner satisfaction, as well as significant decrements in general health status, including aspects of mental and physical health.

A 5-question diagnostic screening tool for HSDD, the Decreased Sexual Desire Screener (DSDS), has been recently validated and found to be easy to use by clinicians who are not experts in sexual health, with an accuracy rate of greater than 85% compared with an expert clinician interview.[36,37]

FEMALE SEXUAL AROUSAL DISORDER

The central diagnostic feature of female sexual arousal disorder (FSAD) as defined by DSM-IV-TR criteria is the inability to achieve, or maintain during sexual activity, an adequate genital lubrication-swelling response.[38] As discussed earlier, arousal in women has 2 parts: a central/cognitive sense of excitement and genital lubrication-swelling. This physiologic arousal response in women consists of vasocongestion of the pelvic vasculature, vaginal lubrication, and expansion and swelling of the external genitalia and breast tissues. If dysfunction of both desire and arousal are present, a diagnosis of both HSDD and FSAD should be made.

Quirk and colleagues[39] have recently shown that the Sexual Function Questionnaire (SFQ) is able to discriminate various sexual dysfunctions, including FSAD. The FSFI has also demonstrated discriminant validity for FSD.[40] The rate of FSAD in the general population found in the PRESIDE study was 5.4%.[25]

FEMALE ORGASMIC DISORDER

The critical factor in the making the diagnosis is criterion A: there must be delay or absence of orgasm *following a normal excitement phase*. Although a lack of sexual excitement may, in turn, lead to the inability to achieve orgasm, this would not correctly be diagnosed female orgasmic disorder (FOD). Another important part of criterion A is the clinician's judgment that the woman's orgasmic capacity is "less than should be reasonable for her age, sexual experience…"[38] Data indicate that, unlike men, women typically find it easier to orgasm as they age, which seems to be related to increased sexual experience.[41] Finally, a woman must have adequate stimulation to achieve orgasm. The diagnosis of FOD would not be indicated in a woman whose sexual partner suffers from premature ejaculation, thus depriving her of sufficient stimulation to reach orgasm. As discussed earlier, for orgasmic dysfunction to be diagnosed as FOD it must cause *distress* to fulfill DSM-IV-TR criterion B.

SEXUAL PAIN DISORDERS: DYSPAREUNIA AND VAGINISMUS

Dyspareunia is the occurrence of recurrent or persistent genital pain during intercourse, and, like all FSDs, it must cause distress to be diagnosed.[38] Dyspareunia cannot be due exclusively to the presence of FSAD (ie, an inadequate lubrication-swelling response to subjective arousal) or vaginismus. Dyspareunia is relatively uncommon in premenopausal women (approximately 5%). While the prevalence of dyspareunia is known to increase among postmenopausal women, estimations of the rate vary widely between 12% and 45%.[42]

Vaginismus has been defined by recurrent or persistent involuntary spasm of the musculature of the outer third of vagina. These spasms interfere with, or even prevent, sexual intercourse. This sexual dysfunction must cause distress, must not be due to another Axis I disorder (eg, somatization disorder), and not caused exclusively by the direct physiologic effects of a medical condition.[38] The SFQ, in addition to being able to discriminate between HSDD, FSAD, and FOD, is also able to detect the presence of sexual pain disorders and discriminate between them.

THE INFLUENCE OF CULTURE

The Study of Women's health Across the Nation (SWAN) used phone and clinic-based interviews to establish the rates of sexual dysfunction in 3167 white, African American, Hispanic, Chinese, and Japanese women, aged 42 to 52 years, who were not using hormones.[43] Researchers found that premenopausal women reported less pain with intercourse than perimenopausal women ($P = .01$), but these 2 groups did not differ in frequency of intercourse, desire, arousal, or physical or emotional satisfaction. Relationships factors, the perceived importance of sex, attitudes toward aging, and vaginal dryness were the variables having the greatest association across all outcomes. Controlling for sociodemographic factors such as income, amount of education, and geography, significant ethnic differences were identified. African American women reported higher frequency of sexual intercourse than white women. Hispanic women reported lower physical pleasure and arousal. Both Chinese and Japanese women reported more pain, less desire, and less arousal that white women, although only the difference in arousal was statistically significant.

SEXUALITY THROUGHOUT THE DEVELOPMENTAL CONTINUUM: PERIMENOPAUSAL AND POSTMENOPAUSAL SEXUALITY

The end of the childbearing years often means the end of discussions about reproductive health between patient and provider. Although much has been made of how contraception has impacted women of childbearing age, few physicians have received adequate training in how to monitor a woman's sexual health through the menopausal transition and beyond, much less how to treat the sexual problems that can arise during this time. Apart from the menopause itself, women at mid-life are also subject to the typical diseases of both men and women in this demographic, and sexual functioning may be affected by the pathophysiology of these disease processes, as well as their treatment.

The Transition Defined

Reproductive stages are classified by changes in menstrual patterns and FSH levels.[44] The onset of the menopausal transition begins with fluctuations in GnRH, which alters the release of FSH and LH. Over the course of a woman's life, as ovulation proceeds, there is a steady decline in the number of follicles present in the ovaries. In general, sometime after age 40 years, the number of follicles is low enough to cause changes in menstruation. When increased release of FSH and LH can no longer compensate for the diminishing number of ovarian follicles, several hormonal changes emerge: androgen synthesis decreases in the theca cells (though the adrenals continue to produce a relatively small amount of androgens), estrogen levels decrease, and progesterone synthesis in the corpus luteum is reduced.[45] The final menstrual period (FMP) in the naturally menopausal woman signals ovarian failure.

One year after FMP, a woman is considered to be postmenopausal. The hypothalamus and anterior pituitary gland continue to function throughout a woman's life. In early menopause FSH and LH levels increase to as much as 20 times their premenopausal levels as LH and FSH attempt to stimulate the production of hormones in the follicle-depleted ovaries.[46] FSH and LH levels decline steadily after age 55, and continue to decline until age 70 years.

Decreased estrogen leads to atrophy in genital tissues. The uterus decreases in size, and the vulva and vagina lose thickness and vascularity. Secretions from the cervix and Bartholin glands decrease, contributing to vaginal dryness. Changes in vaginal flora lead to decreased acid production and increased pH. Vaginal atrophy and dryness may lead to pruritus, dyspareunia, and increased rates of infection. Estrogen is essential in maintaining the integrity of pelvic connective tissue, and its withdrawal during menopause can result in decreased strength in pelvic ligaments, increasing the risk of urinary stress incontinence and prolapse of both the uterus and bladder.[47]

The relationship between vaginal atrophy due to diminishing estrogen levels during menopause and the increased occurrence of dyspareunia is also unclear. Postmenopausal dyspareunia is usually thought to result from atrophy of the vaginal wall tissue, leading to difficulty in lubrication. However, a 1997 Danish study found that while decreasing estrogen levels during menopause were significantly associated with vaginal atrophy, there was not an association with vaginal dryness or dyspareunia.[48]

Breast tissues are also sensitive to the withdrawal of estrogen. Many postmenopausal women experience decreased tactile sensitivity in their breasts. Decreased estrogen leads to diminished fat content in the breasts, as well as decreased nipple sensitivity and erection during sexual arousal. These changes mean that greater stimulation is required to achieve sexual excitement.[49]

Decreased levels of bioavailable testosterone may lead to symptoms of androgen insufficiency, characterized by a diminished sense of well-being or dysphoric mood, persistent and unexplained fatigue, and sexual function changes such as decreased libido, diminished sexual receptivity, and reduced pleasure.[50] Overall, these changes in brain and genital function and anatomy may contribute to an increase in the prevalence of sexual disorders among postmenopausal women.

A prevailing myth about the menopausal transition is that the end of a woman's fertility signals the end of her sex life. Although many women experience problems with sexual function, recent advances in the understanding of FSD allow effective interventions for many of these problems. Recent studies have suggested that the prevalence of sexual complaints increases during the menopausal transition, and that hormonal changes that occur during the menopausal transition have a negative impact on sexual function.[51] From early to late in the menopausal transition, the percentage of women with scores on the McCoy Female Sexuality Questionnaire indicating sexual dysfunction was found to increase from 42% to 88%. More severe sexual dysfunction was correlated with decreasing estrogen, but not with level of free testosterone. By the postmenopausal period, significant decline was found in several areas of sexual response, including: sexual excitement and interest, frequency of sexual intercourse, and overall satisfaction with sexual function. Significant increases were reported in vaginal dryness and dyspareunia. Low satisfaction with partner sexual function was also significantly correlated with poor sexual function. Women with low scores on the Sexuality Questionnaire were more likely to report distress about their sexuality.[52]

However, the results of recent trials investigating the role of testosterone in post-menopausal sexual function have not yet yielded concise clinical recommendations. A recent Australian study of 1021 women aged 18 to 75 years seen in a community-based setting examined the role of multiple androgens in female sexual function. A low PFSF domain score for sexual responsiveness for women aged 45 years or older was associated with higher odds of having a serum dehydroepiandrosterone sulfate (DHEAS) level below the 10th percentile for this age group (odds ratio 3.90, $P = .004$). However, the majority of women with low DHEAS levels did not have low sexual function. No single androgen level, including free testosterone, was found to be predictive of sexual function.

To better examine the role of relationship factors in women's sexual functioning at mid-life, a recent Australian study interviewed 438 women ages 45 to 55 years who were still menstruating at the time of their baseline interview.[53] Eight years of longitudinal data were available for 336 of these women, none of whom underwent surgical or medication-induced menopause. Sexual response was found to be predicted by prior level of sexual function, change in partner status, feelings for partner, and estrogen level. Significant predictors of dyspareunia included premenopausal history of dyspareunia and, contrary to the 1997 Danish study cited earlier, estrogen levels. Frequency of sexual activity was predicted by prior level of sexual function and response, change in partner status, and feelings for partner. In all, prior sexual function and relationship factors were found to be more important than hormonal determinants of sexual function in perimenopausal women.

INTERVENTIONS
Psychological Treatment

For both the contemporary clinician and women suffering from FSD, the most important first step is education about anatomy, physiology, and expectations. Disparities in sexual desire between partners can be addressed in couple's therapy, and should not necessarily be interpreted as a problem with low desire. Duration of sexual activity is an important factor in determining if a woman has received adequate stimulation. For women that have never, or rarely, been able to experience orgasm, either alone or with a partner, directed masturbation (DM) is a technique that has been shown to be highly effective,[54] with success rates of greater than 65%.[55] Other women are able to orgasm while masturbating, but find the pressure of a sexual encounter with their partner too anxiety provoking. Masters and Johnson addressed this problem with *sensate focus* (SF), which dictated programmatic, progressive levels of touching, starting with nonsexual touching, progressing to more sexual touching, and eventual intercourse or other direct genital stimulation. Various other techniques have attempted to reduce the anxiety surrounding sexual encounters, falling under the moniker of systematic desensitization (SD), which entails exposure to sexually explicit material.

Some women experience pervasive anxiety, or other mood symptoms, that are also manifest during sexual activity. Cognitive-behavioral therapy (CBT) uses thought records to capture the cognitions that accompany these emotions. McCabe found that the use of CBT in conjunction with SF, SD, and DM reduced anorgasmia in a sample of sexually dysfunctional women from 66% to 11%.[56]

Lubricants

Lubricants can clearly help with vaginal dryness and resulting dyspareunia, and subsequently improve orgasmic function without any long-term safety concerns. In addition, lubricants can be used in combination with other treatments for sexual dysfunction associated with the menopausal transition. The primary objection to this intervention is displeasure with the mechanical interruption to sexual activity required for vaginal application.

Pharmacotherapy

Various agents have been tested to address FSD, and some have shown a degree of preliminary success. The vasoactive agent, sildenafil, demonstrated efficacy in the treatment of FOD, though larger subsequent studies failed to demonstrate separation from placebo.[57] In a recent study, 50 to 100 mg/d of sildenafil was found to be superior to placebo in effects on arousal and orgasmic dysfunction in premenopausal women with SSRI-induced arousal or orgasmic problems. Better results were seen in women with higher levels of thyroxine and testosterone, which enhances NO function. Despite more than 80% of the women complaining of decreased desire at study baseline, low desire was unaffected by sildenafil treatment.[58]

The non-SSRI bupropion has been studied in women with FSD, and has been found superior to placebo in improving sexual desire and decreasing distress in nondepressed premenopausal women with HSSD.[59,60] Results with bupropion in FOD were less robust.[61] Studies of women with SSRI-induced sexual dysfunction have demonstrated statistical improvements in desire, and clinical improvements in arousal and orgasm with bupropion SR 300 to 400 mg/d.[62] Some of the difficulties in demonstrating superiority of new treatments to placebo may be related to difficulties in defining the study population, lack of validation of outcome measures, and problems obtaining long-term safety data. Unfortunately, Food and Drug Administration (FDA)-approved treatments for FSD remain an unaccomplished goal of medical science.

Hormones

The increase in vasomotor symptoms and FSD during menopause is due, in part, to decreasing levels of available sex steroids. Providing an exogenous source for these hormones is the most straightforward approach to ameliorating these symptoms, with a goal of returning a woman's body to an endocrine milieu closer to its premenopausal state. A meta-analysis of 192 randomized controlled trials showed that estrogen therapy, alone or in a combination form, remains the most reliable, effective therapy for relieving the vasomotor symptoms of menopause, as well as, the associated sexual dysfunction.[63]

However, controversy stemming from the publication of the Women's Health Initiative (WHI) findings has led to concerns that a small percentage of women who use hormone replacement therapy (HRT) may suffer an increased rate of cardiovascular disease, cerebrovascular disease, blood clots, and breast and ovarian cancers.[64–66] Since the publication of the WHI, many clinicians and patients have determined that the increased risk of these serious side effects is small for the individual patient, and in some cases the severity of postmenopausal symptoms may warrant the use of exogenous hormones as a treatment, at least through the perimenopause.[67]

Although several trials have reported that estrogen replacement therapy (ERT) leads to increased desire for sex in postmenopausal women,[68] there have been few randomized placebo-controlled trials in this cohort.[69] A Danish study showed that long-term HRT positively and significantly affected hot flushes, sleep difficulties, sexual problems of decreased libido and dyspareunia, and blood pressure.[70] Libido and problems with mood swings improved in the HRT group more than in the placebo group.

For women experiencing vaginal atrophy and who do not wish to take systemic estrogen, topical estrogen creams may be a solution. Limited randomized controlled trials have shown that low-dose local vaginal estrogen delivery as treatment for vaginal atrophy is effective and well tolerated.[71] All approved vaginal estrogen products in the United States seem equally effective at the doses recommended in their labeling.

Transdermal delivery is another effective route of estrogen administration. Pharmacodynamic differences between oral and transdermal routes of estrogen administration suggest that transdermal estrogen exerts minimal effects on the concentrations of total and bioavailable testosterone, thyroxine, and cortisol, compared with oral estrogen.[72] In particular, free testosterone levels were higher by 16.4% with transdermal estrogen.

Although putative natural progestin-containing creams are efficacious in the treatment of menopausal symptoms when combined with estrogen, patients should be cautioned that these creams may increase sex hormones to levels seen with oral preparations. Although it is unlikely that topical estrogen preparations will affect serum estrogen levels to the same degree as oral HRT, perhaps due to differences in first-pass metabolism with these 2 routes of administration, care should still be taken to avoid using these products in women who should not be exposed to any exogenous sources of estrogen (eg, women with a history of estrogen-receptor positive breast cancer).

A testosterone patch was studied in the early 2000s for the treatment of HSDD in surgically menopausal women. A randomized placebo-controlled study found statistically significant increases in sexual desire and frequency of satisfying sexual encounters among the group of women received the 300 µg/d dose.[73] The 150 µg/d dose showed no significant improvement in either of these outcomes, whereas the 450 µg/d showed no improvement in these outcomes greater than those achieved at the 300 µg/d dose. Another study assessed the efficacy and safety of the 300 µg/d testosterone patch during 24 weeks of administration in surgically menopausal women with HSDD on concomitant estrogen therapy.[74] In this cohort, the 300 µg/d patch was found to significantly increase satisfying sexual activity and sexual desire, and decrease personal distress. Although the incidence of adverse events was similar in both groups ($P>.05$), the incidence of androgenic adverse events (eg, acne, hirsutism) was higher in the testosterone group, though most were mild. While being approved for use in postmenopausal women in the European Union, the testosterone patch failed to gain FDA approval in 2004 due to concerns over long-term safety.

Tibolone

Tibolone is a synthetic steroid sex hormone with estrogenic, androgenic, and progestogenic effects, available in the European Union. In a recent study, 48 postmenopausal women were randomized to tibolone versus estrogen-progesterone HRT for a 3-month treatment period.[75] Based on subjective qualitative scores on the Greene Climacteric Scale (GCS) and McCoy Female Sexuality Questionnaire, tibolone treatment was found to be at least as effective as HRT in improving quality of life. Tibolone was superior to HRT in perceived improvement of sexual performance, including general sexual satisfaction, sexual interest, sexual fantasies, sexual arousal, and orgasm, with decreased frequency of vaginal dryness and dyspareunia. Another study compared tibolone to transdermal estradiol (E2)/norethisterone (NETA) (50 µg/120 µg) in naturally postmenopausal women with FSD.[76] Self-reported FSFI scores, and FSDS scores indicated that both treatments resulted in improved overall sexual function, evidenced by increased frequency of sexual events, and reduction in sexuality-related personal distress. A significantly larger increase in FSFI total scores was seen in the tibolone group compared with the E2/NETA group, with nonsignificant group differences in FSDS scores, although decreases in distress were found in both groups.

SUMMARY

Problems with desire, arousal, and orgasmic function are common in women, but associated distress reduces the rates of sexual disorders to less than 10% of the general population. Comorbid sexual disorders and medical/psychiatric conditions may complicate diagnosis and treatment, particularly in peri- and postmenopausal women. Currently available interventions include psychotherapy, targeted sexual therapies, and pharmacologic treatments. Further research into diagnosis and potential treatments for sexual disorders in women are anticipated to enhance sexual function and satisfaction throughout women's lives.

REFERENCES

1. Kinsey A. Sexual behavior in the human female. Philadelphia: Saunders; 1953.
2. Sand M, Fisher WA. Women's endorsement of models of female sexual response: the nurses' sexuality study. J Sex Med 2007;4:708–19.
3. Braunstein GD. Androgen insufficiency in women: summary of critical issues. Fertil Steril 2002;77(Suppl 4):S94–9.
4. Hull EM, Eaton RC, Moses J, et al. Copulation increases dopamine activity in the medial preoptic area of male rats. Life Sci 1993;52:935–40.
5. Segraves RT. Effects of psychotropic drugs on human erection and ejaculation. Arch Gen Psychiatry 1989;46:275–84.
6. Lee AW, Pfaff DW. Hormone effects on specific and global brain functions. J Physiol Sci 2008;58(4):213–20.
7. Done CJ, Sharp T. Evidence that 5-HT2 receptor activation decreases noradrenaline release in rat hippocampus in vivo. Br J Pharmacol 1992;107:240–5.
8. Frolich PF, Meston CM. Evidence that serotonin affects female sexual functioning via peripheral mechanisms. Physiol Behav 2000;71:383–93.
9. Watson NV, Gorzalka BB. Concurrent wet dog shaking and inhibition of male rat copulation after ventromedial brainstem injection of the 5-HT2 agonist DOI. Neurosci Lett 1992;141:25–9.
10. D'Amati G, di Gioia CRT, Bologna M, et al. Type 5 phosphodiesterase expression in the human vagina. Urology 2002;60:191–5.
11. Palle C, Bredkajer HE, Ottesen B, et al. Vasoactive intestinal polypeptide in human vaginal blood flow: comparison between transvaginal and intravenous administration. Clin Exp Pharmacol Physiol 1990;17:61–8.
12. Marin R, Escrig A, Abreu P, et al. Androgen-dependent nitric oxide release in rat penis correlates with levels of constitutive nitric oxide synthetase isoenzymes. Biol Reprod 2002;61:1012–6.
13. Giuliano F, Allard J, Compagnie S, et al. Vaginal physiological changes in a model of sexual arousal in anesthetized rats. Am J Physiol Regul Integr Comp Physiol 2001;281(1):R140–9.
14. Kruger TH, Hartmann U, Schedlowski M. Prolactinergic and dopaminergic mechanisms underlying sexual arousal and orgasm in humans. World J Urol 2005; 23(2):130–8.
15. Stahl SM. The psychopharmacology of sex, part 2, effects of drugs and disease on the 3 phases of human sexual response. J Clin Psychiatry 2001;62(3):147–8.
16. Clayton A, Ramamurthy S. The impact of physical illness on sexual dysfunction. In: Balon R, editor. Sexual Dysfunction: the brain body connection. Adv Psychosom Med. Basel: Karger; 2008. p. 70–88.

17. Montejo AL, Llorca G, Izquierdo JA, et al. Incidence of sexual dysfunction associated with antidepressant agents: a prospective multicenter study of 1022 outpatients. J Clin Psychiatry 2001;62(Suppl 3):10–21.
18. Clayton AH, Pradko JF, Croft HA, et al. Prevalence of sexual dysfunction among newer antidepressants. J Clin Psychiatry 2002;63:357–66.
19. Clayton A, Kornstein S, Prakash A, et al. Changes in sexual functioning associated with duloxetine, escitalopram and placebo in the treatment of patients with major depressive disorder. J Sex Med 2007;4:917–29.
20. American Psychiatric Association. Diagnostic and statistical manual of mental disorders. Text revision. 4th edition. Washington, DC: American Psychiatric Association; 2000.
21. Nusbaum MRH, Helton MR, Ray N. The changing nature of women's sexual health concerns through the midlife years. Maturitas 2004;49:283–91.
22. Bancroft J, Loftus J, Long JS. Distress about sex: a national survey of women in heterosexual relationships. Arch Sex Behav 2003;32:193–208.
23. Derogatis LR, Burnett AL. The epidemiology of sexual dysfunctions. J Sex Med 2008;5(2):289–300.
24. Hayes RD, Dennerstein L, Bennett CM, et al. Relationship between hypoactive sexual desire disorder and aging. Fertil Steril 2007;87(1):107–12.
25. Shifren JL, Monz BU, Russo PA, et al. Sexual problems and distress in United States women. Obstet Gynecol 2008;112(5):970–8.
26. Arnow BA, Millheiser L, Garrett A, et al. Women with hypoactive sexual desire disorder compared to normal females: a functional magnetic resonance imaging study. Neuroscience 2009;158:484–502.
27. Georgiadis JR, Kortekaas R, Kuipers R, et al. Regional cerebral blood flow changes associated with clitorally induced orgasm in healthy women. Eur J Neurosci 2006;24:3305–16.
28. Komisaruk BR, Whipple B, Crawford A, et al. Brain activity (fMRI and PET) during orgasm in women, in response to vaginocervical self-stimulation. Abstr Soc Neurosci 2002;841:17.
29. Dunn KM, Cherkas LF, Spector TD. Genetic influences on variation in female orgasmic function: a twin study. Biol Lett 2005;1(3):260–3.
30. Dawood K, Kirk KM, Bailey JM, et al. Genetic and environmental influences on the frequency of orgasm in women. Twin Res Hum Genet 2006;9(4):603–8.
31. Wallen K, Lloyd EA. Clitoral variability compared with penile variability supports nonadaptation of female orgasm. Evol Dev 2008;10(1):1–2.
32. Bishop JR, Moline J, Ellingrod VL, et al. Serotonin 2A-1438 G-A and G-protein beta3 subunit C825T polymorphisms in patients with depression and SSRI-associated sexual side effects. Neuropsychopharmacology 2006;31:2281–8.
33. Bishop JR, Ellingrod VL, Akroush M, et al. The association of serotonin transporter genotypes and selective serotonin reuptake inhibitor (SSRI)-associated sexual side effects: possible relationship to oral contraceptives. Hum Psychopharmacol 2009;24:207–15.
34. Ben Zion IZ, Tessler R, Cohen L, et al. Polymorphisms in the dopamine D4 receptor gene (DRD4) contribute to individual differences in human sexual behavior: desire arousal, and sexual function. Mol Psychiatry 2006;11(8):782–6.
35. Leiblum SR, Koochaki PE, Rodenberg CA, et al. Sexual desire disorder in postmenopausal women: US results from the Women's International Study of Health and Sexuality (WISHeS). Menopause 2006;13(1):46–56.
36. Clayton AH, Goldfischer ER, Goldstein I, et al. Validation of the decreased sexual desire screener (DSDS): a brief diagnostic instrument for generalized acquired female hypoactive sexual desire disorder (HSDD). J Sex Med 2009;6:730–8.

37. Goldfischer ER, Clayton AH, Goldstein I, et al. Decreased sexual desire screener (DSDS) for diagnosis of hypoactive sexual desire disorder in women. Obstet Gynecol 2008;111:109.
38. American Psychiatric Association. Diagnostic and statistical manual of mental disorders. 4th edition, text revision. Washington, DC: American Psychiatric Association; 2000. p. 543, 549, 556, 558.
39. Quirk F, Haughie S, Symonds T. The use of the sexual function questionnaire as a screening tool for women with sexual dysfunction. J Sex Med 2005;2:469–77.
40. Sand M, Rosen R, Meston C, et al. The female sexual function index (FSFI): a potential "gold standard" measure for assessing sexual function in women, Poster 24, 3rd International Consultation on Sexual Medicine, Paris, July 10–13, 2009.
41. Levin RJ. Sexual desire and the deconstruction and reconstruction of the human female response model of Masters and Johnson. In: Everaerd W, Laan E, Both S, editors. Sexual appetite, desire and motivation: energetics of the sexual system. Amsterdam (The Netherlands): Royal Netherlands Academy of Arts and Sciences; 2001. p. 63–93.
42. Gregersen N, Jensen PT, Giraldi AGE. Sexual dysfunction in the peri- and postmenopause. Status of incidence, pharmacological treatment and possible risks. A secondary publication. Dan Med Bull 2006;53(3):349–53.
43. Avis NE, Zhao X, Johannes CB, et al. Correlates of sexual function among multiethnic middle-aged women: results from the Study of Women's Health Across the Nation (SWAN). Menopause 2005;12(4):385–98.
44. Arroyo A, Yeh J. Understanding the menopause transition and managing its clinical challenges. Sex Reprod Menopause 2006;3:12–7.
45. Weismiller D. The perimenopause and menopause experience: an overview. Clin Geriatr Med 2003;20:565–70.
46. Hall J. Neuroendocrine physiology of the early and late menopause. Endocrinol Metab Clin North Am 2004;33:637–59.
47. Wilson MM. Menopause. Clin Geriatr Med 2003;19(3):483–506.
48. Laan E, van Lunsen RH. Hormones and sexuality in postmenopausal women: a psychophysiological study. J Psychosom Obstet Gynaecol 1997;18(2):126–33.
49. Phillips NA. Female sexual dysfunction: evaluation and treatment. Am Fam Physician 2000;62(1):127–36, 141–2.
50. Bachmann G, Bancroft J, Braunstein G, et al. Female androgen insufficiency: the Princeton consensus statement on definition, classification, and assessment. Fertil Steril 2002;77(4):660–5.
51. Bachmann GA, Leiblum SR. The impact of hormones on menopausal sexuality: a literature review. Menopause 2004;11:120–30.
52. Dennerstein L, Alexander JL, Kotz K. The menopause and sexual functioning: a review of the population-based studies. Annu Rev Sex Res 2003;14:64–82.
53. Dennerstein L, Lehert P, Burger H. The relative effects of hormones and relationship factors on sexual function of women through the natural menopausal transition. Fertil Steril 2005;84(1):174–80.
54. Heiman JR. Orgasmic disorders in women. In: Leiblum SR, Rosen RC, editors. Principles and practice of sex therapy. 3rd edition. New York: Guildford Press; 2000. p. 84–123.
55. McMullen S, Rosen RC. Self-administered masturbation training in the treatment of primary orgasmic dysfunction. J Consult Clin Psychol 1979;47:912–8.
56. McCabe MP. Evaluation of a cognitive behavioral therapy program for people with sexual dysfunction. J Sex Marital Ther 2001;27:259–71.
57. Shields KM, Hrometz SL. Use of sildenafil for female sexual dysfunction. Ann Pharmacother 2006;40(5):931–4.

58. Nurnberg HG, Hensley PL, Heiman JR, et al. Sildenafil treatment of women with antidepressant-associated sexual dysfunction: a randomized controlled trial. JAMA 2008;300(4):395–404.
59. Segraves RT, Croft H, Kavoussi R, et al. Bupropion sustained release (SR) for the treatment of hypoactive sexual desire disorder (HSDD) in nondepressed women. J Sex Marital Ther 2001;27(3):303–16.
60. Modell JG, May RS, Katholi CR. Effect of bupropion-SR on orgasmic dysfunction in nondepressed subjects: a pilot study. J Sex Marital Ther 2000;26(3):231–40.
61. Seagraves RT, Clayton AH, Croft H, et al. A multicenter, double-blind, placebo-controlled study of bupropion XL in females with orgasm disorder. Abstracts of the 19th Annual U.S. Psychiatric & Mental Health Congress, November, 2006.
62. Clayton AH, Warnock JK, Kornstein SG, et al. A placebo-controlled trial of bupropion SR as an antidote for selective serotonin reuptake inhibitor-induced sexual dysfunction. J Clin Psychiatry 2004;65:62–7.
63. Nelson H, Haney H, Miller J, et al. Management of menopause-related symptoms: summary. (Evidence Rep Technology Assessment No. 120, AHQR Publ. No. 05-E016-1), Rockville (MD): agency for Healthcare Research and Quality. As cited by Petersen M. In: Tepper MS, Owens AF, editors. Menopause and sexuality in sexual health. Westport (CT): Praeger Press; 2007.
64. Rossouw JE, Prentice RL, Manson JE, et al. Postmenopausal hormone therapy and risk of cardiovascular disease by age and years since menopause. JAMA 2007;297(13):1465–77.
65. Wassertheil-Smoller S, Hendrix SL, Limacher M, et al. Effect of estrogen plus progestin on stroke in postmenopausal women: the Women's Health Initiative: a randomized trial. JAMA 2003;289(20):2673–84.
66. Rossouw JE, Anderson GL, Prentice RL, et al. Risks and benefits of estrogen plus progestin in healthy postmenopausal women: principal results from the Women's Health Initiative randomized controlled trial. JAMA 2002;288(3):321–33.
67. Dennerstein G. Re: hormones down under: hormone therapy use after the women's health initiative. Aust N Z J Obstet Gynaecol 2006;47(1):80.
68. Modelska K, Cummings S. Female sexual dysfunction in postmenopausal women: systematic review of placebo-controlled trials. Am J Obstet Gynecol 2003;188(1):286–93.
69. Sherwin BB. The impact of different doses of estrogen and progestin on mood and sexual behavior in postmenopausal women. J Clin Endocrinol Metab 1991; 72:336–43.
70. Vestergaard P, Hermann AP, Stilgren L, et al. Effects of 5 years of hormonal replacement therapy on menopausal symptoms and blood pressure—a randomised controlled study. Maturitas 2003;46(2):123–32.
71. North American Menopause Society. The role of local vaginal estrogen for treatment of vaginal atrophy in postmenopausal women: 2007 position statement of The North American Menopause Society. Menopause 2007;14(3 Pt 1):355–69.
72. Shifren JL, Desindes S, McIlwain M, et al. A randomized, open-label, crossover study comparing the effects of oral versus transdermal estrogen therapy on serum androgens, thyroid hormones, and adrenal hormones in naturally menopausal women. Menopause 2007;14(6):985–94.
73. Braunstein GD, Sundwall DA, Katz M, et al. Safety and efficacy of a testosterone patch for the treatment of hypoactive sexual desire disorder in surgically menopausal women: a randomized, placebo-controlled trial. Arch Intern Med 2005; 165(14):1582–9.

74. Buster JE, Kingsberg SA, Aguirre O, et al. Testosterone patch for low sexual desire in surgically menopausal women: a randomized trial. Obstet Gynecol 2005;105:944–52.

75. Wu MH, Pan HA, Wang ST, et al. Quality of life and sexuality changes in postmenopausal women receiving tibolone therapy. Climacteric 2001;4(4):314–9.

76. Nijland EA, Weijmar Schultz WC, Nathorst-Boos J, et al. Tibolone and transdermal E2/NETA for the treatment of female sexual dysfunction in naturally menopausal women: results of a randomized active-controlled trial. J Sex Med 2008;5(3): 646–56.

Women and Tobacco Dependence

Virginia C. Reichert, NP[a],*, Vicki Seltzer, MD[b],
Linda S. Efferen, MD[c,d], Nina Kohn, MBA, MA[e]

KEYWORDS

• Nicotine addiction • Carbon monoxide • Gender discrepancies

Millions of American girls and women have been drawn to smoking by an industry that has been clearly and systematically targeting women of all ages and life circumstances. Tobacco marketing strategies skillfully link cigarette use to typical female values: independence; self-reliance; weight control; stress management; social progress and popularity; personal attractiveness; autonomy; self-fulfillment; youth; happiness; personal success; health; and active, vigorous, and strenuous lifestyles. Biologically speaking, women are especially vulnerable to the legion of health problems of tobacco use. Smoking is a critical hazard for women in their reproductive years, particularly when they are pregnant.[1]

More than 1 billion people smoke worldwide, and 200 million of them are women. Cigarette smoking is the leading cause of preventable death in the United States and women's share of tobacco-related disease has risen dramatically over the past half century. The point is underscored by the 600% increase since 1950 in women's death rates for lung cancer, a disease that is primarily attributable to smoking. Lung cancer accounted for only 3% of all female cancer deaths in 1950, whereas in 2000 it accounted for an estimated 25%.[2] In fact, more women are estimated to have died of lung cancer in the year 2000 than of cancers of the breast, uterus, and ovary combined. Of course, lung cancer is but one of the many diseases for which risk is greater among smokers than nonsmokers.

The World Health Organization estimates that the number of women smoking will almost triple over the next generation to more than 500 million.[3] Of these, more

---

This article is an updated version of the article "Women and Tobacco Dependence," that appeared in *Medical Clinics of North America* (Volume 88, Issue 6, November 2004).

[a] Stony Brook University Medical Center, Stony Brook, NY 11790, USA

[b] Obstetrics and Gynecology, North Shore University Hospital and Long Island Jewish Medical Center, 36 Bacon Road, Old Westbury, NY 11568, USA

[c] Department of Medicine, Albert Einstein College of Medicine, New York, NY, USA

[d] South Nassau Community Hospital, Oceanside, NY, USA

[e] Biostatistics Unit, North Shore Long Island Jewish Research Institute, 1129 Northern Boulevard, Suite 302, Manhasset, NY 11030, USA

* Corresponding author.

E-mail address: virginia.reichert@stonybrook.edu (V.C. Reichert).

doi:10.1016/j.ogc.2009.10.003
0889-8545/09/$ – see front matter © 2009 Elsevier Inc. All rights reserved.

than 200 million will die prematurely of smoking-related diseases. The biggest rise in female smoking will be in less developed countries, where the current rate of approximately 7% is projected to increase to 20% by 2025. There can be no complacency about the lower level of global tobacco use among women; it does not reflect health awareness, but rather social traditions and women's low economic resources.[4]

It is generally thought that the cessation rate for female smokers is lower than for male smokers. It is not clear, however, whether this is because women are less likely to attempt to quit or because they are less likely to remain abstinent when they do quit. The study by Zhu and colleagues[5] used four population surveys (three cross-sectional and one longitudinal) to show that women are neither less likely to try to quit than men, nor less likely to stay abstinent after they do quit than men.

Another study by Gonzales and colleagues[6] on the effects of gender on relapse prevention in smokers treated with bupropion sustained release found there to be no significant differences by gender within treatment groups. In addition, median time to relapse was also equal for men and women within treatment groups in that study.

Other researchers, however, have observed conflicting results in gender discrepancies related to the cessation of smoking. Bohadana and colleagues[7] found women to be less successful than men at quitting. In this study, male versus female complete abstinence rates, regardless of assigned treatment groups, were significantly different and less impressive among women at all measured time points over the 1-year follow-up.

In addition, Perkins[8] found that although women may be at greater risk of smoking-related diseases than men, women tended to have less success than men in quitting smoking. The difference in cessation rates for women versus men may be even greater in trials of nicotine-replacement therapies. This difference suggests that women benefit less from nicotine-replacement therapies relative to men, although it may depend on the particular form of nicotine-replacement therapy (eg, inhaler vs gum). Some of the non–nicotine-replacement therapy medications may reverse the poorer outcome of women producing quit rates in women comparable with those of men. In addition, gender differences in outcome and overall success rates with nicotine-replacement therapies and some of the non–nicotine-replacement therapy medications seem to be enhanced when treatment includes substantial behavioral counseling. The US Food and Drug Administration–approved medications for treating tobacco dependence are discussed elsewhere in this issue.

Since 2001, over 1460 smokers were treated for tobacco dependence at North Shore University Hospital's Center for Tobacco Control, part of the North Shore–Long Island Jewish Health System in New York. Participants had a mean age of 45.2 for men versus 48.6 for women ($P<.01$). Men had an average of 33 pack-years smoking versus 27 pack-years for women ($P<.01$). There was no difference between the genders in respect to age at the time of their first cigarette (16 years); Fagerstrom score, a validated instrument used to assess nicotine addiction (6.1 out of maximum of 10); or in the number (two) of previous quit attempts (**Table 1**).

Men and women differ in their reasons for smoking (**Table 2**). The questions listed in **Table 2** only reflect those questions adapted from the "Why do you smoke" questionnaire of the American Academy of Family Physicians that reflected significant discrepancies between the genders.[9]

Although men and women differ in their reasons for smoking, contrarily it was discovered that very few discrepancies existed between the genders in citing reasons for wanting to quit. Overwhelmingly, "concern for their health" was the most frequently cited reason for quitting by both groups. Despite being highly addicted to nicotine, only one third of the smokers cited that cigarettes controlled their lives (**Table 3**).

Table 1
Additional demographics of smokers from NS-LIJ health system

NS-LIJ Participant's Demographics	Males[a] N (%)	Females[a] N (%)	P Value[b]
Smokes light brand cigarettes	280 (63.1)	419 (71.9)	<.01
Doctor has advised to quit smoking	398 (87.1)	562 (91.5)	<.05
Believes that nicotine causes cancer	152 (59.4)	222 (71.8)	<.01
High readiness to quit=>7 of 10	319 (76)	404 (72.1)	NS
All comers quit success at 30 d	285 (59.1)	361 (54.9)	NS

The group program of the Center for Tobacco Control is a clinical program and the primary emphasis of which is to help smokers quit. Because the research aim is secondary, analysis is based on observation of the cohort of subjects who chose to attend the class, which resulted in potential bias in interpretation of data. As the program and data collection evolved, interim data collection questionnaires were added. This evolution is reflected in the changeable sample sizes of the various tables. In calculating the all-comer quit rate, however, dropouts were assumed to be smoking.
Abbreviation: NS, not significant.
[a] Total sample sizes vary from 256–482 (males) and 309–657 (females) because of nonresponse or changes in questionnaire over time.
[b] Chi-square test.

Two prominent obstacles to quitting smoking (and common reasons for relapse) for many American women are the management of day-to-day stress and fear of weight gain. Pomerleau and colleagues[10] looked at short-term weight changes (over 1 week) in women smokers and found the abstaining smokers (N = 7) gained 3.1 pounds, compared with 0.3 pounds in the women who continued to smoke (N = 13). In addition, weight gain in the women abstainers in the luteal phase of the menstrual cycle exceeded that in women abstainers in the follicular phase, a significant finding not seen in the group of women who continued to smoke.

It was also found that the identification of perceived obstacles before quitting helps smokers to anticipate difficult situations that may arise during the quitting process. Former participants have revealed that addressing these issues with behavioral modification was of help (**Table 4**).

For women who want to quit, timing the attempt according to their menstrual cycle may influence their success. Allen and colleagues[11] focused on the effects of a trans-dermal nicotine patch in women during acute smoking abstinence when tested in different phases of their menstrual cycle. Results showed that nicotine craving and premenstrual pain and water retention symptoms were diminished in women on the transdermal patch and that this effect was greatest in the late luteal phase. During short-term smoking abstinence in women, transdermal nicotine seemed to have a more pronounced effect in the late luteal phase than in the follicular phase in reducing craving and certain premenstrual symptoms.

For women in particular, tobacco-related diseases represent a cadre of preventable disease. The negative health effects of tobacco exposure are far reaching and extend from the impact of in utero exposure on fetal development and subsequent predisposition to the expression of lung disease, to an effect of tobacco exposure on many other disease processes.

Table 2
Significant gender discrepancies

NS-LIJ Health System Tobacco Dependence Program "Why do You Smoke?"	Smokers Who Responded "Always" or "Frequently"		
	Males (N = 261[a]) N (%)	Females (N = 336[a]) N (%)	P Value[b]
Smoking cigarettes is pleasant and relaxing	158 (62.9)	241 (74.4)	<.01
I light up a cigarette when I am upset about something	201 (77.3)	303 (90.2)	<.01
When I run out of cigarettes I find it unbearable until I can get more	143 (55.4)	242 (72.7)	<.01
Part of my enjoyment of smoking comes from the steps I take to light up	24 (9.2)	54 (16.4)	<.05
When I feel uncomfortable or upset about something, I light up a cigarette	190 (73.4)	305 (91)	<.01
When I feel down or want to take my mind off cares and worries, I smoke a cigarette	122 (46.9)	237 (70.5)	<.01
I get a real gnawing hunger for a cigarette when I haven't smoked for a while	165 (64)	255 (76.6)	<.01
I worry that my smoking has given or will give me cancer	167 (64.5)	249 (75)	<.01
I often feel guilty about my smoking	161 (61.7)	257 (77.2)	<.01

[a] Total sample sizes vary from 251–61 (males) and 324–36 (females) because of nonresponse.
[b] Chi-square test.
Data from American Academy of Family Physicians. Why do you smoke quiz. Available at: http://familydoctor.org. Accessed August 16, 2001.

ADVERSE EFFECTS OF SMOKING ON FERTILITY

Smoking has been demonstrated to have potential adverse effects on several independent components of reproductive function including tubal function, ectopic pregnancy risk, ovulatory function, oocyte depletion, and risk for spontaneous abortion. Clinical effects have been demonstrated with an increased risk for ectopic pregnancy and spontaneous abortion.

The risk for ectopic pregnancy may be doubled in women who smoke.[12] In animal studies nicotine was shown to have an effect on fallopian tube motility, which may contribute to the increased risk for ectopic pregnancy in smokers.

The risk for spontaneous abortion may be significantly greater in women who smoke. This increased risk has been demonstrated in two studies of women who were undergoing in vitro fertilization. In one study, the incidence of spontaneous abortion was 73% in smokers and 24% in nonsmokers.[13] In another study, the spontaneous abortion rate was 42.1% in smokers and 18.9% in nonsmokers.[14] This difference was despite the fact that the number of eggs retrieved, fertilization rate, and implantation rate were controlled.

Table 3
Why are you quitting smoking?

NS-LIJ Participant's Reasons for Quitting	Males[a] N (%)	Females[a] N (%)	P Value[b]
Pressure from family friends	181 (41.9)	216 (37.6)	NS
General health concerns	373 (80.9)	500 (80.8)	NS
Pressure from their doctor	76 (17.6)	124 (21.6)	NS
A recent change in health status	70 (16.1)	109 (18.8)	NS
Expense of cigarettes	162 (37.4)	245 (42)	NS
Smell: odor from tobacco	104 (24.1)	193 (33.4)	<.01
Cigarettes control my life	156 (36.2)	219 (38.2)	NS

Abbreviation: NS, not significant.
[a] Total sample sizes vary from 431–61 (males) or 574–619 (females) because of nonresponse or changes in questionnaire over time.
[b] Chi-square test.

Smoking may have an adverse effect on a woman's ovulatory function. Regular menstrual cycles are directly correlated with regular ovulation. One large study found that heavy smokers had a 67% higher likelihood of having abnormal vaginal bleeding than nonsmokers.[15] Smoking may result in oocyte depletion because smokers have an earlier onset of menopause.[16]

ADVERSE EFFECTS OF SMOKING ON PREGNANCY OUTCOME

Smoking during pregnancy is associated with an overall increased risk for perinatal mortality.[17] Carbon monoxide and nicotine are the main components in smoking that are responsible for adverse effects on fetal outcome.[17]

Smoking during pregnancy has been associated with an increased risk for placenta previa,[18] placental abruption,[19] premature rupture of the membranes,[20] low birth weight,[21] intrauterine growth restriction,[21] and prematurity.[22] A variety of histologic changes have been found more commonly in the placentas of smokers. These

Table 4
Perceived obstacles to this quit attempt

NS-LIJ Participants' Perceived Obstacles to Quitting	Males[a] N (%)	Females[a] N (%)	P Value[b]
Smoke for stress relief	242 (55)	369 (63.1)	<.01
Live with someone who still smokes	71 (16.5)	117 (20.5)	N.S.
Fear of weight gain	63 (14.6)	238 (41.1)	<.01
Unbearable cravings	196 (45.5)	234 (41)	NS
Fear of failure	46 (10.7)	101 (17.5)	<.01
Social situations	62 (17.7)	116 (24.3)	<.05
Enjoyment: I like smoking	168 (48)	219 (45.8)	NS

Abbreviation: NS, not significant.
[a] Total sample sizes vary from 350–440 (males) or 578–85 (females) because of nonresponse or changes in questionnaire over time.
[b] Chi-square test.

changes are ones that are often associated with ischemia and chronic oxygen deprivation.

During the past decade there has been an increasing amount of data available on the adverse effects of smoking on pregnancy outcome. Physicians and the entire health care community have become quite knowledgeable about these adverse effects. Yet, in the United States today, approximately 21% of women smoke cigarettes. Although pregnant women often try to stop smoking, smoking rates for pregnant teenagers are the highest among groups of pregnant women, with 19% of pregnant 18- to 19-year olds smoking.[23] In addition, self-reported smoking cessation rates during pregnancy may be substantially inflated, as is suggested by comparing self-reporting with cotinine salivary testing (**Box 1**).[17]

ADVERSE EFFECTS OF SMOKING ON THE INFANT

Smoking during pregnancy increases the likelihood of sudden infant death syndrome, and postnatal exposure of the infant to tobacco smoke further increases this risk.[24] Infants who have household exposure to cigarette smoke have a higher incidence of acute and chronic respiratory illnesses and may have an increased risk for ear infections.

If a woman who is breast feeding is a cigarette smoker, nicotine is passed to the newborn in the breast milk.[25] Dempsey and Benowitz[25] report that 95 minutes is the mean elimination half-life of nicotine from breast milk, and that there are higher levels of nicotine in the breast milk depending on how many cigarettes were smoked since the last breast feeding and the interval between the last cigarette smoked and breast feeding. Even though nicotine levels in breast milk may be lower if fewer cigarettes are smoked and there is an increased smoke-free time interval before breast feeding, there is still nicotine in breast milk if a woman smokes.

SMOKING AND CANCER RISK

During the past few decades, the very strong causal relationship between cigarette smoking and lung cancer has been proved. This is the malignancy that is most commonly associated with smoking and is the leading cause of cancer death in women. Cigarette smoking, however, is associated with many other cancers in women, including cancer of the bladder, bronchus, cervix, esophagus, kidney, lung, oropharynx, and pancreas.[26]

Box 1
Possible adverse effects of smoking on pregnancy outcome

- Intrauterine growth restriction
- Low birth weight
- Perinatal mortality
- Placental abruption
- Placenta previa
- Premature rupture of membranes
- Prematurity
- Spontaneous abortion

Approximately 12,800 women in the United States develop cervical cancer each year, and many times that number develop preinvasive cervical disease. Smoking seems to be an independent risk factor for preinvasive and invasive cervical cancer.

Pancreatic cancer is one of the five leading causes of cancer death in women in the United States. Pancreatic cancer is difficult to diagnose and cure rates are very poor, even with aggressive therapy. Cigarette smoking is associated with an increased risk for developing this very aggressive malignancy.

Although there has been an occasional report suggesting that there may possibly be a weak association between cigarette smoking and breast cancer,[27] most reports have failed to substantiate this association.[28] A recent article in the *Journal of the National Cancer Institute* is cause for increased concern, however, that active smoking may play a role in breast cancer etiology.[29] In this study, more than 100,000 women with no previous breast cancer diagnosis prospectively reported their smoking status. During the course of the study, 2005 of the women were newly diagnosed with invasive breast cancer. The incidence of breast cancer was higher among current smokers than among those who never smoked (**Box 2**).

CARDIOVASCULAR RISKS FOR WOMEN WHO SMOKE

Exposure to cigarette smoke and environmental tobacco smoke is a strong risk factor for cardiovascular disease in men and women. Along with hypercholesterolemia and hypertension, smoking represents one of the major acquired risk factors for the development of atherosclerotic disease. Cigarette smoking is clearly associated with an increased risk for atherosclerosis of the coronary, cerebral, and peripheral arteries. The precise mechanism by which coronary and cerebrovascular disease risk is increased is not completely understood. Endothelial cell dysfunction, lipid abnormalities, increase in thrombosis, and the antiestrogenic effect of cigarette smoking may all be related.

Smoking is also a major risk factor for acute coronary thrombosis[30] and sudden cardiac death. The risk for acute coronary heart disease is estimated to be approximately two times higher in smokers than in nonsmokers and it seems that smoking has a much larger detrimental effect on women than men despite the overall higher incidence of events in men compared with premenopausal women.[31] Current smoking has been associated with a higher risk for myocardial infarction in women compared with men in several studies; the effect seems to be more pronounced in women less

---

Box 2
Smoking and cancer risk

- Bladder
- Breast (controversial)
- Bronchus
- Cervix
- Esophagus
- Kidney
- Lung
- Oropharynx
- Pancreas

than 45 years of age[32] and to be related to the quantity of tobacco smoked,[33,34] Similarly, the relative risk for coronary death per cigarettes smoked has been shown to be higher in women than men.[35] In younger women, cigarette smoking has been identified as the predominant risk factor for sudden cardiac death,[36,37] which is in contradistinction to the more traditional risk factors, such as hypertension, hypercholesterolemia, and diabetes in older women. The mechanism of acute thrombosis and sudden coronary death in women seems to vary with age. Plaque erosion was seen most frequently as the underlying pathogenic mechanism in smokers who were younger and had less luminal narrowing than the coronary lesions present in the older age group, who more typically presented with plaque rupture.[38]

Cigarette smoking has also been associated with an increased risk for stroke in men and women. A dose-dependent increase has also been demonstrated for stroke risk in men and women without differences observed between the sexes.[31]

The impact of passive smoking on atherosclerotic disease is considered to be smaller than that associated with active smoking, but is an important risk factor for cardiovascular disease. The risk for death caused by ischemic heart disease in nonsmokers exposed to secondhand smoke is increased by approximately 30%.[38] As with active smoking, the effect seems to be dose related, and the detrimental effect may be greater on women than men.[31]

The acute effect of passive smoking on coronary circulation has been evaluated in nonsmokers and asymptomatic active smokers by evaluating the coronary flow velocity reserve, a measure of endothelial function in the coronary circulation.[39] A statistically significant difference at baseline was present between smokers and nonsmokers, before exposure to passive smoke, with nonsmokers having a higher coronary flow velocity reserve. Following passive smoke exposure, the coronary flow velocity reserve decreased significantly in the nonsmoking group and there was no longer any significant difference between the two groups. The results of this study were thought to provide direct evidence that the mechanism whereby passive smoking is a risk factor for cardiac disease morbidity and mortality in nonsmokers occurs by endothelial dysfunction of the coronary circulation.[39]

OSTEOPOROSIS AND SMOKING

Peak bone density is generally fully achieved by the beginning of the fourth decade of life after which there is a gradual bone loss of approximately 0.5% per year. Genetic and environmental factors affect peak bone mass and the rate of bone loss. Osteoporosis, a disease characterized by increased bone fragility and risk for fracture, is extremely common. Many risk factors for osteoporosis have been identified, most of which are predictors for low bone mineral density and include female sex, age, estrogen deficiency, and white or Asian race. The risk for fracture increases with age and is particularly pronounced in postmenopausal women. Other factors, including current cigarette smoking, increase the risk for fractures independent of bone mineral density.

Cigarette smoking is associated with a decrement in sex hormone concentrations and body weight, early menopause, increased bone-turnover markers, decreased calcium absorption and bone mineral density, and up to an 80% increase in risk for fracture.[40] Several case-control studies have demonstrated a several-fold increase in the likelihood of osteoporotic fracture in smokers compared with nonsmokers.[41] Although cigarette smoking has been clearly linked to osteoporosis and osteoporotic fractures, the effect of smokeless tobacco use, which is quite common in certain populations, remains to be further defined, although animal studies provide cause for concern,[42,43] In the human literature it is well established that any tobacco use increases bone loss within the oral cavity.

Smoking cessation should be encouraged for all smokers regardless of sex. As a lifestyle modification, this can help improve peak bone mass, minimize bone loss, and reduce fracture rates.

LUNG CANCER IN WOMEN

Lung cancer is the leading cause of cancer death in the United States in men and women. The lung cancer death rate in women rose from 2.5 cases per 100,000 in 1930 to over 30 per 100,000 in 1990, paralleling the rise in smoking prevalence in women.[44] Indeed, although lung cancer incidence seems to have stabilized in men it has continued to rise in women up to the mid-1990s.[45] Given the lag time between smoking exposure and lung cancer development it is possible that lung cancer rates among women may exceed that in men over the next decades.

Epidemiologic evidence suggests that after adjusting for exposure dose and body habitus women are more susceptible to tobacco's carcinogenic effects than men,[46–54] Dose-response odds ratios were 1.2- to 1.7-fold higher in women compared with men, an effect that was more pronounced for small cell and adenocarcinoma than squamous or epidermoid carcinoma.[45] Biochemical and genetic data further support a male/female difference in tobacco-related lung cancer susceptibility. The gene encoding expression of the gastrin-releasing peptide receptor is located on the distal end of the p arm of the X chromosome. This area has been shown to escape X inactivation; women may have two actively transcribed alleles compared with one in men.[55] Evidence suggesting a role of the gastrin-releasing peptide receptor–ligand system in lung carcinogenesis has been presented.[56] Nicotine induces the gastrin-releasing peptide receptor gene. The gastrin-releasing peptide receptor gene is expressed more frequently in women than in men in the absence of smoking and at an earlier age in response to tobacco exposure.[55] This increased frequency may represent a potential risk factor for the development of lung cancer in women.

Gender differences at the cellular level have also been identified in other studies, including higher levels of DNA adducts, and G-to-T transversion mutations in the p53 gene.[57] DNA adducts, stable complexes of tobacco carcinogens and DNA, are believed to be an early step in cancer induction.[58] Higher DNA adduct burdens have been demonstrated in current and former smokers. In the latter group the age at smoking start was associated with DNA adduct levels, whereas for current smokers recent smoking intensity was the most important factor determining DNA adduct levels. The authors suggest that younger smokers may be more susceptible to the formation of DNA adducts than individuals who start smoking later on in life. This may be particularly applicable to women because there is less of a gender difference in smoking rates between adolescent girls and boys compared with adults.[59]

Gender differences in lung cancer histology have been noted with an increased likelihood of adenocarcinoma in women. There may also be gender-associated differences in presentation and prognosis with non-small cell carcinoma. The K-*ras* gene encodes a protein that when mutated or overexpressed has oncogenic potential. After adjustment for carcinogen exposure, women were found to have a significantly greater likelihood of having a mutation at codon-12 compared with men (odds ratio 3.3; 95% CI 1.3–7.9) and a statistically significant association between K-*ras* mutation and survival for stage I tumors ($P = .002$).[60] A possible role of estrogen exposure in either the selection or initiation of K-*ras* mutant clones in adenocarcinoma has been postulated. Similarly, a genetic susceptibility to the development of lung cancer in women who never smoked but were exposed to environmental tobacco smoke has been proposed.[61]

TOBACCO SMOKE EXPOSURE DURING CHILDHOOD

There are many adverse effects of smoking on pregnancy outcome and the infant. The effect of involuntary tobacco smoke exposure on childhood asthma has been the subject of numerous studies. The preponderance of evidence indicates that involuntary tobacco smoke exposure increases the incidence of wheezing, cough, and phlegm, and that household exposure to environmental tobacco smoke can cause exacerbations in asthma. Evaluation of the effect of in utero exposure on the occurrence of asthma and wheeze, independent of environmental tobacco smoke exposure, has yielded conflicting reports. The Children's Health Study[62] provided an opportunity to investigate the effects of involuntary tobacco smoke exposure on asthma and wheezing in children. Consistent with other reports, the findings in 161 women who reported smoking while pregnant but successful smoking cessation before giving birth indicated an effect from in utero exposure, greater than postnatal exposure, as an independent predictor of wheezing and asthma.[63] There is increasing evidence that in utero exposure adversely affects lung function and increases the incidence of asthma.[64] Lower lung function, increased bronchial hyperreactivity, and inappropriate persistence of a TH2-dominant response pattern may lead to the development of persistent wheezing and asthma.[65] Recent morphometric analyses of infants exposed to cigarette smoke in utero only and in utero and postnatally demonstrated abnormalities compared with those without exposure to cigarette smoke.[66] The altered airway structure may account for the symptoms and abnormal lung function seen in the postnatal period. Although sex differences from in utero exposure have not been evaluated, the effects of cigarette smoking on the lung function of adolescent boys and girls[67] and lung vulnerability to tobacco smoking in adults[68] support a greater vulnerability to the effects of smoking on females than males. Maternal genotypes may modify the association between maternal cigarette smoking and fetal growth.[69]

SUMMARY

When significant resources have been devoted to the implementation of evidence-based tobacco cessation strategies, the results have been dramatic for the population overall, and for women in particular. For example, in California, which has had a comprehensive tobacco control program for 13 years, smoking prevalence declined throughout the 1990s at rates two or three times faster than in the rest of the country. Furthermore, lung cancer incidence rates decreased by 4.8% among women in California, but increased by 13% among women in other parts of the United States. These promising findings indicate that although tobacco-related diseases have become a women's health issue of epidemic proportions, there is the ability to reverse these trends.[70]

Further studies are needed to decipher the most effective combination of existing cessation strategies, in addition to the development of new modalities, for effective treatment of tobacco dependence. In particular, several issues pertaining to women's tobacco usage and treatment need further attention. For instance, little impact has been made in the rate of relapse of women who quit smoking while pregnant, only to start again soon after delivery. Additional funding is needed to address these issues as tobacco usage continues to take its toll on all aspects of women's health care needs.

REFERENCES

1. Christen AG, Christen JA. The female smoker: from addiction to recovery. Am J Med Sci 2003;326:231–4.
2. Ries LAG, Eisner MP, Kosary CL, et al. SEER cancer statistics review, 1973–1997. Bethesda (MD): National Cancer Institute; 2000.
3. Deland K, Lewis K, Taylor AL. Developing a public policy response to the tobacco industry's targeting of women and girls: the role of the WHO framework convention on tobacco control. J Am Med Womens Assoc 2000;55:316–9.
4. Mackay J. Women and tobacco: international issues. J Am Med Womens Assoc 1996;51:48–51.
5. Zhu SH, Billings S, Sun J, et al. Is it harder for women to quit smoking? Available at: http://www.srnt.org/abstracts99. Accessed June 12, 2004.
6. Gonzales D, Bjornson W, Durcan MJ, et al. Effects of gender on relapse prevention in smokers treated with bupropion SR. Am J Prev Med 2002;22:234–9.
7. Bohadana A, Nilsson F, Rasmussen T, et al. Gender differences in quit rates following smoking cessation with combination nicotine therapy: influence of baseline smoking behavior. Nicotine Tob Res 2003;5:111–6.
8. Perkins KA. Smoking cessation in women: special considerations. CNS Drugs 2001;15:391–411.
9. American Academy of Family Practitioners. Why do you smoke? [quiz]. Available at: http://familydoctor.org. Accessed August 16, 2001.
10. Pomerleau CS, Pomerleau OF, Namenek RJ, et al. Short-term weight gain in abstaining women smokers. J Subst Abuse Treat 2000;18:339–42.
11. Allen SS, Hatsukami D, Christianson D, et al. Effects of transdermal nicotine on craving, withdrawal and premenstrual symptomatology in short-term smoking abstinence during different phases of the menstrual cycle. Nicotine Tob Res 2000;2:231–41.
12. Chow W, Daling JR, Weiss NS, et al. Maternal cigarette smoking and tubal pregnancy. Obstet Gynecol 1988;71:167–70.
13. Maximovich A, Beyler SA. Clinical assisted reproduction: cigarette smoking at time of in vitro fertilization cycle initiation has negative effect on in vitro fertilization–embryo transfer success rate. J Assist Reprod Genet 1995;12:75–7.
14. Pattinson HA, Taylor PJ, Pattinson MH. The effect of cigarette smoking on ovarian function and early pregnancy outcome of in vitro fertilization treatment. Fertil Steril 1991;55:780–3.
15. American College of Obstetricians and Gynecologists. Smoking and women's health. ACOG educational bulletin 240. Washington, DC: American College of Obstetricians and Gynecologists; 1997.
16. Seltzer V. Smoking as a risk factor in the health of women. Int J Gynaecol Obstet 2003;82:393–7.
17. Hegaard HK, Kjaergaard H, Moller LF, et al. Multimodal intervention raises smoking cessation rate during pregnancy. Acta Obstet Gynecol Scand 2003;82:813–9.
18. Williams MA, Mittendorf R, Lieberman E, et al. Cigarette smoking during pregnancy in relation to placenta previa. Am J Obstet Gynecol 1991;165:28–32.
19. Naeye RL. Abruptio placenta and placenta previa: frequency, perinatal mortality, and cigarette smoking. Obstet Gynecol 1980;55:701–4.
20. Hadley CB, Main DM, Gabbe SG. Risk factors for preterm premature rupture of the fetal membranes. Am J Perinatol 1990;7:374–9.

21. Haworth JC, Ellestad-Sayed JJ, King J, et al. Fetal growth retardation in cigarette-smoking mothers is not due to decreased maternal food intake. Am J Obstet Gynecol 1980;137:719–23.
22. Lieberman E, Ryan KJ, Monson RR, et al. Risk factors accounting for racial differences in the rate of premature birth. N Engl J Med 1987;317:743–8.
23. Queenan JT. Smoking: the cloudy, smelly plague. Obstet Gynecol 2003;102:893–4.
24. Blair PS, Fleming PJ, Bensley D, et al. Smoking and sudden infant death syndrome. BMJ 1996;313:195–8.
25. Dempsey DA, Benowitz NL. Risks and benefits of nicotine to aid smoking cessation in pregnancy. Drug Saf 2001;24:277–322.
26. Seltzer V. Cancer in women: prevention and early detection. J Womens Health 2000;9:483–8.
27. Brownson RC, Blackwell CW, Pearson DK, et al. Risk of breast cancer in relation to cigarette smoking. Arch Intern Med 1988;148:140–4.
28. Collaborative group on hormonal factors in breast cancer. Alcohol, tobacco and breast cancer–collaborative reanalysis of individual data from 53 epidemiological studies, including 58,515 women with breast cancer and 96,067 women without the disease. Br J Cancer 2002;18:1234–45.
29. Reynolds P, Hurley S, Goldberg DE, et al. Active smoking, household passive smoking, and breast cancer: evidence from the California teachers study. J Natl Cancer Inst 2004;96:29–37.
30. Hung J, Lam J, Lacoste L, et al. Cigarette smoking acutely increases platelet thrombus formation in patients with coronary artery disease taking aspirin. Circulation 1995;92:2432–6.
31. Bolego C, Poli A, Paoletti R. Smoking and gender. Cardiovasc Res 2002;53:568–76.
32. Njolstad I, Arnesen E, Lund-Larsen PG. Smoking, serum lipids, blood pressure, and sex differences in myocardial infarction: a 12-year follow-up of the finnmark study. Circulation 1996;93:450–6.
33. Nyboe J, Jensen G, Appleyard M, et al. Smoking and the risk of first acute myocardial infarction. Am Heart J 1991;122:438–47.
34. Willett WC, Green A, Stampfer MJ, et al. Relative and absolute excess risks of coronary heart disease among women who smoke cigarettes. N Engl J Med 1987;317:1303–9.
35. Tverdal A, Thelle D, Stensvold I, et al. Mortality in relation to smoking history: 13 years' follow-up of 68,000 Norwegian men and women 35–49 years old. J Clin Epidemiol 1993;46:475–87.
36. Burke A, Farb A, Malcom G, et al. Effect of risk factors on the mechanism of acute thrombosis and sudden coronary death in women. Circulation 1998;97:2110–6.
37. Oparil S. Pathophysiology of sudden coronary death in women: implications for prevention. Circulation 1998;97:2103–5.
38. Taylor AE, Johnson DC, Kazemi H. Environmental tobacco smoke and cardiovascular disease: a position paper from the council on cardiopulmonary and critical care, American Heart Association. Circulation 1992;86:699–702.
39. Otsuka R, Watanabe H, Hirata K, et al. Acute effects of passive smoking on the coronary circulation in healthy young adults. JAMA 2001;286:436–41.
40. Follin SI, Hansen LB. Current approaches to the prevention and treatment of postmenopausal osteoporosis. Am J Health Syst Pharm 2003;60:883–904.
41. Spangler JG, Quandt S, Bell RA. Smokeless tobacco and osteoporosis: a new relationship? Med Hypotheses 2001;56:553–7.

42. Galvin RJ, Ramp WK, Lenz LG. Smokeless tobacco contains a non-nicotine inhibitor of bone metabolism. Toxicol Appl Pharmacol 1988;95:292–300.
43. Paulson R, Shanfield J, Sachs L, et al. Effect of smokeless tobacco on the development of the CD-1 mouse fetus. Teratology 1989;40:483–94.
44. Baldini EH, Strauss GM. Women and lung cancer: waiting to exhale. Chest 1997; 112:229S–34S.
45. Zang EA, Wynder EL. Differences in lung cancer risk between men and women: examination of the evidence. J Natl Cancer Inst 1996;88:183–92.
46. Lubin JH, Blot WJ. Assessment of lung cancer risk factors by histologic category. J Natl Cancer Inst 1984;73:383–9.
47. McDuffie HH, Klaassen DJ, Dosman JA. Female-male differences in patients with primary lung cancer. Cancer 1987;59:1825–30.
48. McDuffie HH, Klaassen DJ, Dosman JA. Men, women and primary lung cancer: a Saskatchewan Personal Interview Study. J Clin Epidemiol 1991;44: 537–44.
49. Zang EA, Wynder EL. Cumulative tar exposure: a new index for estimating lung cancer risk among cigarette smokers. Cancer 1992;70:69–76.
50. Brownson RC, Chang JC, Davis JR. Gender and histologic type variations in smoking-related risk of lung cancer. Epidemiology 1992;3:61–4.
51. Risch HA, Howe GR, Jain M, et al. Are female smokers at higher risk for lung cancer than male smokers? A case-control analysis by histologic type. Am J Epidemiol 1993;138:281–93.
52. Osann KE, Anton-Culver H, Kurosaki T, et al. Sex differences in lung cancer risk associated with cigarette smoking. Int J Cancer 1993;54:44–8.
53. Begg CB, Zhang ZF, Sun M, et al. Methodology for evaluating incidence of second primary cancers with application to smoking-related cancers from SEER. Am J Epidemiol 1995;142:653–65.
54. Dwyer T, Blizzard L, Shugg D, et al. Higher lung cancer rates in younger women than young men: Tasmania, 1983 to 1992. Cancer Causes Control 1994;5:351–8.
55. Shriver SP, Bourdeau HA, Gubish CT, et al. Sex-specific expression of gastrin-releasing peptide receptor: relationship to smoking history and risk of lung cancer. J Natl Cancer Inst 2000;92:24–33.
56. Siegfried JM, DeMichele MA, Hunt JD, et al. Expression of mRNA for gastrin-releasing peptide receptor by human bronchial epithelial cells: association with prolonged tobacco exposure and responsiveness to bombesin-like peptides. Am J Respir Crit Care Med 1997;156:358–66.
57. Kure EH, Ryberg D, Hewer A, et al. p53 Mutations in lung tumors: relationship to gender and lung DNA adduct levels. Carcinogenesis 1996;17:2201–5.
58. Wiencke JK, Thurston SW, Kelsey KT, et al. Early age at smoking initiation and tobacco carcinogen DNA damage in the lung. J Natl Cancer Inst 1999;91: 614–9.
59. Surgeon General's Report. Women and smoking 2001: executive summary. Available at: http://www.cdc.gov/tobacco/sgr/sgr_forwomen/Executive_Summary.htm. Accessed December 2, 2003.
60. Nelson HH, Christiani DC, Mark EJ, et al. Implications and prognostic value of K-ras mutation for early-stage lung cancer in women. J Natl Cancer Inst 1999; 91:2032–8.
61. Bennett WP, Alavanja MCR, Blomeke B, et al. Environmental tobacco smoke, genetic susceptibility, and risk of lung cancer in never-smoking women. J Natl Cancer Inst 1999;91:2009–14.

62. Peters JM, Avol E, Navidi W, et al. A study of twelve Southern Californian communities with differing levels and types of air pollution: I. Prevalence of respiratory morbidity. Am J Respir Crit Care Med 1999;159:760–7.
63. Gilliland FD, Li YF, Peters JM. Effects of maternal smoking during pregnancy and environmental tobacco smoke on asthma and wheezing in children. Am J Respir Crit Care Med 2001;163:429–36.
64. Cook DG, Strachan DP. Health effects of passive smoking: 3. Parental smoking and prevalence of respiratory symptoms and asthma in school age children. Thorax 1997;52:1081–94.
65. Holt PG, Macaubas C, Stumbles PA, et al. The role of allergy in the development of asthma. Nature 1999;402:B12–7.
66. Elliot JG, Carroll NG, James AL, et al. Airway alveolar attachment points and exposure to cigarette smoke in utero. Am J Respir Crit Care Med 2003;167:45–9.
67. Gold DR, Wang X, Wypij D, et al. Effects of cigarette smoking on lung function in adolescent boys and girls. N Engl J Med 1996;335:931–7.
68. Langhammer A, Johnsen R, Gulsvik A, et al. Sex differences in lung vulnerability to tobacco smoking. Eur Respir J 2003;21:1017–23.
69. Wang X, Zuckerman B, Pearson C, et al. Maternal cigarette smoking, metabolic gene polymorphism, and infant birth weight. JAMA 2002;287:195–202.
70. Kelly A, Blair N, Pechacek TF. Women and smoking: issues and opportunities. J Womens Health Gend Based Med 2001;10:515–8.

Substance Abuse Among Reproductive Age Women

Brittany B. Albright, BS*, William F. Rayburn, MD, MBA

KEYWORDS

- Substance abuse • Women • Gender differences
- Epidemiology

There are more deaths, illnesses, and disabilities from substance abuse than from any other preventable health condition. Currently, one in four deaths is attributable to alcohol, tobacco, or illicit drug use.[1] A substantial proportion of reproductive-age women consume one or more of these, thereby increasing their risks for unhealthy outcomes, and if pregnant, adverse pregnancy outcomes.[2] Rates of substance abuse are modifiable by public health interventions, with tobacco use and substance abuse (alcohol and/or illicit drugs) being listed among the 10 major public health concerns for the US population in *Healthy People 2010*.[3]

Although prevalence and incidence studies continue to find that males use substances more than females (except among adolescents where use rates are similar), they clearly show that a large number of women abuse substances.[4] The 2006 National Survey on Drug Use and Health reports that of females age 12 years or older in the United States, approximately 41% used an illicit drug(s) at some point in their lives and that currently, 6% use illicit drugs, 23% use tobacco, and 45% use alcohol (3% use alcohol heavily and 15% are binge drinkers).[5] A total of 6% met criteria for substance abuse or dependence in the past year. In contrast, 50% of males report using an illicit drug(s) at some point in their lifetime and 11% currently use illicit drugs, 36% use tobacco, and 57% use alcohol (11% use alcohol heavily and 31% use alcohol in binges). Twelve percent of males met criteria for substance abuse or dependence during the past year.

Prevention and treatment strategies for women should encompass gender-specific differences and implement approaches that address their specific needs.[4] The disparity between society's response to women's and men's substance abuse

This is an updated version of the article "Maternal and Fetal Effects from Substance Use," which appeared in *Clinics in Perinatology* (Volume 34, Issue 4, December 2007).

University of New Mexico School of Medicine, MSC 10 5580, 1 University of New Mexico, Albuquerque, NM 87131, USA

* Corresponding author.

E-mail address: balbright@salud.unm.edu (B.B. Albright).

Obstet Gynecol Clin N Am 36 (2009) 891–906

doi:10.1016/j.ogc.2009.10.008

0889-8545/09/$ – see front matter © 2009 Elsevier Inc. All rights reserved.

obgyn.theclinics.com

remains an ever-present obstacle to the development of needed interventions and viable and effective policies on behalf of women. Care of substance-using women is complex, difficult, and often demanding. Providers must be aware of their unique psychological and social needs, and the related legal and ethical ramifications surrounding maternal substance use.

Focusing on reproductive-age women, this article discusses gender differences in substance abuse, the identification of substance use, comprehensive substance abuse management, and principles of substance abuse treatment. The article also reviews perinatal substance abuse, teratogenic risks, and treatment of substance disorders during pregnancy. Cigarette smoking is beyond the scope of this article and readers should refer to the article, "Women and Tobacco Dependence" in this issue for advice about counseling patients about tobacco dependence and smoking cessation.

GENDER DIFFERENCES

There are variations in the etiology, vulnerability, and consequences of substance abuse between women and men.[4] Research suggests that women are more susceptible than men to substance-related interpersonal difficulties, trauma, and medical consequences, heightening their risk of morbidity and mortality.[6] Males have greater opportunity and access to use drugs, and given equal opportunity, females are equally likely to use drugs and develop associated problems and dependency.[4,7]

A 3-year study sponsored by the National Center on Addiction and Substance Abuse[8] indicated that girls and young women are more vulnerable to abuse and addiction; they become dependent faster and suffer the consequences sooner than boys and young men. Women, in general, experience physiologic consequences related to alcohol misuse more rapidly than do men. Violence and victimization are associated with women's substance use, including adult experience of domestic violence and rape as well as childhood sexual abuse, physical abuse, or neglect.[9–11]

Mental health problems such as depression, anxiety, and posttraumatic stress disorders are associated with substance abuse among women.[12,13] According to epidemiologic data, women with substance use disorders present higher rates of psychiatric comorbidity than men (72% versus 57% in the National Comorbidity Study).[14,15] Comorbid diagnoses more often precede the substance-related disorder in women, whereas the opposite occurs with men.[14,16] For example, among women, major depression is more often primary to the substance use disorder (with the opposite occurring in men); it is therefore less likely to improve with abstinence from psychoactive substances alone and often requires specific treatment.[17]

Consequences associated with heavy drinking may be accelerated in women.[6] Despite overall lower alcohol consumption than men, women tend to experience more associated medical sequelae and progress from onset of drinking to late stages of alcohol dependence more rapidly. For example, heavily drinking women (four or more standard alcoholic drinks per day) died significantly earlier compared with non–alcohol-dependent women (those who consumed fewer than four standard alcoholic drinks per day). There was also a trend toward earlier mortality rates compared with the heavily drinking men (eight standard alcoholic drinks per day).[18] Heavy drinking has been associated with a number of gynecologic problems, including amenorrhea, anovulation, luteal phase dysfunction, and early menopause.[14,19]

Women who abuse substances are often judged more harshly for their behavior than are men, because women are the bearers and primary caretakers of children.[4] The effect of their substance use extends to their unborn and live children. Women who use alcohol or other drugs during pregnancy place their unborn children at heightened risk for developmental delays and disabilities as well as physical and neurologic deficits.[20–22] Children of a parent(s) who misuses substances are at higher risk for a host of behavioral, psychological, and emotional problems.[23,24]

Last, women are often more responsible for contraception than men. Contraception is a primary method to prevent the problems of substance abuse and pregnancy. However, certain forms of contraception pose specific health risks when used by women who abuse substances. As an example, clinicians should assess liver function in women using oral contraceptive pills or patches who also abuse alcohol. Because cocaine and opiate use is associated with prostitution, women who abuse these substances and use an IUD without a barrier contraceptive should be assessed for sexually transmitted diseases.

IDENTIFICATION OF SUBSTANCE USE

The obstetrician-gynecologist may be the only primary care provider for many women. Patients often come for a myriad of health needs that may or may not be related to their substance abuse, including routine physical examinations, prenatal care, psychiatric conditions, and sexual problems.[6] Discussions about infertility, pregnancy, or birth control provide the obstetrician-gynecologist with an opportunity to inquire about patients' alcohol, smoking, or drug habits. From a public health and clinical perspective, this presents an enormous opportunity to screen for, initially counsel, and refer these patients to appropriate treatment as indicated.

Clinical Screening Techniques

A combination of medical, obstetric, and behavioral characteristics should be considered when identifying women with substance use problems (**Table 1**).[25] Questions about substance use are encouraged at the initial visit. A history of past and present substance use should be obtained in a nonjudgmental manner and questions should be limited to frequency and amount of specific substances in addition to the consequences of their substance use.

Substance intake is usually established using patient self-reports. A focus on drinks or substances per occasion, not average substances per day, may be more useful for identifying problem and/or binge drinking and substance use. Providers also need to question about recreational use of illicit drugs and prescription drugs. An inherent problem with the use of prescription records is difficulty in demonstrating whether the potentially addictive drugs were actually taken by the women and not, for example, sold to raise cash to purchase other illicit substances.

Multiple screening instruments exist to assess patients for substance use disorders. **Table 2** summarizes criteria of American Psychiatric Association for the diagnosis of substance abuse and dependence.[26] An efficient general intake screening tool is the Addiction Severity Index (ASI).[1] It effectively assesses a patient's status in several areas, and the composite score measures how a patient's need for treatment changes over time. A screening assessment specific for alcohol abuse is the Alcohol Use Disorders Identification Test (AUDIT) (**Table 3**).[1] It is a 10-item screening questionnaire with three questions on the amount and frequency of drinking, three questions on alcohol dependence, and four on problems caused by alcohol. AUDIT is more effective at capturing binge drinking than the cut-annoyed-guilty-eye Questionnaire.

Medical professionals should assess for signs of drug intoxication, overdose, and withdrawal. Unusual behavior, agitation, dilated or constricted pupils, elevated or decreased blood pressures, rapid or slow heart rates or respiratory rates, and altered

Table 1
Medical, obstetric, and behavior patterns in women suggestive of substance use

Medical

Anemia	Lymphedema
Arrhythmias	Myocardial ischemia or infarction
Bacterial endocarditis	Pancreatitis
Cellulitis, abscesses, or phlebitis	Poor dental hygiene
Cerebrovascular accident	Poor nutritional status
Drug overdose or withdrawal	Septicemia
Hepatitis B, C, and D	Sexually transmitted diseases
HIV seropositivity	Tuberculosis

Behavioral and Personal

Alcohol or substance using partner	Frequent emergency department visits
Bizarre or inappropriate behavior	Incarceration
Child abuse or neglect	Incoherent speech
Chronic unemployment	Noncompliance with appointments
Difficulty concentrating	Poor history
Domestic violence	Prostitution
Family history of substance use	Psychiatric history
	Restless, agitation, demanding

Obstetric

Abruptio placentae	Preterm labor and delivery
Birth outside hospital	Preterm rupture of the membranes
Fetal alcohol syndrome	Reduced fetal growth
Fetal distress	Spontaneous abortion
Neonatal abstinence syndrome	Stillbirth
No, sporadic, or late prenatal care	Sudden infant death syndrome

reflexes are sought. **Table 4** summarizes common drug and alcohol effects.[27] These effects should not be confused with adaptive changes of pregnancy.

Laboratory Testing

In conjunction with questioning, substance testing is occasionally of value in the recent user, although such testing can measure neither the chronicity of her disorder nor the patient's willingness to recover. Toxicology screening with informed consent is recommended, especially among pregnant women with (1) self-reporting of substance use; (2) multiple characteristics suggesting substance use, to facilitate referral to a comprehensive care program; or (3) compliance requirements with treatment recommendations. Random testing during pregnancy raises several legal issues, including the right to privacy, lack of probable cause, and admissibility of test results.[28]

Toxicology testing should be performed during labor for the following clinical scenarios: history of substance abuse during the pregnancy, preterm labor, placental abruption, and/or behavior consistent with acute intoxication. There are variations in state laws regarding toxicology screening during pregnancy. Some states mandate reporting of positive drug screens; others encourage it as a civil commitment. Mandatory drug screen reporting remains controversial depending on the state's approach: public health versus criminal.

Table 2
DSM-IV criteria for substance use disorders

Substance Abuse

When any one of A and both B and C are "yes," a definite diagnosis of abuse is made

A. Has the client experienced the following?   N o   Y e s
   1. Recurrent failure to meet important responsibilities due to use?
   2. Recurrent use in situations when this is likely to be physically
      dangerous?
   3. Recurrent legal problems arsing from use
   4. Continued to use despite recurrent problems aggravated by the
      substance use:

B. These symptoms have occured within a 12 month period   Yes

C. Client had *never* met the criteria for dependence   Yes

Substance Dependence

When any three of A a n d B are "yes," a definite diagnosis of dependence is made

A. Has the client experienced the following?   N o   Y e s
   1. Tolerance (needing more to become intoxicated or discovering
      less effect with same amount
   2. Withdrawal (characteristic withdrawal associated with type of
      drug)
   3. Using more or for longer periods than intended?
   4. Desire to or unsuccessful efforts to cut down?
   5. Considerable time spent in obtaining the substance or using, or
      recovering from its effects?
   6. Important social, work, or recreational activities given up
      because of use?
   7. Continued use despite knowledge of problems caused by or
      aggravated by use.

B. Are three or more of the above positive?   Yes

C. Have these positive items been present during the same 12 month period?   Yes

Courtesy of Project Cork, 2002. DSM-IV criteria for substance use disorders. Available at: http://www.
projectcork.org/clinical_tools/pdf/DSM-IVDxCriteriaSubstanceUseDisorders.pdf.

Urine is the preferred source for drug testing because it is easily available and in large quantities. Urine drug screening is usually performed using an immunoassay technique. Approximate durations of detectability of substances and their metabolites in the urine are shown in **Table 5**.[25] Except for marijuana, most substances are measurable in urine for less than 96 hours after use. Therefore, substances may not be identified unless urine specimens are tested frequently.[29] In the evaluations for cocaine and opiate exposure, hair analysis is also effective. For pregnant women,

Table 3
Alcohol Use Disorders Identification Test (AUDIT)

1. How often do you have a drink containing alcohol?
    (Never, 0)   (Monthly or less, 1)   (Two to four times a month, 2)
    (Two to three times a week, 3)   (Four or more times a week, 4)
2. How many drinks containing alcohol do you have on a typical day when you are drinking?
    (1 or 2 drinks, 0)   (3 or 4 drinks, 1)   (5 or 6 drinks, 2)
    (7 to 9 drinks, 3)   (10 or more, 4)
3. How often do you have six or more drinks on one occasion?
    (Never, 0)   (Monthly or less, 1)   (Two to four times a month, 2)
    (Two to three times a week, 3)   (Four or more times a week, 4)
4. How often during the last year have you found that you were not able to stop drinking once you had started?
    (Never, 0)   (Monthly or less, 1)   (Two to four times a month, 2)
    (Two to three times a week, 3)   (Four or more times a week, 4)
5. How often during the last year have you failed to do what was normally expected from you because of drinking?
    (Never, 0)   (Monthly or less, 1)   (Two to four times a month, 2)
    (Two to three times a week, 3)   (Four or more times a week, 4)
6. How often during the last year have you needed a first drink in the morning to get yourself going after a heavy drinking session?
    (Never, 0)   (Monthly or less, 1)   (Two to four times a month, 2)
    (Two to three times a week, 3)   (Four or more times a week, 4)
7. How often during the last year have you had a feeling of guilt or remorse after drinking?
    (Never, 0)   (Monthly or less, 1)   (Two to four times a month, 2)
    (Two to three times a week, 3)   (Four or more times a week, 4)
8. How often during the last year have you been unable to remember what happened the night before because you had been drinking?
    (Never, 0)   (Monthly or less, 1)   (Two to four times a month, 2)
    (Two to three times a week, 3)   (Four or more times a week, 4)
9. Have you or someone else been injured as a result of your drinking?
    (No, 0)   (Yes, but not in the last year, 2)   (Yes, during the last year, 4)
10. Has a relative or friend, or a doctor or other health worker been concerned about your drinking, or suggested you cut down?
    (No, 0)   (Yes, but not in the last year, 2)   (Yes, during the last year, 4)

Scoring.
o   The number for each response is the number of points.
o   Answers for each question range from 0 to 4.
o   There is no set cut-off point indicating harmful use.
o   A score of 2 or more indicates some level of harmful use.
o   The particular score that warrants a further evaluation, depends in part on the situation, e.g. a score of 3 for someone scheduled for surgery would clearly warrant further evaluation, although this might not be as critical for the healthy individual who is seen during a routine annual physical. However, patient education/harm reduction efforts are indicated for anyone who scores over a 1.

Courtesy of Project Cork. AUDIT. Available at: http://www.projectcork.org/clinical_tools/html/AUDIT.html.

Table 4
Summary of drug and alcohol effects in adults

DRUG CLASS	DRUG	COMMON OR BRAND NAME	DEPENDENCE POTENTIAL PHYSICAL	PSYCHOLOGICAL	DESIRED OR IMMEDIATE EFFECTS	UNDESIRED AND LONG-TERM EFFECTS	OVERDOSE EFFECTS
TOBACCO	Nicotine	Tobacco, Cigarettes, Cigars, Beedies / Smokeless, Snuff, Dip, Chew / Patches, Gum	High / High / Moderate	High / High / Moderate	Relaxation / Concentration, Stimulation	Chronic Withdrawal / Emphysema, Lung Cancer / Cardiovascular Disease	Anxiety
ALCOHOL	Ethanol	Beer, Ale / Wine, Wine Coolers / Whiskey, Liquor / Liqueurs	High / High / High / High	High / High / High / High	Euphoria / Reduced Inhibitions / Impaired Judgment / In-coordination / Slurred Speech / Impaired Memory-Learning	Liver Damage, Brain Damage / Heart Damage, Nerve Damage / Esophageal Hemorrhage, Pancreatitis / Victimization (Rape) / Fetal Alcohol Syndrome / Effects / Withdrawal Seizures, D.T.'S,	Depressed Breathing / Abnormal Heart Beat / Amnesia / Coma / Death
CANNABIS	Marijuana / Hashish, Hash Oil	Grass, Pot, Weed, Dope, Sensimilla, Reefer, Ganja, Herb, Blunts / Hash, Tar, Oil	Low / Low / Low	Moderate / Moderate / Moderate	Euphoria, Hilarity / Altered Perceptions / Reduced Inhibitions / Hunger, Increased Pulse / Impaired Judgment, Red Eyes / Paranoia, Impaired Memory	Accidents, Mistakes / Lung Damage / Memory Impairment / Motivation Loss	Hallucinations / Panic / Agitation / Delirium
STIMULANTS	Cocaine / Amphetamine / Methylphenidate / Methcathinone / MDMA, MDA, MDEA, PCP	Coke, Crack / Dexedrine, Adderall, Uppers, Speed, Ice / Ritalin / Cat / Ecstasy, X, Adam, Eve, Dust	Possible / Possible / Possible / Unknown / Unknown	High / High / High / Possible / Possible	Alertness - Concentration / Excitation - Euphoria / Appetite Loss / Insomnia / Grandiosity	Tolerance / Dehydration, Weight Loss / Brain Damage, Nerve Death / Psychosis / Agitated Delirium / "Crash" Withdrawal	Agitation, Paranoia, Panic / Fever, Hallucinations / Seizures / Heart Attack, Stroke / Fatal Heart Rhythms / Sudden Death
OPIOIDS	Opium / Morphine / Codeine / Heroin / Meperidine / Hydromorphone / Oxycodone / Hydrocodone / Fentanyl	Chinese molasses, dreams, gong, O / Morphine sulfate, M.S., MSO4 / Tylenol #3 cough syrup / H, horse, smack, mojo, China white / Demerol / Dilaudid / Percocet, Percodan / Vicodin, Tussinex / Sublimaze	High / High / High / High / High / High / High / High / High	High / High / High / High / High / High / High / High / High	Euphoric Rush / Pain Relief / Constricted Pupils / Sleepiness	Poor Appetite, Weight Loss / Constipation / IV Use Infections: AIDS, Hep B/C / Addiction - Withdrawal	Respiratory Depression / Respiratory Arrest / Coma / Death
SEDATIVES	Barbiturates / Benzodiazepines / Methaqualone / GHB / Chloral Hydrate	Phenobarb, Seconal, Nembutal, Amytal / Valium, Ativan, Xanax, Tranxene, Restoril / Rohypnol, Roofies / Quaalude, Ludes, Sopor / Gamma-hydroxybutyrate / Noctec, Somnos, Felsules, Micky	High / High / High / Unknown / Moderate	High / High / High / Unknown / Moderate	Relaxation / Drowsiness / Dizziness / Incoordination / Slurring Words	Addiction - Withdrawal / Memory Impairment / Delirium / Victimization (Rape)	Respiratory Depression / Possible Coma or Death if combined, especially with Alcohol / Opioids
HALLUCINOGENS	LSD / Psilocibin / Mescaline / Phencyclidine / Ketamine / DMT, MDMA, MDA, MDEA / Belladonna Alkaloids	Acid, Blotter, Sunshine / Shrooms, Magic Mushrooms / Peyote, Buttons, Mescalito, Mesc / PCP, Angel Dust, Dust, T / Special K, K / Businessman Special, Ecstasy, X, Eve / Atropine, Nightshade, Jimsonweed	Possible / Possible / Possible / Possible / Unknown / Unknown / None	Unknown / Unknown / Unknown / Unknown / Unknown / Unknown / None	Sense of Insight / Integration or Detachment / Altered Perceptions / Visual Hallucinations, Delusions / Jitteriness, Fast or Slow Pulse, Chills / Intense Fear, Anxiety, Paranoia, Panic	Flashbacks / Unpredictable Behavior / Delirium / PCP Psychosis, Violence	PCP lethal in overdose esp. comb. with alcohol, sedatives / Belladonna alkaloids most dangerous comb. with stims.
INHALENTS	Butyl, Amyl Nitrates / Nitrous Oxide / Petroleum Distillates / Chloro-alkenes alkanes	Poppers, Rush, Locker Room Odorizers / Laughing Gas, Whippets, Whipped Cream / Glues, Solvents Toluene, Acetone, Gasoline / Cleaning Agents, Adhesives	Unknown / Unknown / Unknown / Unknown	Unknown / Unknown / Unknown / Unknown	Euphoria / Reduced Inhibitions / Impaired Judgment / In-coordination, Slowed Reflexes	Lethargy, Hangover, Contusion / Nerve Damage / Kidney Failure / Abnormal Heart Rhythms	Suffocation / Coma / Death

Courtesy of Grass W. 2001. Project cork. Available at: http://www.projectcork.org/clinical_tools/pdf/Summary_Chart.pdf.

Table 5
Time intervals before drug elimination in urine

Drug	Detectable in Urine
Alcohol	<12 h
Amphetamines	<48 h
Barbiturates	
Short-acting	<48 h
Long-acting	<7 d
Benzodiazepines	<72 h
Therapeutic use	<72 h
Chronic use	<4–6 wk
Cocaine	<96 h
Marijuana	
Single use	<7 d
Chronic use	<30 d
Opiates	
Morphine, heroin	<48 h
Methadone	<96 h

the expanded plasma volume, increased renal clearance, and transplacental passage of drugs may shorten the duration of detection.[25]

COMPREHENSIVE CARE

Women are underrepresented in traditional substance abuse treatment settings.[6,30] This may be partly because women tend to pursue avenues of treatment other than traditional substance abuse programs, such as mental health or primary care services.[6] The intense social stigma and related shame and guilt feelings also prevent women with substance-related disorders from seeking treatment as often as men.[14] Moreover, many professionals in nonaddiction treatment settings feel more uncomfortable asking female patients about their substance use as compared with male patients. Thus, the opportunity for early diagnosis and proper referral of these clients is missed.[14,31] Care needs to be taken not to stigmatize and shame women who misuse substances or neglect the need to understand and care for them in the process of addressing the effect of their substance use on their children.[4]

Other reasons that substance abusing women do not receive treatment include financial barriers, lack of access, stigma associated with use during pregnancy, or denial of having a substance-related disorder. Young, poor women are often afraid of the medical and social welfare system because they are unaware of the system's resources or have had negative experiences within the system. Pregnant and postpartum women who consume alcohol or other drugs are more stigmatized than women who consume alcohol or other drugs but are not pregnant. These women may, therefore, deny their drug habit, not acknowledge its possible harmful effects, and therefore, not seek help.

Obstetrics-gynecology Clinics

Obstetrics and gynecology clinics are excellent sites for preventive care and sometimes primary care. Many women with a recent history of substance abuse, especially with prescription medications, seek care promptly but do not desire specialized clinics for persons with ongoing substance use problems. Benefits from primary care settings relate to their accessibility, availability, and the established credibility of health care practitioners. Prevention services in prenatal clinics avoid the stigma attached to specialized substance use services.

Available encounters with providers should be used to educate women and to focus on substance use prevention, given that many women in the reproductive-age group could be at risk for having unintended pregnancies and may be experiencing mental or physical distress and engaging in substance use.[32]

Several reports exist about substance abuse treatment in multidisciplinary settings, especially for persons with ongoing substance use. These studies suggest that during pregnancy, even minimal drug interventions (such as methadone maintenance) and counseling, combined with prenatal care, can lead to better maternal and infant outcomes.[33] Although comprehensive interventions such as this show promise for reducing substance use and harm to the fetus, few prenatal clinics are solely dedicated to screening, assessing, and treating pregnant addicts.

Community Rehabilitation Programs

The most common complaint by health care professionals is the feeling of ineffectiveness, because certain patients are unmotivated or too difficult to deal with to retain in treatment.[34] Involving patients in the treatment of their substance use is not a guarantee that they will seek regular care. Certain persons either "kick the habit" or feel that their habit is too infrequent for multidisciplinary care. These patients must be counseled that even a small amount of drug use is not desirable for their health.

Most communities have rehabilitation programs for alcohol, opioid, and stimulant addiction. The Substance Abuse & Mental Health Services Administration lists drug and alcohol abuse treatment programs for each state at http://dasis3.samhsa.gov/. Referral to a rehabilitation program is intended to promote not only the cessation of alcohol, tobacco, and other substances, but also to effect change in patients' lifestyles in a holistic sense. Substance abuse involves not only the woman, but affects the family and the whole community. Professionals willing to work with this population must tackle the many issues associated with substance use: poverty, lack of education and job training, poor parenting skills, domestic violence in the form of physical and sexual abuse, child abuse, family and other personal relations, communicable disease, child development, and such psychiatric disorders as depression, anxiety, and psychosis.

A multidisciplinary team is essential for rehabilitation.[35,36] Favorable outcomes relate directly to the time dedicated to the program. As the patient becomes more involved, a strong and more positive relation develops between patient and staff. The ability to be flexible and to provide an environment that is safe, improves self-esteem, and fosters interpersonal growth is essential.

PRINCIPLES OF TREATMENT

Dependence on substances of abuse remains a major public health problem in the United States because of the high relapse rates and poor treatment responses. Psychological and pharmacologic treatments are intertwined in managing female patients with chemical dependence. Supportive psychotherapy includes counseling, group therapy, lifestyle change training, exercise, and self-help groups such as local chapters of Alcoholics Anonymous and Narcotics Anonymous. Treatment should be conducted by professionals with expertise and training in the area of substance use. Relapse prevention methods, which use peer support and learning principles, are directed toward avoiding situations that elicit conditioned cravings and toward developing better coping skills. Supportive psychotherapy and relapse prevention need further evaluation in women, especially during pregnancy.

Behavioral Treatment

Behavioral treatment approaches include relaxation training, skills training, self-management procedures, and contingency contracting. Contingency contracting involves rearranging that individual's environment so that positive consequences follow desired behavior, while either negative or neutral consequences follow undesired behaviors. These techniques require reinforcement from others, such as spouses, other family members, employers, or health care providers. Individuals admitting to a relapse of substance use or having positive urine drug screening are subject to negative consequences.

Psychopathology among substance abusers is so common that it is difficult to ascertain whether it contributed to or was a result of the substance use. In many instances, abstinence from substance use results in an amelioration of psychiatric disorders. Specific pharmacotherapy may result in resolution of both the psychiatric disorder and the substance use among women whose psychiatric disorder either antedated the substance use or coexisted with the addiction.[37]

Drug Therapy

Select pharmacologic therapy with extensive counseling is an important modality that is beyond the scope of a typical obstetrician-gynecologist's practice. Benzodiazapines and phenobarbital are used to withdraw women who abuse alcohol and sedative-hypnotics. A prime example of replacement therapy is methadone, which has been used widely for years in treating opiate dependence. Opiate addiction leads to receptor system dysfunction and affects the ability of a patient to remain abstinent. Daily methadone maintenance reduces the risk of relapse and enhances retention in treatment.[38] Methadone treatment among opiate-dependent pregnant women has been shown to improve perinatal outcome.[34,35]

Buprenorphine, commonly combined with naloxone and marketed as Suboxone, is an alternative to methadone for opiate addiction and can be prescribed outpatient by obstetrician-gynecologists. To dispense buprenorphine, physicians must complete an 8-hour course, which can be accessed from the American Academy of Addiction Psychiatry at http://www2.aaap.org/buprenorphine. Buprenorphine is useful where methadone maintenance programs are unavailable. For pregnant women, buprenorphine alone (marketed as Subutex) is safe and effective for both mother and newborn, with a diminished neonatal abstinence syndrome compared with methadone.[39,40] However, there is no role for changing pregnant women on methadone to buprenorphine.

Cocaine blocks the reuptake of neurotransmitters such as dopamine, norepinephrine, and serotonin, leading to their depletion.[25] Pharmacologic treatment with dopamine agonists, such as bromocriptine and amantadine, has been advocated to replenish neurotransmitters. Further research is needed to conclude whether these agents are effective and safe at decreasing cocaine use. Drug trials for cocaine addiction have included the use of tricyclic antidepressants, dopamine agonists, lithium, amino acids, and vitamins. None is universally effective in substance users.

STRATEGIES DURING PREGNANCY

Reproductive-age women who abuse substances may conceive at any time. Chronic substance use may affect menstrual cycles, but these effects are reversible with discontinuation of the drug or after tolerance develops. Some studies have reported that the chronic use of certain substances (eg, marijuana) may decrease plasma testosterone and result in subsequent decreases in sperm count, concentration, and motility. These effects on spermatogenesis appear to be reversible and do not cause increased reproductive failure in men. Delivery of a substance or metabolite by the sperm to the oocyte may be associated with developmental toxicity, although toxicity has not been demonstrated in human beings. The authors are unaware of any evidence that men using a specific illicit or licit substance impart an increased risk of an unfavorable pregnancy outcome.

Substance abuse is prevalent among pregnant women, although use rates are lower compared with nonpregnant women. Combined 2002 to 2007 data show that past month alcohol use among women aged 18 to 44 was highest for those who were not pregnant and did not have children living in the household (63.0%) but comparatively low for women in the first trimester of pregnancy (19.0%), and even lower for those in the second (7.8%) or third trimester (6.2%); similar patterns were seen with marijuana, cigarette, and binge alcohol use.[41]

Even though a reduction in substance use may occur during pregnancy, some women may not alter their drug use patterns until pregnancy is diagnosed. For these reasons, a large number of fetuses are exposed to illicit substances in utero Patient interviews and urine toxicologic testing at the initial prenatal visit and at delivery suggest that substance use during pregnancy ranges from 0.4% to 27.0%, depending on the population surveyed.[42–44]

Strategies to encourage women to seek prenatal care and to enroll in treatment programs before and after delivery include the following[45]:

- Educate physicians, midwives, and other health professionals about local treatment resources and the importance of identifying substance-using women within their patient populations.
- Develop and advertise specific services for pregnant and postpartum women. Materials should include information about the program's social services and child care provisions offered at or through the treatment program.
- Provide education on the importance of seeking treatment before delivery.
- Develop and show videotaped stories of other pregnant women who successfully completed substance abuse treatment.
- Conduct outreach activities in places such as Women, Infants and Children (WIC) programs, obstetrics and gynecology clinics, family planning centers, well-baby clinics, departments of social services, Head Start offices, and La Leche League chapters.

Government agencies, as well as the public, are concerned about the use of both legal and illegal drugs by pregnant women.[45] Punitive actions (including jail sentences) against substance-using women who are either pregnant or of childbearing age or hospitals reporting pregnant women suspected of heavy alcohol and other substance use to local public health authorities or to the criminal justice system may cause women to be even more wary of acknowledging their problem. Such persons may resist seeking prenatal care and hospital delivery, particularly if they have children who are in the custody of Child Protective Services or are living with relatives. In many states, protective services, foster care placements, and review boards base their decisions on whether to return a child to the mother on the length of time in which the child is away from the mother. These decisions serve as deterrents to women seeking effective long-term treatment if child care is unavailable.

PERINATAL SUBSTANCE USE AND TERATOGENIC RISKS

Virtually any substance unbound to proteins passes freely from the maternal compartment, across the placenta, and into the fetal compartment, generally within minutes. Concentrations in the fetal circulation can be nearly the same or higher than in the maternal serum. Effects from any substance on the developing embryo and fetus also depend on gestational timing and the extent of drug distribution. Little doubt exists that passage of the drug or metabolite into the fetal central nervous system is unimpeded.

Toxic or teratogenic effects may be expressed as fetal demise, dysmorphism, growth restriction, or behavioral changes. Substances of abuse may be intentionally or inadvertently taken at toxic doses. Moreover, the impurity of most illicit drugs, and the common practice of using multiple substances, makes it difficult to ascribe specific effects to a certain drug. Accurate evaluation of dosage and the exact period of exposure are rarely possible. Behavioral effects from in utero exposure to substances are usually insidious, variable, and not easily recognized. Social, cultural, environmental, and genetic factors may be influential, so tests for altered behavior in previously exposed children may not only measure teratogenic effects of substances but also parental influences on behavior.

Table 6 lists effects in human beings from in utero exposure to certain substances.[46] This list was compiled using data from two or more reports in humans. Although this table serves as a guideline, counseling about absolute risk is unreasonable. The risk of structural anomalies is not increased in most cases of substance exposure, although the background risk of birth defects is 3% in the general pregnancy population.[47] Except for fetal alcohol syndrome, birth defect syndromes are not universally accepted for other substances. Therefore, fetal ultrasound examinations are recommended periodically. Other effects of maternal substance use place the fetus at risk for such problems as low birth weight, small head circumference, prematurity, and other developmental complications.

In the case of illicit drugs, evidence is either insufficient or inconsistent to identify with reasonable certainty those substances that produce neurobehavior effects (visual memory, integration, executive functioning, and so forth) and at what levels. Guidelines for newborn screening include obtaining a detailed maternal substance use history, performing neonatal urine toxicology screening for a history of substance abuse during pregnancy, preterm labor, placental abruption, unexplained neonatal depression, seizures, jitteriness, and possible neonatal abstinence syndrome.[40] Evidence to untangle the environmental factors (such as poverty and the corresponding poor nutrition and lack of access to prenatal care) from substance use–related factors is limited, conflicting, or nonexistent.

SUBSTANCE USE AFTER PREGNANCY

Substance abuse continues to afflict women after pregnancy. Data from 2002 to 2007 suggest that use of substances such as marijuana, cigarettes, and alcohol increases following childbirth.[41] For example, marijuana use was higher for recent mothers with children younger than 3 months old in the household (3.8%) than for women in the third trimester of pregnancy (1.4%), suggesting resumption of use among mothers in the first 3 months after childbirth. There is also an increased

Table 6
Impact of in utero exposure to specific substances on the fetus and newborn infant

Substance	Impact
Alcohol	Microcephaly; growth deficiency; CNS dysfunction including mental retardation and behavioral abnormalities; craniofacial abnormalities (ie, short palpebral fissures, hypoplastic philtrum, flattened maxilla); behavioral abnormalities; abortion,[a] still birth.[a]
Cigarettes	No anomalies; reduced birthweight (200 g lighter); preterm birth; placenta previa, placental abruption; reduced risk of preeclampsia; spontaneous abortion.[a]

Cannabis
  Marijuana
  Tetrahydrocannabinol
  (THC)
  Hashish
	No anomalies; reduction of 0.8 weeks in length of gestation, corresponding decrease in birth weight; subtle behavioral alterations, impaired executive functioning,[a] ventricular septal defect.[a]

Central Nervous System (CNS) sedatives
  Barbiturates
  Diazepam
  Flurazepam
  Meprobamate
  Methaqualone
	Cleft palate[a]; depression of interactive behavior; neonatal withdrawal.

CNS stimulants
  Antiobesity drugs
  Amphetamines
  Cocaine
  Methylphenidate
  Phenmetrazine
	Abortion[a]; excess activity in utero; congenital anomalies (heart,[a] biliary atresia[a]); depression of interactive behavior; urinary tract defects; symmetric growth restriction; placental abruption; cerebral infarction; brain lesions; cranial defects[a]; fetal death; neonatal necrotizing enterocolitis; shortened labor.

Hallucinogens
  Lysergic acid
  diethylamide (LSD)
  Ketamine
  Mescaline
  Dimethyltryptamine
  Phencyclidine (PCP)
	No anomalies; chromosomal breakage[a] (LSD); dysmorphic face; behavioral problems; possible increase in spontaneous abortions.

Narcotics
  Buprenorphine
  Codeine
  Heroin
  Hydromorphone
  Hydrocodone
  Meperidine
  Methadone
  Morphine
  Opium
  Pentazocine (and
  tripelennamine)
	Absent birth defect syndrome; intrauterine withdrawal with increased fetal activity; depressed breathing movements; preterm delivery; preterm rupture of the membranes; fetal growth restriction; meconium-stained amniotic fluid; perinatal mortality; neonatal abstinence syndrome; sudden infant death.[a]

Inhalants
  Gasoline
  Glue
  Paint
	Similar to the fetal alcohol and fetal hydantoin syndromes[a]; growth restriction; preterm labor; increased risk of leukemia in children; impaired heme synthesis.

[a] Conflicting reports in human literature.

incidence of postpartum depression among women who abuse substances. Consequently, clinicians should recommend a social work/child protective services follow-up after delivery.

A desire to breastfeed may be a stimulus to discourage any substance use. Guidelines should be recommended to breastfeeding patients who abuse substances. Tobacco and methadone are not contraindications to breastfeeding. Breastfeeding should be discouraged in women with recent cocaine and amphetamine use. Women who breastfeed are also encouraged to abstain from marijuana and alcohol.

Teenage pregnant women who abuse substances often seek help when giving birth to their first child.[33,48] Counseling and medical treatment are critical before delivery. Being reunited with her newborn infant is often an incentive for a mother of any age to enter treatment. Under supervision, mothers can learn effective parenting skills, become drug-free, and experience improved relationships with their children. This reunification model also unburdens foster care systems by ensuring the safety of the child in a therapeutic milieu.

SUMMARY

- Screen all reproductive age women for substance abuse problems by history, examination, and possibly select urine testing.
- Tobacco and alcohol are the most significant substance abuse problems among women.
- Determine whether there is psychiatric comorbidity, especially depression and anxiety.
- Access and refer to local specialized and residential programs for opiate, cocaine, and stimulant addiction.
- Preconception counseling is the ideal venue for substance abuse treatment.
- Strategies are proposed for management during and after pregnancy.

REFERENCES

1. National Institutes of Health. National institute on drug abuse. Medical consequences of drug abuse: mortality. Available at: http://www.drugabuse.gov/consequences/mortality/. Accessed July 1, 2008.
2. Floyd RL, Jack BW, Cefalo R, et al. The clinical content of preconception care: alcohol, tobacco, and illicit drug exposures. Am J Obstet Gynecol 2008;199: S333–9.
3. Thacker SB, Ikeda RM, Gieseker KE, et al. The evidence base for public health informing policy at the centers for disease control and prevention. Am J Prev Med 2005;29:227–33.
4. Wiechelt S. Introduction to the special issue: international perspectives on women's substance use. Subst Use Misuse 2008;43:973–7.
5. Substance Abuse and Mental Health Services Administration. Results from the 2006 National survey on drug use and health. (Office of Applied Studies, NSDUH Series H-32, DHHS Publication No. SMA 07–4293). Rockville (MD): National Findings; 2007. Available at: http://oas.samhsa.gov/p0000016.html.
6. Greenfield S, Manwani S, Nargiso J. Epidemiology of substance use disorders in women. Obstet Gynecol Clin North Am 2003;30:413–46.
7. Zickler P. Gender differences in prevalence to drug abuse traced to opportunities to use. [Electronic version]. NIDA Notes, 15,(4). Available at: http://www.nida.nih.gov/NIDA Notes/NNVol15N4/Prevalence.html. Accessed September 25, 2007.

8. National Center on Addiction and Substance Abuse at Columbia University. The formative years: pathways to substance abuse among girls and young women ages 8–22. Available at: http://www.casacolumbia.org/pdshopprov/files/151006. pdf. Accessed July 1, 2007.

9. Fals-Stewart W, Golden J, Schumacher JA. Intimate partner violence and substance use: a longitudinal day-to-day examination. Addict Behav 2003; 28(9):1555–74.

10. Kendler KS, Bulik CM, Siberg J, et al. Childhood sexual abuse and adult psychiatric and substance use disorders in women: an epidemiological and co-twin control analysis. Arch Gen Psychiatry 2000;57(10):953–9.

11. Miller BA, Downs WR. Violence against women. In: Goldman MB, Hatch MC, editors. Women and health. San Diego (CA): Academic Press; 2000. p. 527–40.

12. Cottler LB, Nishith P, Compton WM. Gender differences in risk factors for trauma exposure and post-traumatic stress disorder among inner-city drug abusers in and out of treatment. Compr Psychiatry 2001;42(2):111–7.

13. Sonne SC, Back SE, Zuniga CD, et al. Gender differences in individuals with comorbid alcohol dependence and post-traumatic stress disorder. Am J Addict 2001;12:412–23.

14. Zilberman M, Tavares H, Blume S, et al. Towards best practices in the treatment of women with addictive disorders. Addict Disord Their Treat 2002;1:39–46.

15. Kessler RC, McGonagle KA, Zhao S, et al. Lifetime and 12- month prevalence of DSM-III-R psychiatric disorders in the United States: results from the National Comorbidity Survey. Arch Gen Psychiatry 1994;51:8–19.

16. Kessler RC, Crum RM, Warner LA, et al. Lifetime cooccurrence of DSM-III-R alcohol abuse and dependence with other psychiatric disorders in the National Comorbidity Survey. Arch Gen Psychiatry 1997;54:313–21.

17. Zilberman M, Tavares H, Blume S, et al. Substance use disorders: sex differences and psychiatric comorbidities. Can J Psychiatry 2003;48:5–13.

18. Jarque-Lopez A, Gonzalez-Reimers E, Rodriguez-Moreno F, et al. Prevalence and mortality of heavy drinkers in a general medical hospital. Alcohol Alcohol 2001;36(4):335–8.

19. Lex BW. Gender differences and substance abuse. Adv Alcohol Subst Abuse 1991;4:225–96.

20. Chudley AE, Conry J, Cook LL, et al. Fetal alcohol spectrum disorder: Canadian guidelines for diagnosis. CMAJ 2005;172(Suppl 5):S1–21.

21. Coles CD, Black MM. Introduction to the special issue: impact of prenatal substance exposure on children's health, development, school performance, and risk behavior. J Pediatr Psychol 2006;31(1):1–4.

22. Floyd RL, O'Connor MJ, Sokol RJ, et al. Recognition and prevention of fetal alcohol syndrome. Obstet Gynecol 2005;106(5 Part 1):1059–64.

23. Johnson JL, Leff M. Children of substance abusers: overview of research findings. Pediatrics 1999;103(Suppl):1085–99.

24. Lieberman DZ. Children of alcoholics: an update. Curr Opin Pediatr 2000;12(4): 336–40.

25. Rayburn W. Maternal and fetal effects from substance use. Clin Perinatol 2007; 34:559–71.

26. Project Cork. DSM-IV criteria for substance use disorders. Available at: http://www.projectcork.org/clinical_tools/pdf/DSM-IVDxCriteriaSubstanceUseDisorders. pdf. 2002. Accessed August 21, 2009.

27. Grass W. Project cork. Available at: http://www.projectcork.org/clinical_tools/pdf/ Summary_Chart.pdf. 2001. Accessed August 21, 2009.

28. Foley E. Drug screening and criminal prosecution of pregnant women. J Obstet Gynecol Neonatal Nurs 2002;31:133–7.
29. Wolff K, Farrell M, Marsden J, et al. A review of biological indication of illicit drug use, practical considerations and clinical usefulness. Addiction 1999;94:1279–98.
30. Blume S. Addictive disorders in women. In: Frances R, Miller S, editors. Clinical textbook of addictive disorders. 2nd edition. New York: Guilford Press; 1998. p. 413–29.
31. Blume SB, Zilberman ML. Addiction in women. In: Galanter M, Kleber HD, editors. The American psychiatric press textbook of substance abuse. 3rd edition. Washington, DC: American Psychiatric Press, in press.
32. Ahluwalia IB, Mack KA, Mokdad A. Mental and physical distress and high-risk behaviors among reproductive-age women. Obstet Gynecol 2004;104(3): 477–83.
33. Richardson K. Adolescent pregnancy and substance use. J Obstet Gynecol Neonatal Nurs 1999;28(6):623–7.
34. Dashe J, Sheffield J, Jackson G, et al. Relationship between maternal methadone dosage and neonatal withdrawal. Am J Obstet Gynecol 2002;100(6):1244–9.
35. Archie C. Methadone in the management of narcotic addiction in pregnancy. Curr Opin Obstet Gynecol 1998;10(6):435–40.
36. Curet L, Hsi A. Drug abuse in pregnancy. Clin Obstet Gynecol 2002;45(1):73–88.
37. Baurer CR, Shankaran S, Bada HS, et al. The maternal lifestyle study: drug exposure during pregnancy and short-term maternal outcomes. Am J Obstet Gynecol 2002;186(3):487–95.
38. Weaver M, Jarvis M, Schnoll S. Overview of the recognition and management of the drug abuser. Up to Date; 2002. Available at: uptodate.com. Accessed June 8, 2009.
39. Johnson RE, Jones HE, Fischer G. Use of buprenorphine in pregnancy: patient management and effects on the neonate. Drug Alcohol Depend 2003;70: S87–101.
40. Kakko J, Heilig M, Sarman I. Buprenorphine and methadone treatment of opiate dependence during pregnancy: comparison of fetal growth and neonatal outcomes in two consecutive case series. Drug Alcohol Depend 2008;96:69–78.
41. Substance Abuse and Mental Health Services Administration, Office of Applied Studies. (May 21, 2009). The NSDUH report: substance use among women during pregnancy and following childbirth. Rockville (MD). Available at: http://oas.samhsa.gov/2k9/135/PregWoSubUse.htm.
42. Buchi K, Varner M, Chase R. The prevalence of substance abuse among pregnant women in Utah. Am J Obstet Gynecol 1993;81(2):239–42.
43. Chasnoff I, Landress H, Barrett M. The prevalence of illicit drug and alcohol use during pregnancy and discrepancies in mandatory reporting in Pinellas County, Florida. N Engl J Med 1990;322(17):1202–6.
44. Current statewide prevalence of illicit drug use by pregnant women—Rhode Island. MMWR Morb Mortal Wkly Rep 1990;39(14):225–7.
45. USDHS. Outreach to and identification of women: practical approaches in the treatment of women who abuse alcohol and other drugs. Rockville (MD): US Dept Health and Human Services, Public Health Service; 1994. p. 124–6.
46. Reprotox database. Bethesda (MD): Reproductive Toxicology Center; 2007.
47. Cunningham F, Gant N, Leveno K, et al (editors). Teratology, drugs, and medications. In: Williams obstetrics. 22nd edition. New York: McGraw-Hill; 2005 p. 1006–38.
48. Chasnoff IJ, Neuman K, Thornton C, et al. Screening for substance use in pregnancy: a practical approach for the primary care physician. Am J Obstet Gynecol 2001;184(4):752–8.

Understanding and Treating Premenstrual Dysphoric Disorder: An Update for the Women's Health Practitioner

Simone N. Vigod, MD, FRCPC[a,b], Lori E. Ross, PhD[b,c],
Meir Steiner, MD, PhD, FRCPC[d,e,*]

KEYWORDS

• Premenstrual dysphoric disorder • Etiology • Treatment

From ancient times, various facets of women's personalities, capabilities, and moods have been attributed to menstruation,[1] and "instability" resulting from women's reproductive cycles has been used to justify denying women equal access to education and employment.[2]

This is an updated version of the article "A Biopsychosocial Approach to Premenstrual Dysphoric Disorder," which appeared in *Psychiatric Clinics of North America* (Volume 26, Issue 3, September 2003). Dr Vigod is supported by a fellowship from the Ontario Mental Health Foundation and by the Department of Psychiatry, Women's College Hospital, Toronto, Ontario Canada.
Dr Ross is supported by a New Investigator Award from the Canadian Institutes of Health Research and the Ontario Women's Health Council, Award NOW-84656. In addition, support to the Centre for Addiction & Mental Health for salary of scientists and infrastructure has been provided by the Ontario Ministry of Health and Long Term Care. The views expressed here do not necessarily reflect those of the Ministry of Health and Long Term Care.
Dr Steiner is consultant for Wyeth Pharmaceuticals, Bayer Shering Pharmaceuticals, Astra-Zeneca, Azevan Pharmaceuticals, and Servier; has received grant and research support from Canadian Institutes of Health Research, Physicians Services Inc, Wyeth Pharmaceuticals, Astra-Zeneca, and Lundbeck, and received an honorarium from Azevan Pharmaceuticals and Ortho-McNeil. This work was supported in part by the Father Sean O'Sullivan Research Centre, St Joseph's Healthcare, Hamilton, Ontario, Canada.
[a] Department of Psychiatry Women's College Hospital, 76 Grenville Street, Room 944C, Toronto, Ontario, M5S 1B2, Canada
[b] Department of Psychiatry, University of Toronto, Toronto, Ontario, Canada
[c] Social Equity & Health Research Section, Centre for Addiction & Mental Health, 455 Spadina Avenue, Suite 300, Toronto, Ontario M5S 2G8, Canada
[d] Department of Psychiatry & Behavioural Neurosciences, McMaster University, Women's Health Concerns Clinic, St Joseph's Healthcare, Fontbonne Building, 6th Floor, 301 James Street, South Hamilton, Ontario L8P 3B6, Canada
[e] Department of Obstetrics & Gynecology, McMaster University, Women's Health Concerns Clinic, St Joseph's Healthcare, Hamilton, Ontario L8N 4A6, Canada
* Corresponding author. Department of Psychiatry & Behavioural Neurosciences, McMaster University, Women's Health Concerns Clinic, St Joseph's Healthcare, Fontbonne Building, 6th Floor, 301 James Street South Hamilton, Ontario L8P 3B6, Canada.
E-mail address: mst@mcmaster.ca (M. Steiner).

Obstet Gynecol Clin N Am 36 (2009) 907–924
doi:10.1016/j.ogc.2009.10.010
0889-8545/09/$ – see front matter © 2009 Elsevier Inc. All rights reserved.

obgyn.theclinics.com

Over the years, varying definitions of menstrual-related mood symptomatology have been presented. The current position of the American Psychiatric Association, as articulated in the fourth edition of the *Diagnostic and Statistical Manual of Mental Disorders* (DSM-IV), recognizes mood disorders related to the menstrual cycle as a significant mental health issue for some women.[3] However, the label of "disorder" is reserved for those problems that clearly interfere with occupational or social functioning. Premenstrual dysphoric disorder (PMDD) is defined in Appendix B of the DSM-IV-Text Revision (DSM-IV-TR), under axes provided for further study, and is categorized in the text itself as a "depressive disorder not otherwise specified."

The negative impact of PMDD symptoms on daily function and quality of life has been documented,[4] and economic burden, specifically in terms of decreased productivity, has been established.[5] Because of this level of impairment, there is great urgency to understand the biologic and psychosocial underpinnings and treatment options for women who suffer from PMDD. Unfortunately, early medical research did not always take female-specific factors into account, and so for many years, these issues went largely unexplored from a scientific perspective. However, more recently, it has been established that the care of the female patient requires a sophisticated understanding of both reproductive and psychosocial factors across the life span. Mood changes related to the menstrual cycle lie at the interface of obstetrics and gynecology and psychiatry, presenting an important opportunity for collaboration between researchers and practitioners across disciplines.

The purpose of this article is to guide women's health practitioners in issues related to diagnosis and appropriate treatment for PMDD. It will aid non–mental health practitioners in the decision about when to refer to mental health professionals, as well as highlight how psychiatric and other women's health professionals may wish to collaborate on management plans. The review will cover the epidemiology of PMDD and issues related to diagnostic clarification. It will highlight what is known about potential biologic, psychological, and sociocultural etiologic factors, and outline treatment options.

DIAGNOSIS OF PREMENSTRUAL DYSPHORIC DISORDER

The essential features required for diagnosis of PMDD are symptoms of marked and persistent anger/irritability, depressed mood, anxiety, or affective lability, which have regularly occurred during the last week of the luteal phase in most menstrual cycles during the past year. The strict diagnostic criteria of at least 5 of 11 symptoms must be applied to differentiate PMDD from milder symptoms of premenstrual syndrome (PMS). PMDD must also be differentiated from an exacerbation of another physical or mental disorder. However, if criteria for both PMDD and another disorder are clearly met, the DSM-IV-TR states that both can be diagnosed.[3]

Differentiation from Premenstrual Syndrome

In addition to the number of required symptoms, severity of the symptoms is a key component of the diagnosis, in that symptoms must cause significant impairment in the ability to function socially or occupationally during the week before menses. The DSM-IV definition explicitly acknowledges that milder symptoms of PMS, such as mild psychological discomfort, bloating, and breast tenderness, affect up to 70% of women, and so should not be considered to be "disordered."

Physical Disorders as Differential Diagnoses

Physical disorders that may mimic PMDD with premenstrual exacerbations include systemic diseases such as autoimmune disorders, diabetes mellitus, anemia, and hypothyroidism as well as gynecologic conditions such as dysmenorrhea and endometriosis.[6] These can usually be readily differentiated from PMDD by careful history, physical examination, and other relevant investigations including, but not limited to, laboratory testing, imaging, and diagnostic surgical procedures. However, clinicians must hold an index of suspicion for these differential diagnoses.

Psychiatric Disorders as Differential Diagnoses

Premenstrual exacerbations and/or magnification of psychiatric disorders, particularly depression and dysthymic disorder, can be more difficult to tease apart from PMDD[7]; however, this clarification is important because of the implications for treatment. For example, women with an underlying depressive disorder (ie, a woman who has mood symptoms throughout the month), but with increasing severity during the premenstrual period, should be treated for the underlying disorder. With successful treatment of the primary condition, premenstrual symptoms will often remit.[8]

Premenstrual exacerbations of depressive disorders are commonly reported. In the National Institute of Mental Health's Sequenced Treatment Alternatives to Relieve Depression (STAR-D) trial, the first 1500 female participants with major depression were asked whether they experienced a worsening of their depressive symptoms before menses. Of the 433 women who were not taking oral contraceptives, 64% reported worsening symptoms 5 to 10 days pre-menses.[7] In a US community sample, Hartlage and colleagues[9] found that 44% of nondepressed women taking antidepressants reported symptoms premenstrually. This supports the assertion that women who report premenstrual depressive symptoms should be screened for depressive symptoms across all phases of the cycle.

Bipolar disorder is also important to consider on the differential diagnosis of PMDD. Women with underlying bipolar disorder may experience premenstrual exacerbations of depressed mood or irritability.[10] This may be because of the bipolar disorder itself, or to fluctuations in medication levels attributable to pharmacokinetic changes in the premenstrual period. For example, lithium, a commonly used mood stabilizer in the management of bipolar disorder, is a water-soluble drug. Therefore, there is a risk for decreased lithium levels premenstrually owing to increases in the volume of distribution in the premenstrual period, although evidence has been contradictory as to whether this theoretical risk bears out in practice.[11] Once again, if a woman meets full criteria for both bipolar disorder and PMDD, both may be diagnosed. There have been several studies attempting to determine whether women with bipolar disorder are at increased risk of comorbid PMDD. Results have been contradictory and overall do not suggest that women with bipolar disorder are at increased risk for PMDD.[10]

There is also some evidence that women with personality disorders may experience increased irritability and interpersonal difficulties in the premenstrual period.[12] Again, it is important to determine whether a woman meets criteria for PMDD in addition to a personality disorder, as this has implications for treatment.

Prospective Symptom Assessment and Rating Scales

To assist clinicians in making a diagnosis of PMDD, and particularly in the context of psychiatric comorbidity, a DSM-IV-TR diagnosis of PMDD requires a minimum of 2 consecutive months of prospectively daily symptom ratings.[3] Prospective ratings are considered essential, because of debate regarding the extent to which retrospective reports of premenstrual symptoms should be considered reliable.[13] Further, some evidence suggests that owing to mood and cognitive changes, there may be differential symptom reporting depending on the phase of the menstrual cycle in which women are queried.[14,15]

Prospective daily symptom ratings are usually made using Likert or visual analog scales. Validated tools include the Daily Record of Severity of Problems or the Penn Daily Symptom Report (as described in a recent comprehensive review by Pearlstein and Steiner[16]). However, many women, including those without PMDD, report some premenstrual symptoms during the follicular phase. A change in the symptom severity score between the luteal and follicular phases is therefore the most meaningful outcome, and a change of between 30% and 50% has been recommended as an indication of a diagnosis of PMDD.[17]

PREVALENCE AND DEMOGRAPHIC CORRELATES

Estimates of the prevalence of PMDD in community samples are difficult to obtain because of the necessity for strict diagnostic criteria. Most prevalence estimates have relied largely on retrospective data, with variable definitions of "severe" symptoms of PMS. In samples from North America and Europe, prevalence estimates based on DSM-IV-TR diagnostic criteria, but without the requirement for prospective symptom ratings, appear to be in the range of 5% to 6%. A German study of more than 1000 young women aged 14 to 24 yielded a 12-month baseline prevalence of PMDD of 5.8%.[18] A Canadian study of 519 women ages 18 to 55 used the Premenstrual Symptom Screening Tool (PSST) to screen for women who might benefit from treatment for PMDD. Consistent with the previous findings, the authors reported that 5.1% of the women likely suffered from PMDD.[19] Interestingly, a Japanese study of 1152 women ages 15 to 49 in a cancer screening clinic reported a prevalence of only 1.2% using retrospective symptom reporting, indicating possible cultural variability in either prevalence or symptom reporting.[20]

Few studies have estimated the prevalence of PMDD by DSM diagnostic criteria using prospective charting and the resulting prevalence rates appear to depend somewhat on the population being studied. In a study of 217 female university students, 4.6% reported a 30% or greater increase in symptom severity during the premenstrual period using prospective charting over 90 days.[21] In older premenopausal women (aged 36 to 44 years), 6.4% of the women who completed prospective ratings for one cycle met criteria for PMDD.[22] A smaller study in Indian women also reported prevalence of 6.4%,[23] and a Croatian study of young adults aged 18 to 30 reported a prevalence of 5.8% using prospectively collected daily rating scales.[24] Slightly lower rates of PMDD have been found in two prospective studies where samples were representative of the population both with respect to age and sampling frame. Sveindottir and Backstrom[25] studied 83 women sampled from the National Registry of Iceland. Although there was no psychiatric testing to rule out other psychiatric disorders, women filled out 1 month of prospective daily mood charting, revealing a prevalence of PMDD between 2% and 6%. Gehlert and colleagues[26] followed 1246 women (ages 13 to 55) sampled from four geographic regions in the United States. These women underwent psychiatric testing by trained research assistants in their homes and they also completed daily symptom checklists over two menstrual cycles. Using strict DSM-IV-TR criteria, only 1.6% of the women were diagnosed with PMDD.

Few demographic variables are predictive of PMS or PMDD. Younger age has been associated with more severe symptoms of PMDD.[27] There are also data to support a relationship between higher levels of education and reporting of premenstrual symptoms.[28] When women with PMDD and no history of major depressive disorder were compared with women with PMDD and history of depression, the PMDD patients with no depression history were more educated.[29] However, when the total sample of older premenopausal women was considered, PMDD was associated with lower levels of education.[22]

The strict diagnostic criteria for PMDD present substantial methodological difficulties for estimating prevalence. However, the available evidence suggests that there is a small but significant proportion of women, as low as 1% but perhaps as high as 7%, who consistently experience premenstrual symptoms of sufficient severity to cause functional impairment. Younger women may experience more severe symptoms of the disorder and there may be some cross-cultural variation in symptom reporting (discussed further later in this article).

POTENTIAL ETIOLOGIC FACTORS

Over the years, there has been an increasing amount of investigation into understanding the etiology of severe premenstrual dysphoria. As with other psychiatric disorders, PMDD likely has multiple biologic, psychological, and sociocultural determinants. Unfortunately, it is very difficult to study how such factors might interact to produce the clinical picture of PMDD. In all likelihood, the causal pathway is complex, with the potential for multiple pathways to a similar clinical outcome. It is important to distinguish between factors that are associated with increased risk for PMDD and factors that may contribute to the pathophysiology of the disorder. The former factors may be regarded as correlates and are most useful for case identification and epidemiologic description, although they may also ultimately contribute clues to the etiology of the disorder. Potential causal factors may be more useful in guiding prevention and treatment of the disorder.

Biologic Factors

Heritability
One method of investigating the biologic contribution to the etiology of a disorder is to use studies of twin pairs. If twins are reared together, they are presumed to have shared early environments. Therefore, studying concordance rates for a certain disease in mono- and dizygotic twins can help determine the level of genetic contribution to the disorder (ie, the environment is controlled). Twin studies have demonstrated high heritability of premenstrual symptoms: one study of more than 1000 female twins estimated heritability of selected premenstrual symptoms at approximately 56%, with no substantial role for familial environmental factors.[30] Another study of 720 female twin pairs estimated heritability of 44%, although the prevalence of PMDD in this study was extremely high at 24%.[31]

Hormones
Female sex hormones The cyclical nature of PMDD lends itself to the hypothesis that dysfunction in hormonal changes related to the menstrual cycle is a primary biologic determinant of the disorder. However, despite the temporal relationship between symptoms of PMDD and phases of the menstrual cycle, the relationship between female sex hormones and PMDD does not appear to be a simple linear one. The most likely explanation is that women with PMDD are in some way vulnerable to the normal physiologic changes associated with the menstrual cycle. This hypothesis has now been supported in two studies, where women with PMDD showed differential response to women with no premenstrual complaints in response to challenge with physiologic levels of estrogen and progesterone.[32,33] In the first study, women with PMDD had more depressed mood than controls and in the second study, they responded to hormonal challenge with altered gonadotropin levels. Huo and

colleagues[34] recently identified allelic variation in ESR1, the estrogen-alpha receptor gene in women with PMDD, providing preliminary evidence of a possible underlying mechanism for these differential responses.

Providing further support to the hypothesis that some women may be susceptible to the changes associated with the menstrual cycle, there is some evidence that women with PMDD may also be more susceptible to mood disorders in the perinatal period and at perimenopause. This has led researchers to hypothesize that there may be a "reproductive" subtype of depression to which some women are prone.[35] Other hormones besides estrogen and progesterone have also been examined in PMDD patients. Several groups have investigated a potential role for the centrally active progesterone metabolite allopregnanolone. There appears to be a relationship between serum concentrations of allopregnanolone and the severity of symptoms in women with PMDD/PMS.[36,37] It has been hypothesized that differences between women with PMDD and controls are related to differences in sensitivity to allopregnanolone, and not to absolute levels of the neurosteroid.[38] This has been supported in various studies involving the GABA-A receptor, where allopregnanolone acts in the central nervous system. Imaging studies have shown that women with PMDD have differential GABA-A receptor sensitivity,[39] and women with PMDD show differential sensitivity to other compounds with GABA-A activity. PMDD patients are also reported to be more sensitive than control subjects to the anxiogenic effects of the benzodiazepine antagonist flumazenil[40] and less sensitive than controls to a number of benzodiazepines.[41,42] In addition, the severity of symptoms in women with PMDD appears to be related to their sensitivity to GABA steroids.[43] This sensitivity normalizes during treatment with serotonin reuptake inhibitors, possibly because of the drug's modulating effect on allopregnanolone levels, via GABA-A receptors.[44]

Androgens Androgens have also come under investigation in PMDD, in large part because of the prominence of irritability in the PMDD symptom profile. Eriksson and colleagues[45] have observed elevated testosterone levels in women with severe premenstrual irritability. A positive correlation between free testosterone concentrations and irritability has also been observed by our group, but only in patients who reported severe symptoms.[46] One study revealed significantly lower total and free plasma testosterone levels in PMS patients as compared with healthy controls.[47] Some success has been reported in treating PMDD with androgen antagonists.[45]

Other endocrine factors
Other endocrine factors, including cortisol, thyroid hormone, prolactin, melatonin, aldosterone, and endorphins, have also been postulated as contributors to PMS/PMDD. As yet, however, there is little consistent evidence for their involvement.[16,48]

Serotonin
Research investigations using a number of experimental models have also consistently demonstrated an important role for serotonin in the pathophysiology of PMDD. Relationships between serotonin function and secretion of ovarian hormones have also been established, making a complex interaction between hormone secretion and serotonin fluctuation plausible.[49] PMDD patients have lower whole blood serotonin levels[50] and lower platelet serotonin uptake[51] during the premenstrual phase. Melke and colleagues[52] found that women with premenstrual dysphoria had fewer platelet paroxetine binding sites (ie, fewer serotonin transporters) than controls. Differences in brain serotonergic function across the menstrual cycle between women with PMDD and controls have also been identified using positron emission technology

(PET).[53] Challenges with serotonergic agents, such as L-tryptophan, fenfluramine, and buspirone, have similarly provided evidence of serotonin dysfunction in women with PMDD.[54–58]

Several studies have attempted to delineate the genetic basis for differences in serotonin function and metabolism in women with PMDD. Research into AP-2, 5HT transporter, tryptophan hydroxylase, and monoamine oxidase genotypes has mostly been inconclusive.[52,59,60] However, Praschak-Rieder and colleagues[61] found an association between PMDD and 5HTLLPR heterozygosity in women with seasonal affective disorder, and Steiner and colleagues[46] identified a relationship between polymorphism in the serotonin transporter gene and severity of PMDD symptoms.

Finally, the finding that serotonergic drugs, and particularly the selective serotonin reuptake inhibitors (SSRIs) treat PMDD rapidly (see further discussion later in this article), strongly supports the hypothesis that serotonin is involved in the etiology of PMDD. However, it is notable that only 60% of PMDD patients respond to treatment with SSRIs,[62] suggesting that serotonin may not be the only etiologic variable in all PMDD patients.

Psychosocial Factors

Sociocultural factors

As noted previously, a limited number of studies have examined symptoms of PMS and PMDD in non-Western societies. This research has often been plagued by a number of important methodological concerns and, in particular, questionable validity of instruments that have been translated for use in populations other than those in which they were developed. There may be variations in how women respond to questions based on phrasing, expectations, or cultural issues.[63]

As a result of observed cross-cultural differences, the concept of "menstrual socialization" has been proposed as a determinant of premenstrual complaints, suggesting that PMS is a culture-bound syndrome, specific to Western cultures in which most women have been socialized to have negative expectations about menstruation.[64] More specifically, it is argued that North American culture and media perpetuate the idea that the premenstrual period will be associated with negative affect and mood instability,[2] causing women to interpret normal physiologic changes that are essentially neutral in nature to have negative connotations.[65] A role for expectations about menstruation in premenstrual symptom reporting was illustrated in a study where women who viewed a videotape describing the negative consequences of PMS later reported more severe premenstrual symptoms than did women in a control group who watched a neutral video.[66] Similarly, women who were led to believe that they were premenstrual reported significantly more severe physical symptoms than did women who were led to believe that they were not premenstrual.[67] These findings are of particular note in the context of a study that demonstrated that a group intervention designed to positively reframe the experience of menstruation can significantly reduce premenstrual impairment in women with PMDD.[68]

Life stress

Several studies have demonstrated an association between PMS/PMDD and stressful life events,[69–71] and particularly day-to-day stress.[72] Women with premenstrual symptoms also tend to rely more than other women on less effective strategies for coping with stress, such as avoidance or wishful thinking, than on strategies such as problem-focused coping or direct action,[2,73] High levels of state and trait anxiety have been observed in PMS patients.[74,75]

The consistent relationship between life stressors and PMS/PMDD has prompted the suggestion that symptoms may develop as "a learned, legitimate, feminine way of expressing frustration"[65] and, in particular, expressing frustration with the conflict between women's productive and reproductive social roles.[64] This is supported by data from one study that examined personality characteristics of women seeking treatment for premenstrual complaints and found unusually high mean scores on the subscale of the Minnesota Multiphasic Personality Inventory that assesses identification with a traditional feminine social role. This is despite the fact that their sample was highly educated and largely working outside of the home. Further, premenstrual complaints were associated with strong tendencies to overcontrol or repress angry feelings.[76] Further research is needed to elucidate the relationship between traditional gender role socialization and, particularly, silencing one's anger in premenstrual symptoms.

Sexual abuse

Past sexual abuse is reported by a significant proportion of women seeking treatment for PMS: a prevalence of 40% was reported in a population of women seeking treatment at a PMS clinic[77] and 32% among psychiatric inpatients with PMS.[78] This can be compared with a rate of 12.4% in the general population of women.[79] Sexual abuse, and childhood sexual abuse particularly, has lasting effects on both psychological and physiologic responses to stress.[80] Through effects on HPA axis function, past abuse could predispose women to psychiatric disorders, including PMDD. Preliminary evidence suggests that the high prevalence of sexual abuse among women seeking treatment for premenstrual symptoms may account for findings of dysregulated cardiovascular and neuroendocrine responses to laboratory stress in PMDD patients.[81] In fact, Bunevicius and colleagues[82] found that women with PMDD with and without histories of sexual abuse had differential autonomic nervous system response to a challenge with the a-receptor agonist clonidine. In one recent study, more than 80% of women with sexual abuse history seeking treatment for PMS had not previously disclosed the abuse to any health care provider,[83] suggesting that abuse history should be routinely assessed in women with suspected PMDD.

Therefore, overall there is convincing evidence for important roles for biologic and sociocultural variables in the development and interpretation of premenstrual symptoms. A weakness of much of the existing literature is that many of the sociocultural risk factors have largely been investigated in the context of their association with premenstrual symptoms rather than the syndrome of PMDD, and it is not known whether these findings can be generalized. Also, there is very little existing literature investigating how biologic and sociocultural variables may interact in the development of severe PMS and PMDD. For example, childhood sexual abuse has lasting effects on multiple biologic and psychological variables, including endocrine responses to stress and coping styles, which ultimately contribute to a woman's risk for adulthood depression.[84] Further interdisciplinary research into risk factors for PMDD will provide a more complete understanding of the roots of this disorder.

TREATMENT OF PREMENSTRUAL DYSPHORIC DISORDER

Insofar as PMDD has multiple biologic and sociocultural etiologic determinants, its treatment should involve an integrated approach, tailored to each patient's particular set of circumstances. A stepwise approach is recommended, with treatment appropriately reflecting the severity and functional impairment associated with the symptoms. In all cases, treatment should also be provided to address any comorbid psychiatric or medical disorders and issues related to any persistent life stressors or any past or current physical or sexual abuse.

Healthy Lifestyle

For women with mild symptoms, education about the condition, supportive counseling, and general healthy lifestyle measures, such as regular exercise and healthy diet, may be sufficient to result in symptom improvement. Expert opinion is that lifestyle modifications should be the first approach taken in all women presenting with premenstrual complaints, and can be conveniently given a 2-month trial while the patient completes the prospective daily ratings necessary to confirm the diagnosis of PMDD.[85]

Dietary changes can have a noticeable impact on symptom severity: women should be encouraged to reduce or eliminate intake of salty foods, sugar, caffeine (especially coffee), red meat, and alcohol. Increased consumption of fruits, vegetables, legumes, whole grains, and water is also recommended. Finally, eating smaller, more frequent meals that are high in carbohydrates may specifically improve symptoms of tension and depression.[85]

Although evidence for an effect of exercise on PMDD symptoms is largely anecdotal, regular exercise can be advised as part of a healthy lifestyle regimen. Aerobic exercise for 20 to 30 minutes, three to four times per week has been recommended.[86] Reduction of body weight to within 20% of ideal, where possible, is an appropriate goal.[8]

For many women, PMDD is associated with sleep irregularities.[48] To alleviate the associated distress and discomfort, adoption of a regular sleep-wake pattern may be helpful. Women should be encouraged to adhere to consistent bedtimes and waking times during the premenstrual period, and ideally across the menstrual cycle.

Encouraging women to avoid planning stressful activities for the premenstrual period whenever possible can be helpful. This can be facilitated by having women complete symptom assessment forms before, during, and after treatment. Women should be encouraged to review their own daily diaries and identify triggers for symptom exacerbation.

Dietary Supplements

Several dietary supplements are recommended in the lay press for treatment of PMS/PMDD symptoms. Unfortunately, with few exceptions, little scientific evidence is available to support these recommendations.[87] However, so long as they are used at doses that are within the range of recommended daily intake, use of certain dietary supplements need not be discouraged.

Calcium supplementation shows some promise for treatment of PMS/PMDD. One large trial found that 1200 mg of calcium daily reduced symptoms of PMS, including depression, by the second or third treatment cycle.[88] This study has some methodological limitations, in particular the lack of exclusion on the basis of follicular phase symptoms, and thus requires replication. However, increased calcium intake has benefits beyond those associated with reduction of PMS symptoms, particularly with respect to prevention of osteoporosis, and is not associated with any adverse effects so long as doses do not exceed 1500 mg daily.[86]

There is also evidence for efficacy of vitamin B6 (pyridoxine) in treating premenopausal women with depression.[89] This has led to investigation into pyridoxine as a treatment for premenstrual mood symptomatology, although no trials have been done in women with strictly diagnosed PMDD. A recent double-blind placebo-controlled trial of 94 women with premenstrual mood and somatic symptoms revealed a greater decrease in psychiatric symptoms with 80 mg of vitamin B6 compared with placebo.[90] It should be noted that vitamin B6 supplementation is not without risk and higher doses have been associated with peripheral neuropathy.[91]

Although early research suggested that magnesium supplementation was effective for fluid retention in women with PMS, follow-up research has not supported its efficacy for psychiatric symptoms.[92] The effects of complex carbohydrate supplementation have been studied with the rationale that increased tryptophan availability might increase serotonin synthesis. To date, there are two reports of positive effects of a carbohydrate-rich beverage on affective symptoms in women with PMS.[93,94] Soy supplementation also reduced physical but not affective symptoms in a small sample of women with PMS.[95]

Herbal, Complementary, and Other Treatments

Herbal, complementary, and other treatment options have also been addressed in recent reviews, and the strongest evidence appears to be for *Vitex agnus castus* (Chasteberry), which may act as a dopamine agonist to reduce follicle-stimulating hormone (FSH) or prolactin levels, although it may be more beneficial for physical rather than psychological symptoms of PMDD.[16] There are small randomized controlled trials (RCTs) to support saffron and Qi therapy.[96,97]

There have been reports of initial positive RCTs of massage, reflexology, chiropractic manipulation, and biofeedback. Open trials also suggest support for yoga, guided imagery, photic stimulation, and acupuncture.[16] Bright light therapy has been studied as a treatment for PMDD with the rationale that it may induce rapid increase in serotonin (without the side effects of psychotropic medication). Although there has been little evidence to date, a systematic review of four trials suggests that bright light therapy may be an effective option for women with PMDD.[98]

Psychoeducation and Behavioral Treatment

Group psychoeducation can be effective in managing PMS and PMDD. A controlled trial of a psychoeducational group intervention with a focus on positive reframing of women's perceptions of their menstrual cycles found that women with PMDD who received the intervention had reduced premenstrual symptoms and premenstrual impairment, although there were no differences in post-treatment depression or anxiety scores.[68] Several other studies have also noted efficacy of group support in managing symptoms of PMS.[99–101] Relaxation therapy, which is also effective in treating PMS, may be particularly appropriate for women who report a high degree of daily stress.[102,103]

Psychotherapy

Lustyk and colleagues[104] performed a systematic review of the literature to assess the efficacy of cognitive behaviour therapy (CBT) for PMS and PMDD. They identified seven published peer-reviewed studies, of which only five had control groups and only three could be regarded as RCTs. They concluded that on the basis of the existing literature, psychotherapy may provide some benefit; however, effect sizes did not approach those of pharmacotherapy or even behavioral treatments such as relaxation.

Pharmacotherapy for Premenstrual Dysphoric Disorder: Serotonergic Drugs

For women who do not respond to conservative therapies or who have severe symptoms in need of immediate treatment, serotonergic medications, the SSRIs specifically, are the first line of treatment. Over the past several years, the efficacy and safety of using SSRIs in the treatment of PMDD have been well established. As this topic has been comprehensively reviewed in several recent publications[17,105,106] only the relevant conclusions will be summarized here.

Fluoxetine, sertraline, and paroxetine have received Food and Drug Administration (FDA) indications for PMDD, although a Cochrane Database meta-analysis also reveals good evidence of effectiveness for fluvoxamine, citalopram, and the seroto-nergic tricyclic antidepressant clomipramine as well.[106] There has been an RCT supporting the efficacy of the selective serotonin and norepinephrine reuptake inhibitor (SNRI) venlafaxine XR dosed continually across the menstrual cycle and a recent single-blind trial revealing preliminary evidence of effectiveness for the SNRI duloxe-tine.[107,108] For reasons still poorly understood, although SSRIs generally require 2 to 4 weeks for therapeutic effectiveness in depression, they are reported to be effective for PMDD when used either continuously or only in the premenstrual (luteal) phase of the menstrual cycle. Perhaps because of the lack of continued administration, there is no discontinuation syndrome when they are used in this manner. Evidence does indicate that symptoms can recur rapidly when treatment is discontinued, particularly in the women with the most severe symptoms at baseline.[109]

Manipulation of Menstruation

The next line of treatment for severe PMDD involves manipulating the usual hormonal fluctuations associated with the menstrual cycle with the goal of suppressing ovula-tion. Although many hormonal regimens have been suggested for this purpose, few have demonstrated efficacy. Oral contraceptives provide a reasonably safe means of inhibiting ovulation; however, the efficacy of most oral contraceptives in the treatment of PMDD is not well established. The FDA has recently approved a combination of ethinyl estradiol and drospirenone for the treatment of PMDD and a recent Co-chrane Database systematic review supports its efficacy.[110] It is thought that the anti-androgen and anti-mineralocorticoid properties of drospirenone account for the efficacy of this product (as compared with traditional oral contraceptive pills). Likely because the potential for adverse effects with oral contraceptives (eg, deep vein thrombosis, pulmonary embolism) exceeds that of the SSRIs, the FDA indication for this treatment has been limited to women who also wish to use the medication for contraceptive purposes.

The best studied class of drugs for this purpose is the gonadotropin-releasing hormone (GnRH) agonists, such as leuprolide acetate, which have been clearly demon-strated to alleviate symptoms of PMS/PMDD.[62,111] However, GnRH agonists appear to be less effective in treating affective symptoms of PMDD than physical symptoms,[112] and long-term use of GnRH agonists has been associated with a number of unfavorable side effects, including risk for hypoestrogenism and osteoporosis,[9] particularly when the therapy is used for longer than 6 months.[62] Add-back estrogen-progesterone supplementation may prevent some of the undesired side effects of GnRH therapy, but effects of add-back therapy on treatment efficacy may be undesirable.[62] The adverse effects of add-back therapy are purported to be attributable to the use of progesterone; however, estrogen-only add-back therapy is not realistic in premeno-pausal women owing to the increased risk of reproductive cancer. Segebladh and colleagues[113] attempted to discern the optimal hormonal add-back strategy in 27 women with PMDD. The results of their RCT concluded that low-dose estrogen (0.5 mg estrodiol) plus progesterone was superior to high-dose estrogen (1.5 mg estrodiol) plus progesterone in terms of preventing PMDD symptom recurrence.

The synthetic steroid danazol appears to reduce affective and physical symptoms of PMS/PMDD[114]; however, its practical use is limited by the need for concurrent administration of a reliable contraception method. At low doses (200 mg/d), ovulation and thus conception are still possible, and danazol can cause virilization of the fetus. Doses sufficient to inhibit ovulation (600–800 mg/d) have been associated with undesirable side effects, including weight gain, mood changes, and acne.[62]

The final treatment option for women with severe PMDD symptoms and no response to other therapies is permanent suppression of ovulation through oophorectomy. Bilateral oophorectomy with hysterectomy has been reported to be highly effective in permanently eliminating symptoms of PMS.[115] However, because of the extreme nature of this treatment method, it is not recommended even for severe cases. It is possible that the sudden change in hormonal milieu associated with surgical menopause could also be a trigger for mood problems in vulnerable women.

SUMMARY

Existing evidence indicates that there is a small but significant population of women in whom premenstrual symptoms, and particularly affective symptoms, severely impair functioning. Although PMDD is predominantly regarded as a biologically based illness, there is also evidence that variables such as life stress, history of sexual abuse, and cultural socialization are important determinants of premenstrual symptoms. In diagnosing and treating PMDD patients, attention to biologic and sociocultural variables is recommended.

REFERENCES

1. Delaney J, Lupton MJ, Toth E. The curse: a cultural history of menstruation. New York: E.P. Dutton; 1976.
2. Chrisler JC, Johnston-Robledo I. Raging hormones? Feminist perspectives on premenstrual syndrome and postpartum depression. In: Ballou M, Brown LS, editors. Rethinking mental health and disorder: feminist perspectives. New York: Guilford Press; 2002. p. 174–97.
3. American Psychiatric Association. Diagnostic and statistical manual of mental disorders. 4th edition. Text Revision (DSM-IV-TR). Washington, DC: American Psychiatric Association; 2000. p. 771–4.
4. Yang M, Wallenstein G, Hagan M, et al. Burden of premenstrual dysphoric disorder on health-related quality of life. J Womens Health (Larchmt) 2008; 17(1):113–21.
5. Chawla A, Swindle R, Long S, et al. Premenstrual dysphoric disorder: is there an economic burden of illness? Med Care 2002;40:1101–12.
6. Steiner M, Peer M, Soares CN. Comorbidity and premenstrual syndrome: recognition and treatment approaches. Gynaecology Forum 2006;11:13–6.
7. Kornstein SG, Harvey AT, Rush AJ, et al. Self-reported premenstrual exacerbation of depressive symptoms in patients seeking treatment for major depression. Psychol Med 2005;35(5):683–92.
8. Steiner M, Born L. Psychiatric aspects of the menstrual cycle. In: Kornstein SG, Clayton AH, editors. Women's mental health: a comprehensive textbook. New York: Guilford Press; 2002. p. 48–69.
9. Hartlage SA, Brandenburg DL, Kravitz HM. Premenstrual exacerbation of depressive disorders in a community-based sample in the United States. Psychosom Med 2004;66(5):698–706.
10. Kim DR, Gyulai L, Freeman EW, et al. Premenstrual dysphoric disorder and psychiatric co-morbidity. Arch Womens Ment Health 2004;7(1):37–47.
11. Burt VK, Rasgon N. Special considerations in treating bipolar disorder in women. Bipolar Disord 2004;6(1):2–13.

12. Critchlow DG, Bond AJ, Wingrove J. Mood disorder history and personality assessment in premenstrual dysphoric disorder. J Clin Psychiatry 2001;62(9): 688–93.
13. Rubinow DR, Roy-Byrne P, Hoban MC, et al. Prospective assessment of menstrually related mood disorders. Am J Psychiatry 1984;141:684–6.
14. Meaden PM, Hartlage SA, Cook-Karr J. Timing and severity of symptoms associated with the menstrual cycle in a community-based sample in the Midwestern United States. Psychiatry Res 2005;134(1):27–36.
15. Lane T, Francis A. Premenstrual symptomatology, locus of control, anxiety and depression in women with normal menstrual cycles. Arch Womens Ment Health 2003;6(2):127–38.
16. Pearlstein T, Steiner M. Premenstrual dysphoric disorder: burden of illness and treatment update. J Psychiatry Neurosci 2008;33(4):291–301.
17. Smith MJ, Schmidt PJ, Rubinow DR. Operationalizing DSM-IV criteria for PMDD: selecting symptomatic and asymptomatic cycles for research. J Psychiatr Res 2003;37:75–83.
18. Wittchen HU, Becker E, Lieb R, et al. Prevalence, incidence and stability of premenstrual dysphoric disorder in the community. Psychol Med 2002;32:119–32.
19. Steiner M, Macdougall M, Brown E. The premenstrual symptoms screening tool (PSST) for clinicians. Arch Womens Ment Health 2003;6(3):203–9.
20. Takeda T, Tasaka K, Sakata M, et al. Prevalence of premenstrual syndrome and premenstrual dysphoric disorder in Japanese women. Arch Womens Ment Health 2006;9(4):209–12.
21. Rivera-Tovar AD, Frank E. Late luteal phase dysphoric disorder in young women. Am J Psychiatry 1990;147:1634–6.
22. Cohen LS, Soares CN, Otto MW, et al. Prevalence and predictors of premenstrual dysphoric disorder (PMDD) in older premenopausal women. The Harvard study of moods and cycles. J Affect Disord 2002;70:125–32.
23. Banerjee N, Roy KK, Takkar D. Premenstrual dysphoric disorder—a study from India. Int J Fertil Womens Med 2000;45:342–4.
24. Rojnic Kuzman M, Hotujac L. Premenstrual dysphoric disorder—a neglected diagnosis? Preliminary study on a sample of Croatian students. Coll Antropol 2007;31(1):131–7.
25. Sveindottir H, Backstrom T. Prevalence of menstrual cycle symptom cyclicity and premenstrual dysphoric disorder in a random sample of women using and not using oral contraceptives. Acta Obstet Gynecol Scand 2000;79:405–13.
26. Gehlert S, Song IH, Chang CH, et al. The prevalence of premenstrual dysphoric disorder in a randomly selected group of urban and rural women. Psychol Med 2009;39(1):129–36.
27. Freeman EW, Rickels K, Schweizer E, et al. Relationships between age and symptom severity among women seeking medical treatment for premenstrual symptoms. Psychol Med 1995;25:309–15.
28. Marvan ML, Diaz-Erosa M, Montesinos A. Premenstrual symptoms in Mexican women with different educational levels. J Psychol 1998;132:517–26.
29. Soares CN, Cohen LS, Otto MW, et al. Characteristics of women with premenstrual dysphoric disorder (PMDD) who did or did not report history of depression: a preliminary report from the Harvard study of moods and cycles. J Womens Health Gend Based Med 2001;10:873–8.
30. Kendler KS, Karkowski LM, Corey LA, et al. Longitudinal population-based twin study of retrospectively reported premenstrual symptoms and lifetime major depression. Am J Psychiatry 1998;155:1234–40.

31. Treloar SA, Heath AC, Martin NG. Genetic and environmental influences on premenstrual symptoms in an Australian twin sample. Psychol Med 2002; 32(1):25–38.

32. Schmidt PJ, Nieman LK, Danaceau MA, et al. Differential behavioral effects of gonadal steroids in women with and in those without premenstrual syndrome. N Engl J Med 1998;338:209–16.

33. Eriksson O, Backstrom T, Stridsberg M, et al. Differential response to estrogen challenge test in women with and without premenstrual dysphoria. Psychoneuroendocrinology 2006;31(4):415–27.

34. Huo L, Straub RE, Roca C, et al. Risk for premenstrual dysphoric disorder is associated with genetic variation in ESR1, the estrogen receptor alpha gene. Biol Psychiatry 2007;62(8):925–33.

35. Payne JL, Palmer JT, Joffe H. A reproductive subtype of depression: conceptualizing models and moving toward etiology. Harv Rev Psychiatry 2009;17(2):72–86.

36. Freeman EW, Frye CA, Rickels K, et al. Allopregnanolone levels and symptom improvement in severe premenstrual syndrome. J Clin Psychopharmacol 2002;22:516–20.

37. Nyberg S, Backstrom T, Zingmark E, et al. Allopregnanolone decrease with symptom improvement during placebo and gonadotropin-releasing hormone agonist treatment in women with severe premenstrual syndrome. Gynecol Endocrinol 2007;23(5):257–66.

38. Andreen L, Nyberg S, Turkmen S, et al. Sex steroid induced negative mood may be explained by the paradoxical effect mediated by GABAA modulators. Psychoneuroendocrinology 2009;34(8):1121–32.

39. Epperson CN, Haga K, Mason GF, et al. Cortical gamma-aminobutyric acid levels across the menstrual cycle in healthy women and those with premenstrual dysphoric disorder: a proton magnetic resonance spectroscopy study. Arch Gen Psychiatry 2002;59:851–8.

40. Le Melledo JM, Van Driel M, Coupland NJ, et al. Response to flumazenil in women with premenstrual dysphoric disorder. Am J Psychiatry 2000;157:821–3.

41. Sundstrom I, Ashbrook D, Backstrom T. Reduced benzodiazepine sensitivity in patients with premenstrual syndrome: a pilot study. Psychoneuroendocrinology 1997;22:25–38.

42. Sundstrom I, Nyberg S, Backstrom T. Patients with premenstrual syndrome have reduced sensitivity to midazolam compared to control subjects. Neuropsychopharmacology 1997;17:370–81.

43. Sundstrom I, Andersson A, Nyberg S, et al. Patients with premenstrual syndrome have a different sensitivity to a neuroactive steroid during the menstrual cycle compared to control subjects. Neuroendocrinology 1998;67(2):126–38.

44. Sundstrom I, Backstrom T. Citalopram increases pregnanolone sensitivity in patients with premenstrual syndrome: an open trial. Psychoneuroendocrinology 1998;23(1):73–88.

45. Eriksson E, Sundblad C, Landen M, et al. Behavioural effects of androgens in women. In: Steiner M, Yonkers KA, Eriksson E, editors. Mood disorders in women. London: Martin Dunitz; 2000. p. 233–46.

46. Steiner M, Dunn EJ, MacDougall M, et al. Serotonin transporter gene polymorphism, free testosterone, and symptoms associated with premenstrual dysphoric disorder. Biol Psychiatry 2002;51:91S.

47. Bloch M, Schmidt PJ, Su TP, et al. Pituitary-adrenal hormones and testosterone across the menstrual cycle in women with premenstrual syndrome and controls. Biol Psychiatry 1998;43:897–903.

48. Baker FC, Kahan TL, Trinder J, et al. Sleep quality and the sleep electroencephalogram in women with severe premenstrual syndrome. Sleep 2007;30(10): 1283–91.
49. Steiner M, Pearlstein T. Premenstrual dysphoria and the serotonin system: pathophysiology and treatment. J Clin Psychiatry 2000;61(Suppl 12):17–21.
50. Rapkin AJ, Edelmuth E, Chang LC, et al. Whole-blood serotonin in premenstrual syndrome. Obstet Gynecol 1987;70:533–7.
51. Taylor DL, Mathew RJ, Ho BT, et al. Serotonin levels and platelet uptake during premenstrual tension. Neuropsychobiology 1984;12:16–8.
52. Melke J, Westberg L, Landen M, et al. Serotonin transporter gene polymorphisms and platelet [^{3}H] paroxetine binding in premenstrual dysphoria. Psychoneuroendocrinology 2003;28(3):446–58.
53. Jovanovic H, Cerin A, Karlsson P, et al. A PET study of 5-HT1A receptors at different phases of the menstrual cycle in women with premenstrual dysphoria. Psychiatry Res 2006;148(2–3):185–93.
54. Bancroft J, Cook A, Davidson D, et al. Blunting of neuroendocrine responses to infusion of L-tryptophan in women with perimenstrual mood change. Psychol Med 1991;21:305–12.
55. Yatham LN. Is 5HT1α receptor subsensitivity a trait marker for late luteal phase dysphoric disorder? A pilot study. Can J Psychiatry 1993;38:662–4.
56. FitzGerald M, Malone KM, Li S, et al. Blunted serotonin response to fenfluramine challenge in premenstrual dysphoric disorder. Am J Psychiatry 1997; 154:556–8.
57. Steiner M, Yatham LN, Coote M, et al. Serotonergic dysfunction in women with pure premenstrual dysphoric disorder: is the fenfluramine challenge test still relevant? Psychiatry Res 1999;87:107–15.
58. Rasgon N, Serra M, Biggio G, et al. Neuroactive steroid-serotonergic interaction: responses to an intravenous L-tryptophan challenge in women with premenstrual syndrome. Eur J Endocrinol 2001;145:25–33.
59. Magnay JL, Ismail KM, Chapman G, et al. Serotonin transporter, tryptophan hydroxylase, and monoamine oxidase A gene polymorphisms in premenstrual dysphoric disorder. Am J Obstet Gynecol 2006;195(5):1254–9.
60. Damberg M, Westberg L, Berggard C, et al. Investigation of transcription factor AP-2 beta genotype in women with premenstrual dysphoric disorder. Neurosci Lett 2005;377(1):49–52.
61. Praschak-Rieder N, Willeit M, Winkler D, et al. Role of family history and 5-HTTLPR polymorphism in female seasonal affective disorder patients with and without premenstrual dysphoric disorder. Eur Neuropsychopharmacol 2002;12(2):129–34.
62. Mitwally MF, Kahn LS, Halbreich U. Pharmacotherapy of premenstrual syndromes and premenstrual dysphoric disorder: current practices. Expert Opin Pharmacother 2002;3:1577–90.
63. Halbreich U, Alarcon RD, Calil H, et al. Culturally-sensitive complaints of depressions and anxieties in women. J Affect Disord 2007;102(1–3):159–76.
64. Johnson TM. Premenstrual syndrome as a Western culture-specific disorder. Cult Med Psychiatry 1987;11:337–56.
65. Anson O. Exploring the bio-psycho–social approach to premenstrual experiences. Soc Sci Med 1999;49:67–80.
66. Marvan ML, Escobedo C. Premenstrual symptomatology: role of prior knowledge about premenstrual syndrome. Psychosom Med 1999;61:163–7.
67. Ruble DN. Premenstrual symptoms: a reinterpretation. Science 1977;197:291–2.

68. Morse G. Positively reframing perceptions of the menstrual cycle among women with premenstrual syndrome. J Obstet Gynecol Neonatal Nurs 1999;28:165–74.

69. Beck LE, Gevirtz R, Mortola JF. The predictive role of psychosocial stress on symptom severity in premenstrual syndrome. Psychosom Med 1990;52:536–43.

70. Warner P, Bancroft J. Factors related to self-reporting of the pre-menstrual syndrome. Br J Psychiatry 1990;157:249–60.

71. Fontana AM, Palfai TG. Psychosocial factors in premenstrual dysphoria: stressors, appraisal, and coping processes. J Psychosom Res 1994;38:557–67.

72. Woods NF, Most A, Longenecker GD. Major life events, daily stressors, and perimenstrual symptoms. Nurse Res 1985;34:263–7.

73. Ornitz AW, Brown MA. Family coping and premenstrual symptomatology. J Obstet Gynecol Neonatal Nurs 1993;22:49–55.

74. Picone L, Kirkby RJ. Relationship between anxiety and premenstrual syndrome. Psychol Rep 1990;67:43–8.

75. Christensen AP, Board BJ, Oei TPS. A psychosocial profile of women with premenstrual dysphoria. J Affect Disord 1992;25:251–9.

76. Stout AL, Steege JF. Psychological assessment of women seeking treatment for premenstrual syndrome. J Psychosom Res 1985;29:621–9.

77. Paddison PL, Gise LH, Lebovits A, et al. Sexual abuse and premenstrual syndrome: comparison between a lower and higher socioeconomic group. Psychosomatics 1990;31:265–72.

78. Friedman RC, Hurt SW, Clarkin J, et al. Sexual histories and premenstrual affective syndrome in psychiatric inpatients. Am J Psychiatry 1982;139:1484–6.

79. MacMillan HL, Fleming JE, Streiner DL, et al. Childhood abuse and lifetime psychopathology in a community sample. Am J Psychiatry 2001;158:1878–83.

80. Heim C, Newport DJ, Heit S, et al. Pituitary-adrenal and autonomic responses to stress in women after sexual and physical abuse in childhood. JAMA 2000;284: 592–7.

81. Matsumoto T, Ushiroyama T, Kimura T, et al. Altered autonomic nervous system activity as a potential etiological factor of premenstrual syndrome and premenstrual dysphoric disorder. Biopsychosoc Med 2007;1:24.

82. Bunevicius R, Hinderliter AL, Light KC, et al. Histories of sexual abuse are associated with differential effects of clonidine on autonomic function in women with premenstrual dysphoric disorder. Biol Psychol 2005;69(3):281–96.

83. Golding JM, Taylor DL, Menard L, et al. Prevalence of sexual abuse history in a sample of women seeking treatment for premenstrual syndrome. J Psychosom Obstet Gynaecol 2000;21:69–80.

84. Kendler KS, Gardner CO, Prescott CA. Toward a comprehensive developmental model for major depression in women. Am J Psychiatry. 2002;159:1133–45.

85. Jarvis CI, Lynch AM, Morin AK. Management strategies for premenstrual syndrome/premenstrual dysphoric disorder. Ann Pharmacother 2008;42(7):967–78.

86. Frackiewicz EJ, Shiovitz TM. Evaluation and management of premenstrual syndrome and premenstrual dysphoric disorder. J Am Pharm Assoc 2001;41: 437–47.

87. Bendich A. The potential for dietary supplements to reduce premenstrual syndrome (PMS) symptoms. J Am Coll Nutr 2000;19:3–12.

88. Thys-Jacobs S, Starkey P, Bernstein D, et al. Calcium carbonate and the premenstrual syndrome: effects on premenstrual and menstrual symptoms. Am J Obstet Gynecol 1998;179:444–52.

89. Williams AL, Cotter A, Sabina A, et al. The role for vitamin B-6 as treatment for depression: a systematic review. Fam Pract 2005;22(5):532–7.

90. Kashanian M, Mazinani R, Jalalmanesh S. Pyridoxine (vitamin B6) therapy for premenstrual syndrome. Int J Gynaecol Obstet 2007;96(1):43–4.

91. Wyatt KM, Dimmock PW, Jones PW, et al. Efficacy of vitamin B-6 in the treatment of premenstrual syndrome: systematic review. BMJ 1999;318:1375–81.

92. Khine K, Rosenstein DL, Elin RJ, et al. Magnesium (Mg) retention and mood effects after intravenous mg infusion in premenstrual dysphoric disorder. Biol Psychiatry 2006;59(4):327–33.

93. Sayegh R, Schiff I, Wurtman J, et al. The effect of a carbohydrate-rich beverage on mood, appetite, and cognitive function in women with premenstrual syndrome. Obstet Gynecol 1995;86:520–8.

94. Freeman EW, Stout AL, Endicott J, et al. Treatment of premenstrual syndrome with a carbohydrate-rich beverage. Int J Gynaecol Obstet 2002;77(3):253–4.

95. Bryant M, Cassidy A, Hill C, et al. Effect of consumption of soy isoflavones on behavioural, somatic and affective symptoms in women with premenstrual syndrome. Br J Nutr 2005;93(5):731–9.

96. Agha-Hosseini M, Kashani L, Aleyaseen A, et al. Crocus sativus L. (saffron) in the treatment of premenstrual syndrome: a double-blind, randomised and placebo-controlled trial. BJOG 2008;115(4):515–9.

97. Jang HS, Lee MS. Effects of qi therapy (external qigong) on premenstrual syndrome: a randomized placebo-controlled study. J Altern Complement Med 2004;10(3):456–62.

98. Krasnik C, Montori VM, Guyatt GH, et al. Medically Unexplained Syndromes Study Group. The effect of bright light therapy on depression associated with premenstrual dysphoric disorder. Am J Obstet Gynecol 2005;193(3 Pt 1):658–61.

99. Walton J, Youngkin E. The effect of a support group on self-esteem of women with premenstrual syndrome. J Obstet Gynecol Neonatal Nurs. 1987;16:174–8.

100. Seideman RY. Effects of a premenstrual syndrome education program on premenstrual symptomatology. Health Care Women Int 1990;11:491–501.

101. Taylor D. Effectiveness of professional–peer group treatment: symptom management for women with PMS. Res Nurs Health 1999;22:496–511.

102. Goodale IL, Domar AD, Benson H. Alleviation of premenstrual syndrome symptoms with the relaxation response. Obstet Gynecol 1990;75:649–55.

103. Morse CA, Dennerstein L, Farrell E, et al. A comparison of hormone therapy, coping skills training, and relaxation for the relief of premenstrual syndrome. J Behav Med 1991;14:469–89.

104. Lustyk MK, Gerrish WG, Shaver S, et al. Cognitive-behavioral therapy for premenstrual syndrome and premenstrual dysphoric disorder: a systematic review. Arch Womens Ment Health 2009;12(2):85–96.

105. Steiner M, Pearlstein T, Cohen LS, et al. Expert guidelines for the treatment of severe PMS, PMDD, and comorbidities: the role of SSRIs. J Womens Health (Larchmt) 2006;15(1):57–69.

106. Brown J, O'Brien PM, Marjoribanks J, et al. Selective serotonin reuptake inhibitors for premenstrual syndrome. Cochrane Database Syst Rev 2009;(2):CD001396.

107. Freeman EW, Rickels K, Yonkers KA, et al. Venlafaxine in the treatment of premenstrual dysphoric disorder. Obstet Gynecol 2001;98(5):737–44.

108. Ramos MG, Hara C, Rocha FL. Duloxetine treatment for women with premenstrual dysphoric disorder: a single-blind trial. Int J Neuropsychopharmacol 2009;12(8):1081–8.

109. Freeman EW, Rickels K, Sammel MD, et al. Time to relapse after short- or long-term treatment of severe premenstrual syndrome with sertraline. Arch Gen Psychiatry 2009;66(5):537–44.

110. Lopez LM, Kaptein AA, Helmerhorst FM. Oral contraceptives containing drospir-enone for premenstrual syndrome. Cochrane Database Syst Rev 2009;(2):CD006586.

111. Muse KN, Cetel NS, Futterman LA, et al. The premenstrual syndrome: effects of "medical ovariectomy". N Engl J Med 1984;311:1345–9.

112. Freeman EW, Sondheimer SJ, Rickels K. Gonadotropin-releasing hormone agonist in the treatment of premenstrual symptoms with and without ongoing dysphoria: a controlled study. Psychopharmacol Bull 1997;33:303–9.

113. Segebladh B, Borgstrom A, Nyberg S, et al. Evaluation of different add-back estradiol and progesterone treatments to gonadotropin-releasing hormone agonist treatment in patients with premenstrual dysphoric disorder. Am J Obstet Gynecol 2009;201(2):139.e1–139.e8.

114. O'Brien PMS, Abukhalil I. Randomised controlled trial of the management of premenstrual mastalgia using luteal phase only Danazol. Am J Obstet Gynecol 1999;180:18–23.

115. Cronje WH, Vashisht A, Studd JWW. Hysterectomy and bilateral oophorectomy for severe premenstrual syndrome. Humanit Rep 2004;19(9):2152–5.

Index

Note: Page numbers of article titles are in **boldface** type.

A

Abortion, spontaneous, antidepressants and, 775
Abuse
    sexual, PMDD due to, 914
    substance. See *Substance abuse.*
S-Adenosyl methionine, for depression, 795–797
Androgens, PMDD due to, 912
Antenatal depression, 772–773
Antidepressant(s)
    sedating, for insomnia, 835
    spontaneous abortion due to, 775
    teratogenicity of, 775–776
Antihistamine(s), for insomnia, 835–836

B

Behavior(s), health risk, IPV and, 851
Behavioral therapy
    in PMDD management, 916
    in substance abuse management among reproductive age women, 900
Benzodiazepine(s), for insomnia, 834
Breastfeeding, St. John's wort while, 794–795

C

Cancer(s)
    lung, in women, 885–886
    smoking and, 882–883
Cardiovascular system, smoking effects on, 883–884
Childbearing, depression complicating, **771–788.** See also *Depression, childbearing complicated by.*
Children, IPV effects on, 855–856
Cognitive therapy, for insomnia, 837–838
Community rehabilitation programs, for substance abuse among reproductive age women, 899
Complementary therapies, in PMDD management, 916
Comprehensive women's health centers, physicians in, 748
Cortisol, late sleep increase in, in memory consolidation, 820–821
Culture, as factor in female sexual dysfunction, 867
Culture of medicine, changing, 760–761

Obstet Gynecol Clin N Am 36 (2009) 925–933
doi:10.1016/S0889-8545(09)00114-4
0889-8545/09/$ – see front matter © 2009 Elsevier Inc. All rights reserved.

obgyn.theclinics.com

Moving?

Make sure your subscription moves with you!

To notify us of your new address, find your **Clinics Account Number** (located on your mailing label above your name), and contact customer service at:

Email: journalscustomerservice-usa@elsevier.com

800-654-2452 (subscribers in the U.S. & Canada)
314-447-8871 (subscribers outside of the U.S. & Canada)

Fax number: 314-447-8029

Elsevier Health Sciences Division
Subscription Customer Service
3251 Riverport Lane
Maryland Heights, MO 63043

*To ensure uninterrupted delivery of your subscription, please notify us at least 4 weeks in advance of move.

Printed and bound by CPI Group (UK) Ltd, Croydon, CR0 4YY

03/10/2024

01040453-0001